Neonatology Questions and Controversies
Gastroenterology and Nutrition

Neonatology Questions and Controversies
Gastroenterology and Nutrition
Fourth Edition

Series Editor

Richard A. Polin, MD
William T. Speck Professor of Pediatrics
Executive Vice Chair, Department of Pediatrics
Vagelos College of Physicians and Surgeons
Columbia University

Other Volumes in the Neonatology Questions and Controversies Series

HEMATOLOGY AND TRANSFUSION MEDICINE

RENAL, FLUID AND ELECTROLYTE DISORDERS

INFECTIOUS DISEASE, IMMUNOLOGY, AND PHARMACOLOGY

NEONATAL HEMODYNAMICS

NEUROLOGY

THE NEWBORN LUNG

Neonatology Questions and Controversies

Gastroenterology and Nutrition

Edited by

Josef Neu, MD
Professor
Department of Pediatrics
Division of Neonatology
Gainesville, Florida
United States

Brenda Poindexter, MD, MS
Chief, Division of Neonatology
System Medical Director for Neonatology
Marcus Professor of Pediatrics
Children's Healthcare of Atlanta and Emory
University
Atlanta, Georgia
United States

Consulting Editor

Richard A. Polin, MD
William T Speck Professor of Pediatrics
Executive Vice Chair Department of Pediatrics
Vagelos College of Physicians and Surgeons
Columbia University
New York City, New York
United States

ELSEVIER

Elsevier
1600 John F. Kennedy Blvd.
Ste 1800
Philadelphia, PA 19103-2899

NEONATOLOGY QUESTIONS AND CONTROVERSIES:
GASTROENTEROLOGY AND NUTRITION, FOURTH EDITION

ISBN: 978-0-323-87875-3

Notice

Practitioners and researchers must always rely on their own experience and knowledge in evaluating
and using any information, methods, compounds or experiments described herein. Because of rapid
advances in the medical sciences, in particular, independent verification of diagnoses and drug dosages
should be made. To the fullest extent of the law, no responsibility is assumed by Elsevier, authors, editors
or contributors for any injury and/or damage to persons or property as a matter of products liability,
negligence or otherwise, or from any use or operation of any methods, products, instructions, or ideas
contained in the material herein.

Previous editions copyrighted 2019, 2012 and 2008.

Content Strategist: Sarah E. Barth
Content Development Specialist: Vaishali Singh
Publishing Services Manager: Shereen Jameel
Project Manager: Maria Shalini
Design Direction: Margaret M. Reid

Printed in India

Last digit is the print number: 9 8 7 6 5 4 3 2

Working together
to grow libraries in
developing countries

www.elsevier.com • www.bookaid.org

Contributors

Douglas G. Burrin, PhD
Research Physiologist
USDA/ARS Children's Nutrition Research Center
 Department of Pediatrics
Baylor College of Medicine
Professor Pediatrics
Baylor College of Medicine
Houston, Texas
United States

Kara L. Calkins, MD, MSCR
Associate Professor
Pediatrics
David Geffen School of Medicine at UCLA
Physician
Department of Pediatrics
Mattel Children's Hospital UCLA
Los Angeles, California
United States

Priyanka Verma Chugh, MD, MS
Research Fellow
Department of Surgery
Boston Children's Hospital
Boston, Massachusetts
United States

Diomel de la Cruz, MD
Associate Professor
Department of Pediatrics
Division of Neonatology
University of Florida
College of Medicine
Gainesville, Florida
United States

Donna Tracy Geddes, Post Grad Dip (Sci), PhD
Professor
School of Molecular Sciences
The University of Western Australia
Perth, Western Australia
Australia

Daniel R. Gipson, MD
Neonatology Fellow
Department of Pediatrics
University of Florida
Gainesville, Florida
United States

Rebecca J. Hill, PhD, RNutr
Senior Principal Nutrition Scientist
Nutrition Science
Reckitt/Mead Johnson Nutrition Institute
Evansville, Indiana
United States

Flavia Indrio, MD
Professor
Pediatrcs
University of Salento
Lecce
Italy

Sudarshan Rao Jadcherla, MD, FRCPI, DCH, AGAF
Professor
Department of Pediatrics
The Ohio State University College of Medicine,
 Sections of Neonatology and Pediatric
 Gastroenterology & Nutrition
Attending Neonatologist
Section of Neonatology
Nationwide Children's Hospital
Director
The Neonatal and Infant Feeding Disorders Program
Nationwide Children's Hospital
Principal Investigator
Center for Perinatal Research
The Research Institute at Nationwide Children's
 Hospital
Columbus, Ohio
United States

Tom Jaksic, MD, PhD
W. Hardy Hendren Professor of Surgery
Boston Children's Department of Surgery
Harvard Medical School
Vice Chair Pediatric Surgery
Department of Pediatric Surgery
Boston Children's Hospital
Surgical Director
Center for Advanced Intestinal Rehabilitation (CAIR)
Boston Children's Hospital
Boston, Massachusetts
United States

Sarah E. Mahoney, BS, BA
MD-PhD Candidate
Yale School of Medicine
Yale University
New Haven, Connecticut
United States

Camilia R. Martin, MD, MS
Chief, Division of Neonatology
Department of Pediatrics
Weill Cornell Medicine
Alexandra Cohen Hospital for Women and
  Newborns
New York, New York
United States

Maria Teresa Murguia-Peniche, MD, MPH
Adjunct Clinical Assistant Professor
School of Medicine
Indiana University
Associate Medical Director
Medical Sciences
Reckitt|Mead Johnson
Evansville, Indiana
United States

Emily Kristen Nes, MD
Surgical Research Fellow
Department of Surgery
Boston Children's Hospital
Boston, Massachusetts
United States

Josef Neu, MD
Professor
Pediatrics
University of Florida
Gainesville, Florida
United States

Eric B. Ortigoza, MD, MSCR
Assistant Professor
Division of Neonatal-Perinatal Medicine
Department of Pediatrics
UT Southwestern Medical Center
Dallas, Texas
United States

Mohan Pammi, MD, PhD, MRCPCH
Professor
Pediatrics
Baylor College of Medicine
Houston, Texas
United States

Kristin L. Santoro, MD
Department of Neonatology
Beth Israel Deaconess Medical Center
Instructor
Department of Pediatrics
Harvard Medical School
Boston, Massachusetts
United States

Daniel T. Robinson, MD, MSc
Department of Pediatrics
Northwestern University Feinberg School of
  Medicine
Division of Neonatology
Ann & Robert H. Lurie Children's Hospital of
  Chicago
Chicago, Illinois
United States

Sarah N. Taylor, MD, MSCR
Professor
Department of Pediatrics
Yale University School of Medicine
New Haven Connecticut
United States

Caitlin Elizabeth Vonderohe, DVM, PhD
Instructor
Pediatrics
Baylor College of Medicine
Houston, Texas
United States

Lisa Stinson, PhD, MASM
Research Fellow
School of Molecular Sciences
The University of Western Australia
Perth, Western Australia
Australia

Series Foreword

"To study the phenomena of disease without books is to sail an uncharted sea, while to study books without patients is not to go to sea at all."

"Medicine is learned by the bedside and not in the classroom. Let not your conceptions of disease come from the words heard in the lecture room or read from the book. See and then reason and compare and control. But see first."

William Osler

Before the invention of movable type by Johannes Gutenberg in the 15th century, physicians learned medicine by serving an apprenticeship with individuals considered experienced. There were no printed textbooks, and medical journals were not published until the beginning of the 19th century. By apprenticing oneself to a physician over a period of years, one learned how to be a competent practitioner. Internships in the United States evolved from those apprenticeships in the 18th century. The term *residency* was chosen because the physicians-in-training had a "residence" at the hospital. Modern-day internships began at Johns Hopkins Hospital in 1904. The Johns Hopkins Hospital was cofounded by Osler, William Stewart Halstead, William Henry Welch, and Howard Kelly. Halstead is credited with creating the first surgical residency and coined the phrase "see one, do one, teach one" (SODOTO). That educational philosophy has since been adopted by nearly every specialty in medicine, including neonatology.

Modern-day trainees in neonatology still learn how to care for critically ill infants and how to perform procedures by watching, assisting, and listening to more experienced individuals at the bedside. The SODOTO approach is considered a fundamental educational tool. However, over a three-year period, much of education occurs away from the bedside, during teaching rounds and conferences. The teaching is often more theoretical, and by design, rounds in the nursery and conferences are passive learning exercises. In those settings, trainees listen but do not take an active role in the educational process. Learning is always more effective when the recipient takes an active role in their education. Ideally, they should be questioning what they hear, reading pertinent literature, and when the opportunity arises, teaching others. Unfortunately, much of the information transmitted in those settings is not usually followed by an active phase of questioning and reading by the trainee.

Most graduates of fellowship programs turn out to be excellent practitioners, but once they leave the fellowship program, new information is acquired only intermittently, either at conferences or from journals and textbooks. As a source of new information, journals provide access to the most up-to-date information. However, that information is unfiltered, and the conclusions of a study may not be appropriate (or perhaps may be risky) for a critically ill infant. Textbooks such as those in the *Neonatology Questions and Controversies* series offer practitioners an opportunity to hear from experts in neonatal-perinatal medicine who have synthesized (and filtered) the existing literature and can provide up-to-date recommendations.

As with preceding editions, the fourth edition of the *Neonatology Questions and Controversies* series will include seven volumes. Each volume has been extensively revised, and we have added several new editors: Terri Inder joined Jeffrey Perlman for the Neurology volume; James Wynn joined William Benitz and P. Brian Smith as a coeditor for the Infectious Disease, Immunology and Pharmacology volume; and Patrick McNamara is now a coeditor with Martin Kluckow for the Neonatal Hemodynamics volume. The reader will find many completely new chapters; however, like the preceding edition, each of them is focused on day-to-day clinical decisions encountered by neonatologists. Nothing will replace the teaching that occurs at the bedside when confronted with a critically ill neonate, and the SODOTO educational approach still has an important role in education. Procedures are best learned by simulations and guidance by experienced practitioners at the bedside. However, expertise as a practitioner can only be enhanced by reading and incorporating new information into daily practice, once such information has been proven safe and effective. Perhaps SODOTO should be changed to LQRT (listen, question, read, teach). *Neonatology Questions and Controversies* is a unique source to learn from experts in the field who have been through the LQRT process many times. Osler's quotes at the beginning of this Preface suggest that both bedside teaching and journals/textbooks play a synergistic role in physician education, and that neither one alone is sufficient.

As with all prior editions, I am indebted to an exceptional group of volume editors who chose the content and authors and who edited the manuscripts. I also want to thank Sarah Barth (Publisher), as well as Vasowati Shome and Vaishali Singh (Senior Content Development Specialists) at Elsevier, who have guided the development of this series.

Richard A. Polin, MD

Preface

In the fourth edition of this book, we update the reader with a better understanding of the developmental biology of the gastrointestinal tract and how this relates to optimizing nutrition for the most vulnerable infants. We expand upon the concept that the intestine is not simply an organ for digestion and absorption, but also one of the most important immune organs of the body with a massive surface area that interacts with ingested food as well as a vast array of microbes and antigenic materials. The concept that the gut does not act on its own and that it interacts heavily with other organs such as the brain (the *gut–brain axis*) is emphasized.

In the past decade, studies have focused on associations between the gastrointestinal tract and nutritional health and disease with individual nutrients, microbes, and metabolites. Today questions are being raised about whether certain "diseases," such as what is called "necrotizing enterocolitis," are distinct entities, especially since we have major problems with a definition. This edition delves into this topic and discusses how other poorly defined diagnoses, such as sepsis, bronchopulmonary dysplasia, and central nervous system disorders, relate to a breakdown of homeostasis in the intestinal tract.

We are in an exciting new era in which rapidly emerging technologies such as artificial intelligence and multiomics are transforming the practice of medicine. These technologies show considerable promise for predictive analytics as well as augmenting our understanding of mechanisms of pathophysiology. In addition, they provide an opportunity for us to harvest our newly developing understanding of the dynamic composition of human milk to provide precision nutrition to these infants. How to best understand these new concepts is the focus of considerable research today. Some of the updated and new chapters in this book address these newly developing paradigms.

Contents

Chapter 1

Maturation of Motor Function: Clinical Implications

Sudarshan Rao Jadcherla

Chapter Outline

Key Points

1. Structural and functional development of gut motility in human infants is a process in continuum and varies with birth gestation, postnatal age, nutritional methods, acute illnesses and/or their treatments, comorbidities, and genetic factors. The entire process is complex and is dependent on maturation of the central and enteric nervous systems and gut musculature.

2. Gastrointestinal motility reflexes develop *in utero*, and several are functional at full-term birth while some have limited functions after preterm birth. Postnatal maturation advances the frequency, magnitude, sensitivity thresholds, coordination, cross-system interactions, and adaptation of these reflexes.

3. The developmental aspects of pharyngo-esophageal, gastrointestinal, and colonic motility in human neonates are highlighted. Postnatal maturation of gastrointestinal motility reflexes is dependent on sensory and motor regulation of the intrinsic enteric nervous system integrated and modulated by the central nervous system and autonomic nervous system.

4. In infants with oral and/or enteric feeding difficulties, mechanisms of motility dysfunction can be due to maldevelopment (absence of reflexes), immaturity (lack of progression with postmenstrual age), malfunction (poor transit and clearance reflexes), or maladaptation (abnormal consequences related to contiguous and cross-system reflexes).

Introduction

The neonatal period is a time of rapid growth and development that is critical for the evolution of gastrointestinal motility reflexes. Development is grossly dependent on the infant's maturation both *in utero* and *ex utero*. By 14 weeks gestation the cellular components necessary for coordinated neural and muscular activities exist in the fetal gut. However, maturation of neuromuscular functions occurs during mid- and late gestation. This translates to fully functional coordinated gut motility patterns in the full-term healthy neonate capable of independent feeding, aerodigestive protection, and small and large intestinal peristalsis. After birth, this process continues to evolve *ex utero* and is influenced by the postnatal maturational changes in the central nervous system and enteric nervous system (CNS and ENS), gut muscles, and interstitial cells of Cajal (ICC), as well as by the diet and rapidly changing anatomy and physiology during infancy. In vulnerable high-risk preterm infants, the influences of immaturity, along with other comorbid conditions including neurologic injury, chronic lung disease, hypoxia, inflammation, and sepsis, among others, can complicate and alter the postnatal development of gastrointestinal motility. Coordinated movements of the gut are crucial for the primary function of the neonatal foregut (to facilitate a safe feeding process to steer the feedings away from the airway), midgut (gastrointestinal transit of luminal contents to modulate absorption and propulsion), and hindgut (evacuation of excreta to maintain intestinal milieu homeostasis). In this chapter we will review and summarize the developmental aspects of gut motility (pharyngoesophageal, gastrointestinal, and colonic) to further explain its potential clinical implications and controversies in neonates.

Embryologic Aspects of Motility Development

By the third week of conception, the human gut initially arises as a primitive tube from the endoderm of the trilaminar embryo and later receives contributions from all the germ cell layers.[1-3] The endoderm gives rise to the epithelial lining and glands, the ectoderm gives rise to the oral cavity and the anus, and the mesoderm-derived splanchnic mesenchyme gives rise to the smooth muscle and connective tissue. During week 4, the differentiation of the foregut, midgut, and hindgut occurs. The foregut later develops into the airway and lung buds, pharynx, esophagus, stomach, and proximal portion of the duodenum; the midgut

gives rise to the remainder of the duodenum, small intestine, and portions of the large intestine up to the distal transverse colon; and the hindgut develops into the distal part of the transverse colon, descending colon, rectum, and proximal part of the anal canal.

Smooth muscle is innervated by the intrinsic neurons of the ENS, which consists of interconnected ganglia containing neurons and glial cells.[1-3] The ENS arises from precursor cells derived from the vagal (hindbrain) neural crest that enter the foregut and advances in a rostral-caudal direction. The cells colonize the gut through a complex process of migration, proliferation, and differentiation along defined pathways, and they reach the midgut by week 5 of development and the entire length of the gut by week 7.[2,4-6] A second, more caudal region of the neural crest, that is, the sacral neural crest, also contributes a smaller number of cells that are restricted to the hindgut ENS.[7] The ganglia of the ENS are organized in two plexus layers that span the length of the gut—an outer myenteric plexus situated between the longitudinal and circular muscle layers, and an inner submucosal plexus lying between the circular muscle and the muscularis mucosae.[8,9] Neurons within the myenteric plexus are primarily involved in the control of gut motility, whereas neurons within the submucosal plexus are mainly involved in controlling mucosal functions, such as electrolyte and hormone secretion.[1,3] The ENS neurons may be classified according to their function as afferent sensory neurons, interneurons, and motor neurons.[1,8,9] Activation of afferent neurons is the first step in the triggering of motor reflexes as they translate stimuli from the intestinal lumen into nerve impulses that are transmitted to interneurons and motor neurons. Interneurons form circuitry chains running both orally and aborally within the myenteric plexus. The orally running interneurons activate excitatory motor neurons, resulting in smooth muscle contraction, and the aborally running interneurons activate inhibitory motor neurons, resulting in smooth muscle relaxation. The excitatory motor neurons release acetylcholine and the inhibitory motor neurons release nitric oxide or vasoactive intestinal polypeptide. This sequential enteric reflex pattern of ascending contraction and descending relaxation, called *peristalsis*, forms the basis for Starling's Law of the Intestine[10] (Fig. 1.1), which facilitates bolus propulsion in the peristaltic direction. The

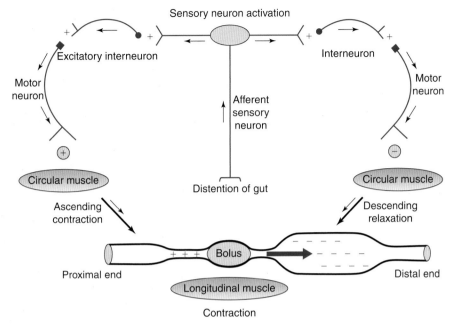

Fig. 1.1 Peristaltic reflexes: Starling's Law of the Intestine. A schematic representation of the afferent and efferent components of the peristaltic reflex, Starling's Law of the Intestine. When luminal stimulation occurs by mechanoreceptor, chemoreceptor, osmoreceptor, or tension receptor activation, there ensues a cascade of proximal afferent and distal efferent activation. This results in sequential proximal excitatory and distal inhibitory neurotransmission, resulting in peristalsis to facilitate gastrointestinal transit. At the level of the esophagus, such sequences also facilitate aerodigestive protection.

initiation and regulation of peristalsis is a complex process that involves pacemaker cells (ICCs) in addition to the smooth muscle cells and enteric nerves. ICCs generate spontaneous electrical slow waves, which constitute the basic electrical rhythm in the gut. ICCs develop independent of neural crest–derived enteric neurons or glia and originate mainly from Kit-positive mesenchymal mesodermal precursors.[2]

The ENS is remarkably independent, but its neuronal activity can be modified or modulated by the CNS via the autonomic nervous system (ANS; parasympathetic and sympathetic nervous systems).[9,11] Much of the parasympathetic innervation to the gut travels via the Vagus nerve and the sacral nerves and is primarily excitatory to gut function by promoting secretion and peristalsis. In contrast, sympathetic innervation travels along the mesenteric blood vessels from the prevertebral ganglia and is primarily inhibitory to gut function by decreasing peristalsis and reducing perfusion of the gut.

The human fetal gut, by week 14, has the longitudinal, circular, and muscularis mucosal layers of smooth muscle, submucosal and myenteric plexuses, and ICC networks that are associated with the ENS.[2] However, the first coordinated gut motility patterns do not occur until birth or about that time.[3] By 11 weeks swallowing ability develops, by 18 to 20 weeks sucking movements appear, and by full-term gestation the fetus can swallow and circulate nearly 500 mL of amniotic fluid. ENS-mediated contractile activity is prominent in function by full-term birth and is essential for propulsive activity. Variations in gut motility and peristaltic patterns occur in prematurely born neonates and are discussed in the latter part of this chapter.

Pharyngo-esophageal Motility Reflexes in Human Neonates

MATURATION OF ESOPHAGEAL PERISTALSIS AND UPPER ESOPHAGEAL SPHINCTER AND LOWER ESOPHAGEAL SPHINCTER FUNCTIONS

In neonates, *deglutition* refers to bolus propulsion from the mouth into the stomach, and it involves complex coordination of rhythmic sequences including sucking, swallowing, and breathing for safe bolus transit. Effective swallowing rhythms require pharyngeal contractions along with well-timed relaxations of the upper and lower esophageal sphincters (UES and LES, respectively) and sequential esophageal contractions.[12] Using micromanometry methods, pharyngeal, UES, esophageal body, and LES functions have been characterized in neonates.[13–15] During basal state, UES and LES maintain a resting tone irrespective of age or activity states, thus providing protective physical barriers against refluxate. With growth and maturation, the muscle mass and therefore the tone and activity of the UES increase. The average resting UES pressure (mean ± standard deviation) in preterm born neonates at 33 weeks postmenstrual age (PMA) was 17 ± 7 mm Hg and in full-term born neonates was 26 ± 14 mm Hg, whereas in adults it was 53 ± 23 mm Hg. Similarly, changes in LES length and tone have been observed with growth.[14,16,17] Additionally, esophageal lengthening occurs in a linear fashion during postnatal growth in both premature and full-term infants.[18]

MATURATION OF BASAL AND ADAPTIVE ESOPHAGEAL MOTILITY

Pharyngeal swallowing and secondary peristalsis constitute the principal methods used to drive the bolus from the oral cavity to the stomach, at the same time protecting the airway from aspiration or penetration. Pharyngeal swallowing may occur spontaneously, termed *primary peristalsis*[19] (Fig. 1.2), or when provoked by direct pharyngeal or esophageal stimulation, termed *pharyngeal reflexive swallow*[20,21] and *esophago-deglutition response*,[22] respectively. Regardless of nomenclature, pharyngeal swallowing is marked by a cascade of sequential reflexes characterized by pharyngeal peristalsis, UES relaxation, esophageal body peristalsis, and LES relaxation reflex (LESRR), to allow for bolus propagation into the stomach.[13,22–24] This sequence is normally associated with a respiratory pause called *deglutition apnea* (inspiratory or expiratory) suggesting cross-communications between the pharynx and the airway. This occurs because of the physical closure of the airway by elevation of the soft palate and larynx, by tilting of the epiglottis, and by the neural suppression of respiration in the brain stem. Evaluation of consecutive spontaneous solitary swallows in preterm infants at 33 weeks, preterm

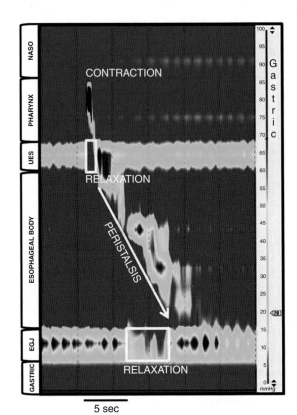

5 sec

Fig. 1.2 An example of primary peristalsis. An example of spontaneous primary esophageal peristalsis in a premature infant evoked upon pharyngeal contraction, upper esophageal sphincter relaxation, forward propagation of esophageal body peristalsis, and lower esophageal sphincter relaxation. Such sequences facilitate swallowing and esophageal clearance.

infants at 36 weeks, full-term infants, and adults has shown significant age-dependent maturational changes in the sphincter kinetics and in the amplitude and velocity of esophageal peristaltic contractions.[13,23] Importantly, primary esophageal peristalsis exists by 33 weeks PMA; however, it undergoes further maturation and differentiation during postnatal growth and is significantly different from that of adults.[13]

The esophagus is a frequent target for retrograde bolus from the stomach as in gastro-esophageal reflux events. Refluxate can trigger esophageal reflexes via stimulation of mechano-, osmo-, or chemo-sensitive esophageal receptors. In neonates, two types of esophageal reflexes exist to clear the luminal contents back into the stomach: (1) by a pharyngeal swallow-dependent *esophago-deglutition response* (as mentioned earlier), or (2) by a more mature pharyngeal swallow-independent peristaltic sequence response called *secondary peristalsis*.[16,22,23] Secondary peristalsis is marked by a coordinated sequence of UES contractile reflex (UESCR), esophageal body peristalsis, and LESRR[16,22,23] (Fig. 1.3). UESCR increases the pressure barrier against entry of refluxate into the pharynx and is mediated by the Vagus nerve.[16,22,23] These reflexes prevent the ascending spread of the bolus and favor descending propulsion to ensure esophageal clearance.

Safe and efficient oral feeding in infants requires synchronization of sucking, swallow processing (pharyngeal swallow and esophageal peristalsis), and breathing.[25–27] In neonates, pharyngeal contractility during bottle-feeding is distinct from basal and adaptive swallowing mechanisms and occurs between distal and proximal regions.[28] It is important to note that infants with feeding failure tend to exhibit poor sucking and pharyngeal rhythms along with poor or failed esophageal peristalsis.[26,27] Consequently, gastrostomy tube feeding is frequently indicated and may result in long-term neurodevelopmental impairment.[29]

Although the nature and composition of the bolus within the pharyngeal or esophageal lumen can vary, peristalsis remains the single most important function that must occur to favor luminal clearance away from the airway. These reflexes advance with maturation in premature infants. For example, in a longitudinal study of healthy premature infants (34 vs. 39 weeks PMA), recruitment frequency of pharyngeal reflexive swallow and LESRR was greater at 39 weeks PMA.[30] Furthermore, secondary peristalsis upon mid-esophageal provocation has been described as occurring as early as 32 weeks PMA.[12,13,22,23] When premature infants were studied at 33 weeks and 36 weeks PMA for esophageal provocation characteristics, the occurrence of secondary peristalsis and the frequency of completely propagated secondary peristalsis were significantly higher at 36 weeks PMA, with increments in dose volumes of air or liquid esophageal provocation. The occurrence of UESCR was also volume dependent, and its characteristics showed improvement with advancing maturation. Similarly, the aerodigestive defense mechanisms during the sleep state also mature with time in preterm infants, as evidenced by the greater ability to remain asleep with less cortical arousal, during esophageal provocation.[31] During this maturation process, the peristaltic response becomes faster and more efficient with faster esophageal clearance and greater intraluminal esophageal pressure.[12] Preterm infants exhibit lesser frequency of pharyngeal contractions and swallowing activity despite more oral feeding experiences, indicating underdeveloped excitatory and inhibitory rhythmic activity even at full-term status.[32] Regardless of adaptive state, all these findings are suggestive of the existence of vago-vagal protective reflex mechanisms that facilitate esophageal clearance in healthy premature neonates and indicate that both gestational

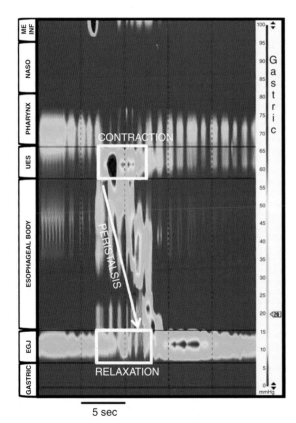

Fig. 1.3 An example of secondary peristalsis. An example of swallow-independent secondary esophageal peristalsis in a premature infant in response to a mid-esophageal infusion. Absence of pharyngeal waveform, presence of propagating esophageal body peristalsis, upper esophageal sphincter contraction, lower esophageal sphincter relaxation, and complete esophageal propagation are also noted. Such sequences are evoked during esophageal provocations and contribute to esophageal and airway protection by facilitating clearance.

and postnatal ages impact development of these reflexes. Functional immaturity in any components, at either an individual level or an integrated level, is associated with oral feeding difficulties. Many components within each of these levels mature at different times and rates and may explain why infants of similar gestation age demonstrate wide variation in oral feeding skills.[25]

Gastrointestinal Motility Reflexes in Human Neonates

Local intestinal contractions are coordinated by neural regulation modulated by the ENS, the ANS, and the CNS. The gut has a network of specialized intrinsic pacemaker muscle cells (ICCs) that also play a role in triggering these coordinated contractions.[33–35] Intestinal myoelectrical activity consists of slow waves and spike bursts. ICCs at the level of the myenteric plexus (ICC-MY) mediate the slow waves whose function is to regulate the maximum rate of muscular contraction.[36] The frequency of slow waves varies along the gut, but each part of the gut has a characteristic frequency. The stomach has the lowest frequency of slow waves (3–5 times/min) whereas the fastest frequency is in the duodenum (9–11 times/min) and then diminishes distally in the midgut (6–8 times/min).[37–39] The spike bursts are fast-action potentials that only appear on the slow-wave plateau when the small intestine contracts and that determine the intensity of the intestinal contractions. Finally, motor function can be modulated by gastrointestinal hormones and peptides, which may exert endocrine or paracrine activity, resulting in inhibitory (e.g., peptide YY, nitrergic, vasoactive intestinal peptide) or excitatory (e.g., cholinergic–muscarinic, cholecystokinin, substance P) modulation.[40] All the neural and muscular elements are present by 32 weeks gestation, but full neural and neuroendocrine integration is not achieved until late in infancy.[40,41]

Gastric Motor Functions

Anatomically, the stomach can be divided into the fundus, corpus (body), antrum, and pylorus. Functionally, the proximal stomach (fundus and proximal corpus) acts as a gastric reservoir, and the distal stomach

(distal corpus and antrum) acts as a gastric pump where the peristaltic waves occur. The gastric fundus accommodates the ingested nutrients by receptive relaxation reflex. This is largely mediated by the Vagus nerve as stimulation of the mechanoreceptors in the mouth and pharynx and of the distal esophagus induces vago-vagal reflexes that cause relaxation of the gastric reservoir by nitric oxide (inhibitory transmitter) pathways.[11,42] Fundus relaxation is a prerequisite for antral contraction and gastric emptying.[11,43] However, receptive relaxation in neonates and infants is not well studied. In contrast to the fundus, the antrum has tonic and phasic activity and is responsible for the churning of nutrients with secretions to initiate early digestion and to empty the stomach contents into the duodenum. Contractile activity in the antrum is coordinated with that in the duodenum to promote emptying of contents into the upper small intestine. Hence the physical and chemical characteristics of the nutrients entering the duodenum trigger feedback signals to the antrum to hasten or slow emptying. Ultrasonographic studies of the fetal stomach detected gastric emptying occurring as early as 13 weeks gestation,[44] and the length of gastric emptying cycles in fetuses increases just before birth.[45] The rate of gastric emptying is not influenced by nonnutritive sucking but is influenced by caloric density and/or osmolality of milk; for example, gastric emptying time may be modified by calorically denser formulas and is dependent on nutrient composition as protein accelerates gastric emptying while carbohydrates and lipids decrease gastric emptying. Additionally, high milk osmolality or extreme stress, such as that caused by the presence of systemic illness, can also delay gastric emptying.[38,46] The administration of drugs for clinical care, such as opioids or mydriatics, may also impair gastrointestinal functioning.[47] Interestingly, bolus feedings appear to delay gastric emptying in some preterm infants, presumably via rapid distention.[48]

Small Intestine Motor Functions

As in the stomach, there is an ICC network located in the intestinal wall between the internal circular and the external longitudinal muscle layers that initiate the slow waves. Peristaltic waves are far spreading and rapid at the proximal small intestine and become shorter and slower toward the distal gut. The intrinsic contractile rhythm of the stomach, duodenum, and small intestine is present as early as 24 weeks gestation. Full neural integration is inadequate at birth, and gastric emptying and the overall intestinal transit are slower in the preterm infant than in the full-term infant. Overall gut transit can vary from 7 to 14 days and depends on gestational maturation.

The small intestine exhibits two basic patterns of motor activity: (1) fed response and (2) fasting response. During fed response, the muscle layers contract in a disorganized fashion, resulting in active, continuous mixing and churning of nutrients and secretions resulting in chyme (Fig. 1.4). The fed response facilitates transport of nutrients distally to facilitate digestion and absorption. Although an adult-like fed response is seen in most full-term infants in response to bolus feeding, only about 50% of the preterm infants exhibit such a response.[49] In contrast, in the fasting state, the small intestine does not stay quiescent, but experiences muscular contractions organized into patterns known as the *interdigestive migrating motor complex* (IMMC) (Fig. 1.5). Depending on the intensity of motor activity, the IMMC cycle can be divided into four periods: phase I, or period of smooth muscle quiescence, during which the intestine is at rest; phase II, or period of random and unorganized motor activity; and phase III (migrating motor complex, MMC), in which bowel contractions occur at maximum frequency and intensity when >90% of slow waves are accompanied by spike bursts. It is usually generated at the duodenum, although it can be generated at any point between the stomach and the ileum.[50] MMCs are responsible for about 50% of the forward movement of nutrients and are considered the "intestinal housekeeper." This robust, well-organized pattern is replaced by randomly occurring contractile waveforms that terminate in the reappearance of quiescence (phase IV). The MMC is interrupted by feeding, and the subsequent fed response is characterized by irregular muscle contractions.

Control of the MMC is complex.[51,52] Vagus nerve control of the MMC seems to be restricted to the stomach, as vagotomy abolishes motor activity in the stomach but leaves periodic activity in the small bowel intact.[52] Phase III MMC of antral origin can be induced with intravenous administration of motilin, erythromycin, or ghrelin, whereas administration of serotonin or somatostatin induces phase III MMC of duodenal origin.[52] Preterm infants exhibit comparable fasting levels of motilin to adults, but motilin fails to cycle MMC in the preterm infant. Motilin receptor agonists, such as antibiotics (e.g., erythromycin/clarithromycin), can trigger initiation of the MMC in preterm infants whose gestational ages exceed 32 weeks (Fig. 1.6).[41,53,54] The MMC is incompletely developed until 32 weeks

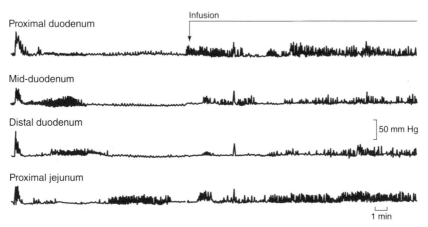

Fig. 1.4 Small intestinal motor activity in term infant (40 weeks gestation) during fasting and progressing through initiation of milk infusion. Presence of the migrating motor complex is followed by a brief period of quiescence before feeding is initiated. Quiescence is replaced by persistent motor activity in all four leads shortly after feeding infusion is begun. Adapted from Berseth CL. Neonatal small intestinal motility: motor responses to feeding in term and preterm infants. *J Pediatr.* 1990;117(5):777-782. doi:10.1016/s0022-3476(05)83343-8.

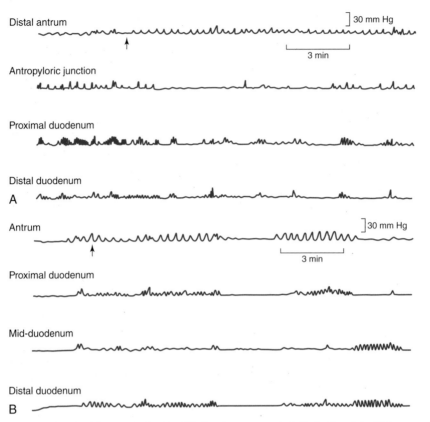

Fig. 1.5 Nonmigrating (A) and migrating (B) gastroduodenal motility in a human neonate in the fasting state. (A) A representative manometric recording depicting nonmigrating activity in a term infant. Fasting motor activity recorded in the antrum is shown in the top line, activity in the antropyloric junction in the second, and duodenum in the third and fourth. (B) A representative manometric recording in the same infant and three duodenal leads. The *arrow* indicates the presence of migrating motor complex, a phenomenon mediated by motilin, serotoninergic system, or vagal parasympathetic system. Adapted from Jadcherla SR, Klee G, Berseth CL. Regulation of migrating motor complexes by motilin and pancreatic polypeptide in human infants. *Pediatr Res.* 1997;42(3):365-369. doi:10.1203/00006450-199709000-00018.

gestation and is highly uncoordinated in infants at 27 weeks gestation.[55] Propagating, cyclical MMCs with clearly defined phases develop between 37 weeks and full term.[56] The absence of the MMC in the very premature infant appears to be the result of overall immaturity of the integration of motor pattern, absence of the motilin receptor, and/or absence of fluctuating levels of motilin.

The method of feeding influences motor patterns during fasting as well as feeding. The provision of small early feedings versus no feeding or nonnutritive feedings (i.e., sterile water) accelerates the maturation of fasting motor patterns,[57–60] which, in turn, are associated with better feeding tolerance. Interestingly,

small feedings (i.e., 20 mL/kg/d) induce maturation of motor patterns that is comparable with that induced by larger feedings.[60] This induction of maturation is likely neurally mediated because hormone release is not as robust in response to small feedings as in response to larger feedings.[58] In one animal model, it was shown that the acceleration of maturation of motor patterns is associated with an increase in nitric oxide neuronal (inhibitory) pathways,[61] both of which may regulate motor activity. Additionally, feeding diluted formula slows the onset and intensity of feeding responses.[59,62] Continuous feeds or transpyloric feeds may change the intestinal motility pattern by suppressing the fasting periods, thus hampering the

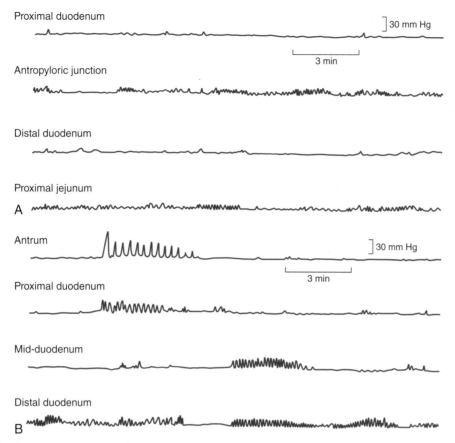

Fig. 1.6 The migrating motor complex results from stimulation of motilin receptors after enteral erythromycin. (A) Example of motility recording in an infant at 26 weeks gestation 30 minutes after the enteral erythromycin. No evidence of migrating motor activity is seen. (B) Example of motility recording in an infant at 33 weeks gestation 30 minutes after the administration of intragastric erythromycin. Phasic contractions appear in the antrum and are temporally coordinated with the occurrence of phasic activity in the three duodenal recording ports. Adapted from Jadcherla SR, Klee G, Berseth CL. Regulation of migrating motor complexes by motilin and pancreatic polypeptide in human infants. *Pediatr Res.* 1997;42(3):365-369. doi: 10.1203/00006450-199709000-00018.

intestinal bacterial clearance.[63,64] There are reports of the beneficial effects of pre- and probiotics to enhance gastrointestinal motility in preterm infants,[64] but the evidence is not strong enough to recommend its routine use in very premature infants.[65]

Development of Colonic Motility in Human Neonates

The large intestine has two main functions: (1) it is a fermenting chamber in which fiber and indigestible nutrients are hydrolyzed by microbes, and (2) it produces feces by absorption of water. To fulfill these functions, the digesta must be intensively mixed and slowly moved aborally. There is significant lack of data on colonic motility in human preterm infants, and this is largely the result of technical limitations, the need for invasive approaches, and ethical concerns. Some evidence can be gleaned from animal studies. Colonic motility is quite distinct from small intestinal motility, and regionalization of contractions occurs. ICC-mediated slow-wave activity causes colonic contractions when the depolarization is of sufficient amplitude. The internal anal sphincter, a specialized thickening of circular muscle, maintains a state of tonic contraction, thus maintaining continence in association with the external sphincter. Distension of the rectum, typically with feces, results in an ENS-dependent reflexive relaxation of the sphincter (recto-anal inhibitory reflex).[66] It is not surprising, then, that the passage of meconium is inversely related to gestational age at birth.[67] Although it is highly likely that the propagating contractile activity that occurs before birth contributes to the propulsion of meconium anally before birth, this has yet to be conclusively demonstrated. It may be postulated that colonic distention results in neural feedback, inhibiting motor function in the upper intestine. An observation study in preterm infants undergoing routine glycerin enema to stimulate meconium passage was associated with better feeding tolerance,[68] but a subsequent randomized trial in preterm infants <32 weeks showed no difference in the time to reach full enteral feeds with daily glycerin suppositories.[69] Short-chain fatty acids (SCFAs), such as butyrate, have been proposed as potential therapeutic agents that can modulate neuronal excitability by increasing the cholinergic-mediated colonic contractions, thereby augmenting colonic transit.[70] However, the generation of SCFAs in the colon induces relaxation of the proximal stomach and the LES via release of polypeptide YY hormone, which can slow the gastric emptying.[71]

Clinical Pathophysiological Considerations at Crib-side Management

Preterm gastrointestinal motility is distinct from full-term gastrointestinal motility. Therefore, when evaluating gastrointestinal motility of neonates, both intra- and extrauterine maturation need to be considered. In healthy full-term born neonates, complete intrauterine maturation occurs wherein complete gastrointestinal structural development and partial development of select functions happen. If the neonate is born full-term and healthy, they are well prepared for extrauterine life and further postnatal maturation of gastrointestinal motility functions. In the absence of structural anomalies, most full-term born neonates do well with feeding milestones. In premature neonates, both gestational age at birth and chronological age, and therefore PMA, need to be considered when evaluating organ maturation. Vagal nerve maturation and aerodigestive functions mature with increasing PMA.

Providers should determine whether mechanisms of motility dysfunction are due to maldevelopment (as indicated by the absence of reflexes over time), immaturity (lack of advancement appropriate for PMA), malfunction (poor propagation and poor clearance reflexes contributing to prolonged stasis), or maladaptation (abnormalities in contiguous and cross-system reflexes and therefore their consequences). Neonates admitted to the ICU should be evaluated for structural anomalies as a high concern. In the presence of any pathologies related to the airway/lungs, CNS, or congenital heart disease, these infants are likely to have maladaptation and/or maldevelopment and malfunction of pharyngo-esophageal motility and aerodigestive reflexes. On the other hand, in a preterm born neonate, large and small bowel motility functions appear and mature first, thus allowing for the ability to provide enteral nutrition so that peristalsis ensues, nutrient digestion and absorption occur, and growth continues in a healthy state. However, in the presence of inflammation or structural bowel disease, these motility functions are impaired, and maturational delays are expected.

Next, upon maturation of gastrointestinal motility and appropriate sphincteric coordination, pharyngo-esophageal motility reflexes evolve, and these are then followed by oral feeding skills. The upstream oral skills are the last to develop and are dependent on the adequacy and appropriate development and function of downstream gastrointestinal milestones. Thus functions guided by the ENS and the CNS develop, in that order. Oropharyngeal coordination and esophageal motility take time to mature, adapt, and develop functional skills. This is further complicated in the presence of structural disease, chronic lung disease, or neurologic sequelae.

Implications and Controversies of Gut Motility in Neonatal Gastrointestinal Therapies

DIAGNOSIS

- Mechanical gastrointestinal functions, such as suck-swallow processing coordination, UES/LES tone, gastric emptying, and intestinal motility, may be immature in preterm infants. It is difficult to determine how these functions are advancing within an individual infant as wide heterogeneity exists regarding *in utero* and *ex utero* maturation and associated comorbidities. Because of immaturity, infants are more prone to oral feeding difficulties, gastroesophageal reflex, gastric residuals, bowel distention, and delayed meconium passage compared with full-term infants.

- The symptoms and signs of feeding intolerance in preterm infants (gastric residuals, abdominal distention, emesis) that are generally an expression of anatomical and functional immaturity of the gut have poor predictive value for both enteral feeding outcomes and pathologic bowel motility. The combination of local and systemic symptoms and signs needs to be considered while interpreting the clinical and prognostic significance of nonspecific symptoms and signs of feeding intolerance.
- Standardized algorithms are lacking for motility assessments owing to multiple factors including heterogeneity of patient populations, nonspecificity of symptoms, and testing methodologies not widely available in the infant population. Personalized and evidence-based strategies have shown to be beneficial.[26,27] Objective metrics of various testing methodologies are being developed,[32,72,73] but they may also benefit from concurrent and multidisciplinary evaluations.[74]

MANAGEMENT

- Management of gastrointestinal motility issues should be tailored around the functional maturity level in an individual infant, rather than being based on their gestational age or PMA.
- Enteral trophic nutrition is associated with acceleration of gut motility patterns. If feeding intolerance limits the ability to provide full feeding volumes to an infant, smaller feeding volumes may be just as capable of inducing maturation.
- Very premature infants have a small gastric capacity and delayed gastric emptying. An infant who is intolerant to bolus feedings may tolerate feedings that are given as slow intermittent gavage over 1 hour. Similarly, an infant who has large

gastric residuals on a 3-hourly feeding regimen may tolerate feeding better with short-interval (2-hourly) feeding with smaller feeding volume.
- As the relative importance of different neurotransmitters to gastrointestinal contractile activity changes significantly during development, drugs that successfully treat motility disorders in adults will not necessarily have similar effects in infants and children.
- Erythromycin, as a prokinetic agent, may be effective in inducing migrating motor complexes in premature infants >33 weeks PMA. However, its safety and efficacy in preterm infants is not completely defined, so use of oral erythromycin should be limited to rescue treatment of severe persistent feeding intolerance.

Summary

Postnatal maturation of the gastrointestinal motility reflexes is dependent on sensory and motor regulation of the intrinsic ENS integrated and modulated by the CNS and the ANS. These reflexes mature in evolution frequency, magnitude, response sensitivity, and associated responses with advanced postnatal maturation. In infants with oral and/or enteric feeding difficulties, mechanisms of motility dysfunction can be due to maldevelopment (absence of reflexes), immaturity (lack of progression with PMA), malfunction (poor transit and clearance reflexes), or maladaptation (abnormal consequences related to contiguous and cross-system reflexes).

REFERENCES

1. Furness JB. Types of neurons in the enteric nervous system. *J Auton Nerv Syst.* 2000;81(1-3):87-96. doi:10.1016/s0165-1838(00)00127-2.
2. Burns AJ, Hofstra RM. The enteric nervous system: from embryology to therapy. *Dev Biol.* 2016;417(2):127-128. doi:10.1016/j.ydbio.2016.08.013.
3. Burns AJ, Roberts RR, Bornstein JC, Young HM. Development of the enteric nervous system and its role in intestinal motility during fetal and early postnatal stages. *Semin Pediatr Surg.* 2009;18(4):196-205. doi:10.1053/j.sempedsurg.2009.07.001.
4. Wallace AS, Burns AJ. Development of the enteric nervous system, smooth muscle and interstitial cells of Cajal in the human gastrointestinal tract. *Cell Tissue Res.* 2005;319(3):367-382. doi:10.1007/s00441-004-1023-2.
5. Zhou Y, James I, Besner GE. Heparin-binding epidermal growth factor-like growth factor promotes murine enteric nervous system

development and enteric neural crest cell migration. *J Pediatr Surg.* 2012;47(10):1865-1873. doi:10.1016/j.jpedsurg.2012.05.008.

6. Metzger M, Caldwell C, Barlow AJ, Burns AJ, Thapar N. Enteric nervous system stem cells derived from human gut mucosa for the treatment of aganglionic gut disorders. *Gastroenterology.* 2009;136(7):2214-2225.e1-3. doi:10.1053/j.gastro.2009.02.048.

7. Wang X, Chan AK, Sham MH, Burns AJ, Chan WY. Analysis of the sacral neural crest cell contribution to the hindgut enteric nervous system in the mouse embryo. *Gastroenterology.* 2011; 141(3):992-1002.e1-6. doi:10.1053/j.gastro.2011.06.002.

8. Costa M, Brookes SJ, Hennig GW. Anatomy and physiology of the enteric nervous system. *Gut.* 2000;47(suppl 4):iv15-iv19; discussion iv26. doi:10.1136/gut.47.suppl_4.iv15.

9. Gallego D, Malagelada C, Accarino A, et al. Nitrergic and purinergic mechanisms evoke inhibitory neuromuscular transmission in the human small intestine. *Neurogastroenterol Motil.* 2014;26(3):419-429. doi:10.1111/nmo.12293.

10. Goyal RK, Hirano I. The enteric nervous system. *N Engl J Med.* 1996; 334(17):1106-1115. doi:10.1056/NEJM199604253341707.

11. Gallego D, Mañé N, Gil V, Martínez-Cutillas M, Jiménez M. Mechanisms responsible for neuromuscular relaxation in the gastrointestinal tract. *Rev Esp Enferm Dig.* 2016;108(11):721-731. doi:10.17235/reed.2016.4058/2015.

12. Singendonk MM, Rommel N, Omari TI, Benninga MA, van Wijk MP. Upper gastrointestinal motility: prenatal development and problems in infancy. *Nat Rev Gastroenterol Hepatol.* 2014;11(9):545-555. doi:10.1038/nrgastro.2014.75.

13. Jadcherla SR, Duong HQ, Hofmann C, Hoffmann R, Shaker R. Characteristics of upper oesophageal sphincter and oesophageal body during maturation in healthy human neonates compared with adults. *Neurogastroenterol Motil.* 2005;17(5):663-670. doi:10.1111/j.1365-2982.2005.00706.x.

14. Omari TI, Miki K, Fraser R, et al. Esophageal body and lower esophageal sphincter function in healthy premature infants. *Gastroenterology.* 1995;109(6):1757-1764. doi:10.1016/0016-5085(95)90741-6.

15. Staiano A, Boccia G, Salvia G, Zappulli D, Clouse RE. Development of esophageal peristalsis in preterm and term neonates. *Gastroenterology.* 2007;132(5):1718-1725. doi:10.1053/j.gastro.2007.03.042.

16. Gupta A, Gulati P, Kim W, Fernandez S, Shaker R, Jadcherla SR. Effect of postnatal maturation on the mechanisms of esophageal propulsion in preterm human neonates: primary and secondary peristalsis. *Am J Gastroenterol.* 2009;104(2):411-419. doi:10.1038/ajg.2008.32.

17. Strobel CT, Byrne WJ, Ament ME, Euler AR. Correlation of esophageal lengths in children with height: application to the Tuttle test without prior esophageal manometry. *J Pediatr.* 1979;94(1):81-84. doi:10.1016/s0022-3476(79)80361-3.

18. Gupta A, Jadcherla SR. The relationship between somatic growth and in vivo esophageal segmental and sphincteric growth in human neonates. *J Pediatr Gastroenterol Nutr.* 2006; 43(1):35-41. doi:10.1097/01.mpg.0000226368.24332.50.

19. Jadcherla SR, Shaker R. Esophageal and upper esophageal sphincter motor function in babies. *Am J Med.* 2001;111(suppl 8A): 64S-68S. doi:10.1016/s0002-9343(01)00848-8.

20. Jadcherla SR, Gupta A, Stoner E, Fernandez S, Shaker R. Pharyngeal swallowing: defining pharyngeal and upper esophageal sphincter relationships in human neonates. *J Pediatr.* 2007;151(6):597-603. doi:10.1016/j.jpeds.2007.04.042.

21. Hasenstab KA, Sitaram S, Lang IM, Shaker R, Jadcherla SR. Maturation modulates pharyngeal-stimulus provoked pharyngeal and respiratory rhythms in human infants. *Dysphagia.* 2018;33(1):63-75. doi:10.1007/s00455-017-9833-z.

22. Jadcherla SR, Hoffmann RG, Shaker R. Effect of maturation of the magnitude of mechanosensitive and chemosensitive reflexes in the premature human esophagus. *J Pediatr.* 2006;149(1):77-82. doi:10.1016/j.jpeds.2006.02.041.

23. Jadcherla SR, Duong HQ, Hoffmann RG, Shaker R. Esophageal body and upper esophageal sphincter motor responses to esophageal provocation during maturation in preterm newborns. *J Pediatr.* 2003;143(1):31-38. doi:10.1016/S0022-3476(03)00242-7.

24. Pena EM, Parks VN, Peng J, et al. Lower esophageal sphincter relaxation reflex kinetics: effects of peristaltic reflexes and maturation in human premature neonates. *Am J Physiol Gastrointest Liver Physiol.* 2010;299(6):G1386-G1395. doi:10.1152/ajpgi.00289.2010.

25. Lau C. Development of suck and swallow mechanisms in infants. *Ann Nutr Metab.* 2015;66 Suppl 5(05):7-14. doi:10.1159/000381361.

26. Jadcherla SR, Stoner E, Gupta A, et al. Evaluation and management of neonatal dysphagia: impact of pharyngoesophageal motility studies and multidisciplinary feeding strategy. *J Pediatr Gastroenterol Nutr.* 2009;48(2):186-192. doi:10.1097/MPG.0b013e3181752ce7.

27. Jadcherla SR, Peng J, Moore R, et al. Impact of personalized feeding program in 100 NICU infants: pathophysiology-based approach for better outcomes. *J Pediatr Gastroenterol Nutr.* 2012;54(1):62-70. doi:10.1097/MPG.0b013e3182288766.

28. Jadcherla SR, Prabhakar V, Hasenstab KA, et al. Defining pharyngeal contractile integral during high-resolution manometry in neonates: a neuromotor marker of pharyngeal vigor. *Pediatr Res.* 2018;84(3):341-347. doi:10.1038/s41390-018-0097-6.

29. Jadcherla SR, Khot T, Moore R, Malkar M, Gulati IK, Slaughter JL. Feeding methods at discharge predict long-term feeding and neurodevelopmental outcomes in preterm infants referred for gastrostomy evaluation. *J Pediatr.* 2017;181:125-130.e1. doi:10.1016/j.jpeds.2016.10.065.

30. Jadcherla SR, Shubert TR, Gulati IK, Jensen PS, Wei L, Shaker R. Upper and lower esophageal sphincter kinetics are modified during maturation: effect of pharyngeal stimulus in premature infants. *Pediatr Res.* 2015;77(1-1):99-106. doi:10.1038/pr.2014.147.

31. Jadcherla SR, Chan CY, Fernandez S, Splaingard M. Maturation of upstream and downstream esophageal reflexes in human premature neonates: the role of sleep and awake states. *Am J Physiol Gastrointest Liver Physiol.* 2013;305(9):G649-G658. doi:10.1152/ajpgi.00002.2013.

32. Prabhakar V, Hasenstab KA, Osborn E, Wei L, Jadcherla SR. Pharyngeal contractile and regulatory characteristics are distinct during nutritive oral stimulus in preterm-born infants: implications for clinical and research applications. *Neurogastroenterol Motil.* 2019;31(8):e13650. doi:10.1111/nmo.13650.

33. Miller JL, Sonies BC, Macedonia C. Emergence of oropharyngeal, laryngeal and swallowing activity in the developing fetal upper aerodigestive tract: an ultrasound evaluation. *Early Hum Dev.* 2003;71(1):61-87. doi:10.1016/s0378-3782(02)00110-x.

34. Gariepy CE. Intestinal motility disorders and development of the enteric nervous system. *Pediatr Res.* 2001;49(5):605-613. doi:10.1203/00006450-200105000-00001.

35. Grundy D, Schemann M. Enteric nervous system. *Curr Opin Gastroenterol.* 2007;23(2):121-126. doi:10.1097/MOG.0b013e3280287a23.

36. Hirst GD, Edwards FR. Generation of slow waves in the antral region of guinea-pig stomach—a stochastic process. *J Physiol.* 2001; 535(Pt 1):165-180. doi:10.1111/j.1469-7793.2001.00165.x.

37. Berseth CL. Gastrointestinal motility in the neonate. *Clin Perinatol.* 1996;23(2):179-190.

38. Berseth CL. Motor function in the stomach and small intestine in the neonate. *NeoReviews.* 2006;7:e27-e33. doi:10.1542/neo.7-1-e28.

39. Berseth CL. Neonatal small intestinal motility: motor responses to feeding in term and preterm infants. *J Pediatr.* 1990;117(5):777-782. doi:10.1016/s0022-3476(05)83343-8.

40. Jadcherla SR, Klee G, Berseth CL. Regulation of migrating motor complexes by motilin and pancreatic polypeptide in human infants. *Pediatr Res.* 1997;42(3):365-369. doi:10.1203/00006450-199709000-00018.

41. Jadcherla SR, Berseth CL. Effect of erythromycin on gastroduodenal contractile activity in developing neonates. *J Pediatr Gastroenterol Nutr.* 2002;34(1):16-22. doi:10.1097/00005176-200201000-00005.

42. Travagli RA, Anselmi L. Vagal neurocircuitry and its influence on gastric motility. *Nat Rev Gastroenterol Hepatol.* 2016;13(7): 389-401. doi:10.1038/nrgastro.2016.76.

43. Kuiken SD, Tytgat GN, Boeckxstaens GE. Role of endogenous nitric oxide in regulating antropyloroduodenal motility in humans. *Am J Gastroenterol.* 2002;97(7):1661-1667. doi:10.1111/j.1572-0241.2002.05824.x.

44. Sase M, Miwa I, Sumie M, Nakata M, Sugino N, Ross MG. Ontogeny of gastric emptying patterns in the human fetus. *J Matern Fetal Neonatal Med.* 2005;17(3):213-217. doi:10.1080/14767050500073340.

45. Sase M, Miwa I, Sumie M, et al. Gastric emptying cycles in the human fetus. *Am J Obstet Gynecol.* 2005;193(3 Pt 2):1000-1004. doi:10.1016/j.ajog.2005.05.044.

46. Pearson F, Johnson MJ, Leaf AA. Milk osmolality: does it matter? *Arch Dis Child Fetal Neonatal Ed.* 2013;98(2):F166-F169. doi:10.1136/adc.2011.300492.

47. Bonthala S, Sparks JW, Musgrove KH, Berseth CL. Mydriatics slow gastric emptying in preterm infants. *J Pediatr.* 2000;137(3):327-330. doi:10.1067/mpd.2000.107842.

48. al Tawil Y, Berseth CL. Gestational and postnatal maturation of duodenal motor responses to intragastric feeding. *J Pediatr.* 1996;129(3):374-381. doi:10.1016/s0022-3476(96)70069-0.

49. Al-Tawil Y, Klee G, Berseth CL. Extrinsic neural regulation of antroduodenal motor activity in preterm infants. *Dig Dis Sci.* 2002;47(12):2657-2663. doi:10.1023/a:1021084517391.

50. Ye-Lin Y, Garcia-Casado J, Prats-Boluda G, Ponce JL, Martinez-de-Juan JL. Enhancement of the non-invasive electroenterogram to identify intestinal pacemaker activity. *Physiol Meas.* 2009;30(9):885-902. doi:10.1088/0967-3334/30/9/002.

51. Takahashi T. Interdigestive migrating motor complex—its mechanism and clinical importance. *J Smooth Muscle Res.* 2013;49:99-111. doi:10.1540/jsmr.49.99.

52. Deloose E, Janssen P, Depoortere I, Tack J. The migrating motor complex: control mechanisms and its role in health and disease. *Nat Rev Gastroenterol Hepatol.* 2012;9(5):271-285. doi:10.1038/nrgastro.2012.57.

53. Jones MP, Wessinger S. Small intestinal motility. *Curr Opin Gastroenterol.* 2005;21(2):141-146. doi:10.1097/01.mog.0000153310.20704.a3.

54. Gokmen T, Ozdemir R, Bozdag S, et al. Clarithromycin treatment in preterm infants: a pilot study for prevention of feeding intolerance. *J Matern Fetal Neonatal Med.* 2013;26(15):1528-1531. doi:10.3109/14767058.2013.794213.

55. Berseth CL. Gestational evolution of small intestine motility in preterm and term infants. *J Pediatr.* 1989;115(4):646-651. doi:10.1016/s0022-3476(89)80302-6.

56. Bisset WM, Watt JB, Rivers RP, Milla PJ. Ontogeny of fasting small intestinal motor activity in the human infant. *Gut.* 1988;29(4):483-488. doi:10.1136/gut.29.4.483.

57. Berseth CL, Nordyke C. Enteral nutrients promote postnatal maturation of intestinal motor activity in preterm infants. *Am J Physiol.* 1993;264(6 Pt 1):G1046-G1051. doi:10.1152/ajpgi.1993.264.6.G1046.

58. Berseth CL, Nordyke CK, Valdes MG, Furlow BL, Go VL. Responses of gastrointestinal peptides and motor activity to milk and water feedings in preterm and term infants. *Pediatr Res.* 1992;31(6):587-590. doi:10.1203/00006450-199206000-00010.

59. Baker JH, Berseth CL. Duodenal motor responses in preterm infants fed formula with varying concentrations and rates of infusion. *Pediatr Res.* 1997;42(5):618-622. doi:10.1203/00006450-199711000-00012.

60. Owens L, Burrin DG, Berseth CL. Minimal enteral feeding induces maturation of intestinal motor function but not mucosal growth in neonatal dogs. *J Nutr.* 2002;132(9):2717-2722. doi:10.1093/jn/132.9.2717.

61. Oste M, Van Ginneken CJ, Van Haver ER, Bjornvad CR, Thymann T, Sangild PT. The intestinal trophic response to enteral food is reduced in parenterally fed preterm pigs and is associated with more nitrergic neurons. *J Nutr.* 2005;135(11): 2657-2663. doi:10.1093/jn/135.11.2657.

62. Koenig WJ, Amarnath RP, Hench V, Berseth CL. Manometrics for preterm and term infants: a new tool for old questions. *Pediatrics.* 1995;95(2):203-206.

63. Goulet O, Olieman J, Ksiazyk J, et al. Neonatal short bowel syndrome as a model of intestinal failure: physiological background for enteral feeding. *Clin Nutr.* 2013;32(2):162-171. doi:10.1016/j.clnu.2012.09.007.

64. Indrio F, Riezzo G, Raimondi F, Bisceglia M, Cavallo L, Francavilla R. Effects of probiotic and prebiotic on gastrointestinal motility in newborns. *J Physiol Pharmacol.* 2009;60(suppl 6):27-31.

65. Viswanathan S, Lau C, Akbari H, Hoyen C, Walsh MC. Survey and evidence based review of probiotics used in very low birth weight preterm infants within the United States. *J Perinatol.* 2017;37(1):104. doi:10.1038/jp.2016.181.

66. Hao MM, Young HM. Development of enteric neuron diversity. *J Cell Mol Med.* 2009;13(7):1193-1210. doi:10.1111/j.1582-4934.2009.00813.x.

67. Weaver LT, Lucas A. Development of bowel habit in preterm infants. *Arch Dis Child.* 1993;68(3 Spec No):317-320. doi:10.1136/adc.68.3_spec_no.317.

68. Shim SY, Kim HS, Kim DH, et al. Induction of early meconium evacuation promotes feeding tolerance in very low birth weight infants. *Neonatology.* 2007;92(1):67-72. doi:10.1159/000100804.

69. Khadr SN, Ibhanesebhor SE, Rennix C, et al. Randomized controlled trial: impact of glycerin suppositories on time to full feeds in preterm infants. *Neonatology.* 2011;100(2):169-176. doi:10.1159/000323964.

70. Soret R, Chevalier J, De Coppet P, et al. Short-chain fatty acids regulate the enteric neurons and control gastrointestinal motility in rats. *Gastroenterology.* 2010;138(5):1772-1782. doi:10.1053/j.gastro.2010.01.053.

71. Cherbut C. Motor effects of short-chain fatty acids and lactate in the gastrointestinal tract. *Proc Nutr Soc.* 2003;62(1):95-99. doi:10.1079/PNS2002213.

72. Martin-Harris B, Carson KA, Pinto JM, Lefton-Greif MA. BaByVFSSImP© a novel measurement tool for videofluoroscopic assessment of swallowing impairment in bottle-fed babies: establishing a standard. *Dysphagia*. 2020;35(1):90-98. doi:10.1007/s00455-019-10008-x.

73. Rayyan M, Omari T, Cossey V, et al. Characterizing esophageal motility in neonatal intensive care unit patients using high resolution manometry. *Front Pediatr*. 2022;10:806072.

74. Jadcherla SR, Hasenstab KA, Osborn EK, et al. Mechanisms and management considerations of parent-chosen feeding approaches to infants with swallowing difficulties: an observational study. *Sci Rep*. 2021;11:19934.

Chapter 2

Intestinal Mucosal Immunity

Josef Neu

Chapter Outline

Key Points

1. In addition to being a digestive absorptive organ, the gastrointestinal tract is also one of the largest immune organs of the body. It is normally inhabited by commensal microbes and is exposed to a prodigious dietary antigen load.

2. Factors that play a role in balancing protection against pathogens and tolerance include a highly efficient mucosal barrier and a specialized multifaceted immune system composed of a large population of scattered immune cells and organized lymphoid tissues.

3. These factors are greatly affected by gestational age, type of feeding, and pharmacologic treatments.

Introduction

Fetal and neonatal intestinal mucosal immune development is pivotal for future health. Maternal and neonatal nutritional and environmental exposures are known to alter the intestinal microbial ecology, which in turn affects the maturational course of the developing mucosal immune system. In this chapter we discuss the various components that comprise the intestinal mucosa interface, factors that affect early development of this integrated system, and the effects of perturbations of this system on subsequent health and disease. Emphasis is placed on infants born at a gestational age of less than 37 weeks.

Components of the Intestinal Mucosal Immune System

The intestinal mucosal immune system constitutes a defensive barrier that is one of the largest surface areas of the body. Three component structures provide these defensive capabilities: (1) the epithelium, (2) the lamina propria, and (3) Peyer's patches.

THE INTESTINAL EPITHELIUM

The first line of defense, the intestinal epithelial surface, comprises several different cell types, the majority of which are absorptive epithelia. Covering the epithelial cells is a layer of mucus that serves as the first line of defense. This mucus is secreted by goblet cells that are interspersed between the absorptive epithelia. These secretory cells synthesize and secrete glycoproteins, sometimes referred to as *mucins* (Fig. 2.1).

As depicted in Fig. 2.1, there is a crypt to villus gradient of epithelial cells, where cells in the crypt migrate to the villus tip. At the very base of the crypt are additional cells called the *Paneth cells*, which secrete antimicrobial peptides that protect against pathogenic agents that are injurious to the intestinal epithelial cells (IECs). These Paneth cells are strategically placed close to the mitotic region in the crypt where their secretions provide protection for the vulnerable but highly mitotically active cells that reside in the crypt region.[1] Cells that migrate to the tip of the villus stop undergoing mitosis, continue to differentiate into functional absorptive epithelia, and are extruded from the tip of the villus in a process called *anoikis*, a form of programmed cell death.[2]

In addition to their absorptive function, IECs directly participate in immune surveillance of the intestine. These cells act as a physical barrier and signal to other components of the mucosal immune system by producing cytokines and chemokines. The IECs express pattern recognition receptors (PRRs).[3] A subset of these PRRs, the toll-like receptors (TLRs), play a vital role in the innate immune system by mediating signaling from microbial cell components such as lipoteichoic acid, flagellin, and lipopolysaccharide in the production of various cytokines and chemokines, which in turn propagates the inflammatory process. The inflammatory response can either protect against these pathogens or cause cellular injury if unregulated.

Another class of cells located in the intestinal epithelium, the innate lymphoid cells (ILCs), can be activated to produce cytokines, which play critical roles in inflammation. When ILCs are activated, they express cytokines that protect epithelial cells from injury.[4]

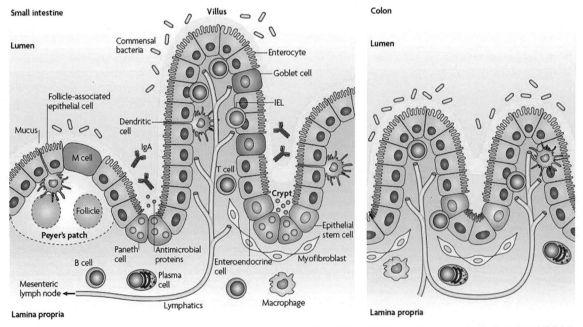

Fig. 2.1 The intestinal epithelial surface comprises several different cell types, the majority of which are absorptive epithelia. From Abreu MT. Toll-like receptor signalling in the intestinal epithelium: how bacterial recognition shapes intestinal function. *Nat Rev Immunol.* 2010;10:131–144. doi:https://doi.org/10.1038/nri2707.

Another unique set of cells, dendritic cells (DCs), recognize and eliminate exogenous pathogens. DCs act as gatekeepers, controlling the passage of antigens through the mucosal barrier to mucosal-associated lymphoid tissue.[5] These cells open interepithelial tight junctions, enter the lumen, and with their branched projections, sense antigenic materials and phagocytose various microbes, including pathogens.[5] DCs also act as messengers between the innate and adaptive immune systems, regulating intestinal immune tolerance by promoting the differentiation of CD4[+] T cells toward regulatory T cells (Tregs).[6]

Proinflammatory T helper (Th) cells eliminate pathogens during a host defense response. This is accomplished by destroying tissue via inducing tissue inflammation. Tregs are involved in immunologic homeostasis, preventing overactive inflammatory responses or loss of tolerance, which is thought to be an important component of autoimmunity such as seen in type 1 diabetes.[7]

LAMINA PROPRIA

The second major line of defense of the mucosal immune system is the lamina propria. This consists of cells that reside in the lower layer of the intestinal epithelium and is composed of B and T cells (Fig. 2.2). The intestinal tract is continuously exposed to a large quantity of antigens, which places the epithelium under considerable stress. The mechanism that provides tolerance to the normal intestinal flora but still has the capability to respond to pathogenic organisms is found in the lamina propria. Imbalances in proinflammatory versus antiinflammatory microorganisms or other stimuli may lead to inflammation, such as seen in various forms of inflammatory bowel disease (IBD).[8]

PEYER'S PATCHES

The third major component of the intestinal mucosal immune system are Peyer's patches. Fig. 2.2 illustrates where the Peyer's patches are found in the intestinal layers. Peyer's patches are organized lymphoid nodules commonly found in the small intestines (inside the oval). Fig. 2.2 depicts the ileum, which is particularly rich in Peyer's patches. Both B cells and plasma cells are found in these nodules.[9] IgA-producing plasma cells are generated from activated B cells in Peyer's patches.[10] Secretory

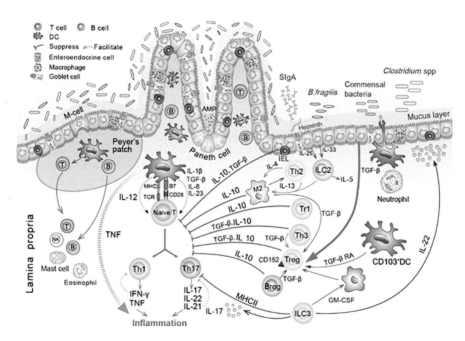

Fig. 2.2 The second major component of the mucosal immune system is the lamina propria. This consists of cells that reside in the lower layer of the intestinal epithelium and comprises B and T cells. The figure shows the location of immune regulatory cells and other immune cells and their signaling cascades in the lamina propria of the gut. The luminal microbiome lies adjacent to the intestinal epithelium.

IgA is a major protective barrier against infections in the infant intestinal tract.

Another cell type found on the intestinal surface are the intestinal microfold (M) cells. These are epithelial cells that most often reside in conjunction with Peyer's patches of the small intestine. Their microfolds are especially suited for shuttling antigens into the Peyer's patch, stimulating appropriate immune responses.

The role of the intestinal microbiota in all these processes is critical. In addition to stimulation of the various immune signaling pathways that may lead to homeostasis, hyperinflammatory states, and tolerization, microbes also produce protective metabolites. These include short-chain fatty acids (SCFAs) such as butyrate and the amino acid tryptophan that can enhance gut integrity.[11]

Factors Affecting the Fetal Intestinal Mucosal Immune System

Interactions between maternal microbiota, stress, and nutrition affect fetal development. These interactions in turn affect both the mother's and the fetus's immune systems.[12] Overnutrition and undernutrition are linked to unhealthy pregnancy.[13,14]

A large quantity of metabolites are produced by microbes residing in the maternal intestine. These can be absorbed and enter the maternal circulation, enter the fetus, and play a role in subsequent immune homeostasis.[15,16]

Microbes may also play a role if they reside in the placenta, amniotic fluid, or fetal intestine. The dogmatic view of a "sterile womb" has come into question in the past several years. A commentary in the journal *Nature* succinctly summarizes this controversy as a scientific "knife fight" discussing various aspects and data on different sides of this controversy.[17] Further studies have supported the existence of a fetal intestinal microbiome, the function of which remains unclear. However, some of the strains have immunomodulatory capability, which may play a role in survival of the fetus.[18]

Despite skepticism about the *in utero* microbiome, maternal intestinal and vaginal microbes and their metabolites and interactions with the fetal immune system certainly exist and likely affect the trajectory of the developing immune system.[19,20] Exposure to large quantities of viral and/or bacterial antigenic material may act synergistically with maternal stress and in turn lead to responses that may trigger preterm labor.[21] These relationships remain hypothetical, but the technology now exists to test these hypotheses.

Microbes in the pregnant woman's intestinal tract differ during the stages of pregnancy.[22] Gut microbiota change dramatically from the first to the third trimesters. The types of microbes present during these stages may become dysbiotic due to various pathologic stressors. This is hypothesized to contribute to pregnancy complications including fetal rejection (causing preterm delivery).[23]

Factors During Perinatal and Postnatal Development Affecting the Intestinal Immune System

At the beginning of extrauterine life, the newborn encounters myriad antigens to which it must selectively and appropriately respond. The conditions during the birth process as well as subsequent early exposures dictate subsequent development.

MODE OF DELIVERY: SURGICAL VERSUS VAGINAL

Cesarean section (C-section) delivery is often lifesaving for both mother and baby. However, there are large discrepancies in the number of these operative procedures. In many areas of the globe this procedure is not readily available, and in others its use exceeds medical necessity. Several studies have suggested that the microbial ecology of the infant gastrointestinal tract may be affected for long periods of time after C-section delivery. In some studies these differences in microbial composition among infants' feces born via C-section versus vaginal delivery have been found to be present for up to 7 years, and on average, recovery to a "normal microbiome" may take several months.[24,25] The reasons for differences in the developing microbiota related to mode of delivery appear to be more than simply the physical passing of the infant through the birth canal, which inoculates a symbiotic intestinal flora into the infant.[26,27] However, it is important to remember that infants born by C-section are more often subjected to peripartum antibiotics, take longer to initiate feedings, and have longer hospital stays with exposures to hospital microbes than their vaginally delivered counterparts, all of which may influence the developing microbiome and immunologic systems. Epidemiologic studies have associated C-section deliveries with increased incidences of food allergy, obesity, asthma, and IBD.[28-30]

ANTIBIOTIC USE

Antibiotic use can markedly affect intestinal microbiota in the mother as well as in the developing infant. Intrapartum antimicrobial prophylaxis (IAP) results in the reduction of potentially protective *Actinobacteria* and *Bacteroidetes* and an abundance of *Proteobacteria* and *Firmicutes* in the fecal microbiomes of babies from treated mothers.

Administration of broad-spectrum antibiotics shortly after birth leads to decreased species richness[31] and delayed colonization of *Bifidobacterium* in the neonate.[32] Wheezing and eczema by 8 years of age as well as IBD and type 2 diabetes mellitus later in life are linked to early antibiotic exposure.[33,34]

POSTNATAL MICROBIOTA AND INTESTINAL DEVELOPMENT IN PRETERM INFANTS

The last trimester of pregnancy represents a critical developmental window for the fetal intestine that is often shortened by preterm birth.[35] If the infant is born preterm, feeding reflexes as well as various functions such as intestinal motility, villus, and crypt anatomy are not yet fully developed. Preterm infants are thus at several disadvantages when forming a postnatal microbiome and a mucosal immune system.[35,36]

The intestinal microbiota is central to neonatal mucosal immunity.[37] Shortly after birth, gut colonization is influenced by microbes from the immediate environment including what kind of enteral nutrition the infant receives. Fresh mother's milk produced shortly after birth, known as *colostrum*, contains microbes and numerous valuable immunologic components. Providing mother's milk soon after birth represents a critical window that is especially important for premature infants. Intestinal microbes promote integrity of the intestinal barrier tight junction proteins between IECs, thus preventing translocation of inflammatory microorganisms, antigens, and potentially other toxic agents into the neonate's circulation.[38] Some commensal microbes in milk stimulate goblet cell secretion, which coats the intestinal surface with mucous, providing a protective barrier. Commensals strengthen interepithelial tight junction integrity, which prevents uptake of large molecules and microbiota. Dysbiotic microbiotas, which still require greater delineation as to their taxonomy and function, are thought to weaken intestinal integrity.

Underdevelopment of the preterm intestine leads to dysbiosis-associated inflammation and microbial translocation and may result in proinflammatory processes that are related to short-term adverse outcomes such as necrotizing enterocolitis, late-onset sepsis (LOS), and chronic lung disease. In these situations microbial diversity is reduced, and the relative abundance of various microbes is very different compared with healthy term infants.[39-44]

NEONATAL NUTRITION AND MICROBIOTA DEVELOPMENT: ROLE OF MOTHER'S MILK

Breastfeeding promotes development of a symbiotic neonatal microbiome (e.g., *Bifidobacterium*-dominant).[44] Breast milk also contains glycans that are not present in commercial formulas and that play a role in selection of commensal bacteria. These are referred to as human milk oligosaccharides (HMOs). Some of these breast milk–derived bioactive components recoup the preterm infant's presumed lack of endogenous intestinal mucin and innate defenses.[45]

The ideal carbohydrate source for infant nutrition is lactose. Despite studies suggesting low intestinal lactase activities in the preterm human intestine, symbiotic bacteria have evolved to prefer lactose as a carbon source. HMOs, which are not absorbed by the intestine, can serve as substrate from microbial metabolism and modulate the composition of the infant microbiota.[46] Both unabsorbed lactose and HMOs are fermentable carbohydrate prebiotics that select for beneficial gut bacteria involved with metabolic and immunologic advantages for the infant. In doing so, they produce beneficial metabolites such as microbial SCFAs and folate (vitamin B9). SCFAs (acetate, propionate, and butyrate) are all critical in maintaining systemic immune homeostasis,[47] and their metabolites dictate immune development in the preterm infant.

Various immunoglobulins and immune cells are unique to the first milk (colostrum) that the mother provides during lactation. Many of these factors are not present in mature breast milk. Thus the consumption of colostrum provides a mechanism of passive immunity transfer from the mother.[48]

Gut closure refers to the development of relative impermeability of the neonatal intestine. Prior to closure, during the open phase, there is passage of large molecules from the intestinal lumen to the blood through tight junctions as well as transport of large immunoglobulin molecules from breast milk. Microchimerism also occurs, wherein maternal cells travel from breast milk through infant mucosa.[49] These maternal cells are thought to aid in tissue repair and regulation of the neonatal immune response, including tolerance. Passive immunity conferred through secretory immunoglobulin A (sIgA) in the breast milk makes up over 90% of all antibodies present in the milk.[50] Newborns lack sIgA at birth and thus are reliant on the mother's milk for sIgA.[50]

Breast milk *exosomes*, nanovesicles containing immunologically relevant components, have generated recent interest. Human milk exosomes contain microRNAs (miRNAs). These originate from the mammary gland and have been found to promote cellular

development and immune function. They also serve in the genetic exchange between cells, including intestinal cells.[51]

In summary, human breast milk is more than a nutrient. Fig. 2.3 summarizes several of the bioactive components found in fresh mother's milk. These include numerous bioactive components that determine the composition of intestinal microbiota, as well as their metabolites that determine the trajectory of lifelong immune responses and modulate disease risk throughout life.[52,53] It should be noted that for pooled donor milk, many of these bioactive components are decreased or lost completely during the pasteurization process. The dynamic qualities of mother's own milk supplied to the infant at specific times via the enteromammary system[54–57] are also lost. Although observational studies suggest a benefit of donor milk in terms of outcomes such as necrotizing enterocolitis (NEC),[58,59] a prospective randomized study did not show a benefit.[60] With the challenges resulting from the lack of a clear definition of NEC (see Necrotizing Enterocolitis Chapter), potential bias in observational compared to prospective randomized studies, the loss

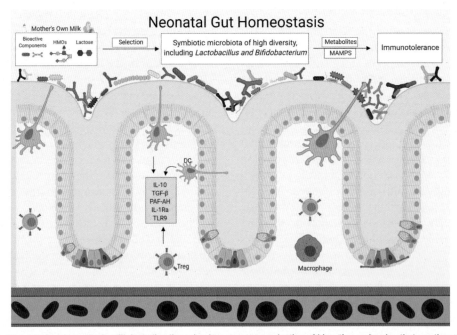

Fig. 2.3 Compositional factors in mother's milk including live microbes promote production of bioactive molecules that are thought to protect the mucosal barrier, promote the growth of commensal bacteria, and provide a balance between pro- and antiinflammatory processes.

of the bioactive components in donor milk,[61] and concerns about growth and neurodevelopmental outcomes with donor milk,[62] enthusiasm that equates donor milk to babies' own mothers' milk should be tempered.

Neonatal Immune System: Preterm Infants

The mucosal immune system in the preterm neonate must respond to foreign antigens and to the baby's own antigens in a homeostatic fashion from birth.[63] The mucosal immune development that elicits such responses begins in the womb.[64] We are still in the early stages of understanding fetal mucosal immune development, especially in humans, but we are learning that prenatal events can modulate the developing fetal immune system toward a proinflammatory state prior to delivery.[65,66]

Considerable information about human fetal immunology can be learned from infants born preterm. Blood leukocytes from preterm human infants differ from their full-term counterparts. Such leukocytes have lower PRR function, reduced bacterial elimination, and hindered endothelial adhesive rolling.[67] The human newborn lacks adult levels of mature B cells and T cells, but the innate immune system including intestinal dendritic cell and macrophage populations function normally.[35] The human neonatal Th2 and Th17 type immune responses can eliminate extracellular pathogens in the gut. However, Th1 defenses against intracellular pathogens are relatively silent in early stages of neonatal development.[68]

At birth, various cytokines such as interleukin (IL)-23, IL-12, IL-1B, IL-6, and tumor necrosis factor alpha (TNF-α) are key proinflammatory messengers of the innate immune system.[67,69] IL-10 derived from T-regulatory cells is the main antiinflammatory cytokine. Studies in humans have associated higher levels of serum IL-10 with NEC, suggesting a futile attempt to dampen inflammation.[70]

TOLL-LIKE RECEPTORS

The innate toll-like receptor (TLR) response is compromised in preterm infants.[69] TLRs in the neonate intestinal epithelium are involved in microbiota-mediated mucosal development. TLR4 responds to lipopolysaccharide, found in high concentrations in gram-negative pathogenic microbes, by signaling an increase of proinflammatory nuclear factor kappa B (NFκB). This process

includes the adapter protein MYD88. Dissociation from inhibitory molecules [inhibitor of nuclear factor kappa B (IkB proteins)] permits NFκB to pass into the nucleus where it stimulates transcription of proinflammatory cytokines and chemokines, as seen in Fig. 2.4. One of the major chemokines induced by this response includes IL-8, which induces migration of neutrophils to the site of infection. This induces TNF-α release and promotes a proinflammatory response.[71]

NEONATAL B AND T LYMPHOCYTES

Vulnerability of the neonatal intestine is due at least in part to an underdeveloped adaptive immune system. In fetal life, germinal centers in Peyer's patches necessary for B cell proliferation, differentiation, and isotype switching are not fully developed.[72,73,74] Thus functional immaturity of B lymphocytes and associated cells and tissues occurs during early infancy. B lymphocytes are present at birth, but functional maturation into sIgA-secreting plasma cells is not complete until approximately 1 year after birth. Therefore, at least in the early phases of neonatal life, the neonate relies on sIgA provided from mother's milk.[75]

Tolerizing components of the immune system also differ between neonates and adults. Adult regulatory T cell products, including IL-10 and TGF-β, are markedly lower in neonates. This causes an enhanced potential for unchecked proinflammatory sequelae.[76] Despite this diminished neonatal Treg function, these cells still likely contribute to preventing proinflammatory neonatal effector T cell responses to commensals.

ABERRATIONS IN NEONATAL IMMUNITY: SOME SELECT PATHOLOGIC CONSEQUENCES

Among the diseases associated with prematurity, NEC and LOS are of high concern. Unfortunately, these are not discrete clinical entities and perhaps should not even be considered defined diseases.[77,78] However, in some patients NEC[79] and LOS do appear to represent a hyperactive immune system that damages the host.

NEC has been the subject of decades of research, but its etiology and definition remain poorly understood. Studies suggest that the time from birth to the onset of NEC is inversely proportional to the length of gestation.[80] The precise reason for this has not yet been determined but may relate to the heterogeneity

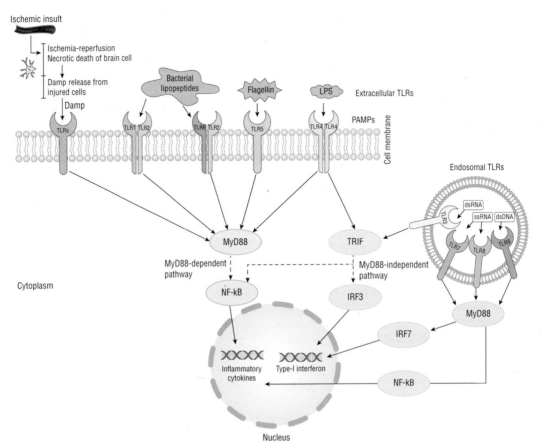

Fig. 2.4 Toll-like receptor signaling affecting NFκB translocation and cytokine production. Adapted from Ashayeri Ahmadabad R, Mirzaasgari Z, Gorji A, Khaleghi Ghadiri M. Toll-like receptor signaling pathways: novel therapeutic targets for cerebrovascular disorders. *Int J Mol Sci.* 2021;22(11):6153. doi:10.3390/ijms22116153.

of what we have been calling "NEC." In the future, we will likely have a better delineation of the various forms of intestinal injury and/or dysfunction in neonates and thus focus on each one of these individually to determine their pathophysiology.

Nevertheless, we have relied on cell culture and animal models in our quest to evaluate specific pathophysiologic mechanisms. Cell cultures may help us better understand basic mechanisms of cellular injury and repair, but it is difficult to relate these to a poorly defined disease.

Rodents and piglets are the most used animal models of NEC. The rationale for the use of these models originated in the 1970s when it was thought that hypoxia was a major antecedent of NEC.[81] However, in

clinical practice hypoxic events usually do not temporally associate with the development of NEC.[82] Therefore the lack of a suitable animal model and the problem of a clear definition are major barriers to understanding the pathophysiology of what is frequently diagnosed as NEC.

There are, however, several variables that may be important in the development of NEC. For example, the microbiome may have a key role in the pathogenesis of NEC. Using non-culture-based microbiome analysis, several studies have found increases in the bacterial phyla *Proteobacteria* and decreases in *Firmicutes* and *Bacteroidetes* prior to NEC onset.[83–85]

Human milk feeding is associated with a lower incidence of NEC.[86] Numerous additional studies support this protective role of mother's milk, but none are prospective and/or randomized, thus allowing for potential bias and numerous confounding factors. Nevertheless, this is a tenable hypothesis at least partially based on numerous protective factors present in baby's own mother's milk.

LOS is a life-threatening diagnosis in neonates that differs from adult sepsis because in neonates the immune response is managed largely by the innate immune system.[87] An abnormal intestinal microbiome has been implicated in the pathogenesis of neonatal LOS.[88] Sampling of stools and blood from LOS preterm infants found that microbes present in the infants' stools were also often isolated from their blood. This suggests bacterial translocation from the intestine as a key for development of LOS.[43,88]

As a component of the intestine-derived sepsis cascade, potentially pathogenic microbes under certain conditions of stress may induce inflammation. After inflammation is induced, there is a disruption of interepithelial tight junction proteins[89,90] causing increased interepithelial permeability leading to bacterial translocation. This increased permeability is associated with increased responses to flagellin, endotoxin, and exotoxins, leading to inflammatory responses in a highly immunoreactive subepithelium.

Summary

It is clear that various factors, especially the microbial environment and diet, are critical in development of mucosal immunity and that early perturbations may have devastating effects, such as inflammation-related intestinal necrosis and LOS. Importantly, it is during these early periods that the microbiome and immune systems codevelop and are most sensitive to interventions.

Public health initiatives involving proper nutrition during pregnancy and breastfeeding should continue to be a top priority for the improvement of neonatal intestinal mucosal immunity. We need to continue multiomic-based studies that will lead to a better understanding of mechanisms that relate to intestinal injury and health. This should ultimately lead to interventional strategies to treat and prevent diseases seen in the neonatal period as well as during adulthood that have their origins in early intestinal mucosal development.

REFERENCES

1. Ayabe T, Ashida T, Kohgo Y, Kono T. The role of Paneth cells and their antimicrobial peptides in innate host defense. *Trends Microbiol.* 2004;12(8):394-398. doi:10.1016/j.tim.2004.06.007.
2. Bertrand K. Survival of exfoliated epithelial cells: a delicate balance between anoikis and apoptosis. *J Biomed Biotechnol.* 2011;2011:534139. doi:10.1155/2011/534139.
3. Akira S, Takeda K, Kaisho T. Toll-like receptors: critical proteins linking innate and acquired immunity. *Nat Immunol.* 2001;2(8):675-680. doi:10.1038/90609.
4. Wang HC, Zhou Q, Dragoo J, Klein JR. Most murine CD8+ intestinal intraepithelial lymphocytes are partially but not fully activated T cells. *J Immunol.* 2002;169(9):4717-4722. doi:10.4049/jimmunol.169.9.4717.
5. Rescigno M, Urbano M, Valzasina B, et al. Dendritic cells express tight junction proteins and penetrate gut epithelial monolayers to sample bacteria. *Nat Immunol.* 2001;2(4):361-367. doi:10.1038/86373.
6. Luciani C, Hager FT, Cerovic V, Lelouard H. Dendritic cell functions in the inductive and effector sites of intestinal immunity. *Mucosal Immunol.* 2022;15(1):40-50. doi:10.1038/s41385-021-00448-w.
7. Vaarala O, Atkinson MA, Neu J. The "perfect storm" for type 1 diabetes: the complex interplay between intestinal microbiota, gut permeability, and mucosal immunity. *Diabetes.* 2008;57(10):2555-2562. doi:10.2337/db08-0331.
8. Varol C, Vallon-Eberhard A, Elinav E, et al. Intestinal lamina propria dendritic cell subsets have different origin and functions. *Immunity.* 2009;31(3):502-512. doi:10.1016/j.immuni.2009.06.025.
9. Reboldi A, Cyster JG. Peyer's patches: organizing B-cell responses at the intestinal frontier. *Immunol Rev.* 2016;271(1):230-245. doi:10.1111/imr.12400.
10. Bemark M, Boysen P, Lycke NY. Induction of gut IgA production through T cell-dependent and T cell-independent pathways. *Ann N Y Acad Sci.* 2012;1247:97-116. doi:10.1111/j.1749-6632.2011.06378.x.
11. McDermott AJ, Huffnagle GB. The microbiome and regulation of mucosal immunity. *Immunology.* 2014;142(1):24-31. doi:10.1111/imm.12231.
12. Valentine G, Chu DM, Stewart CJ, Aagaard KM. Relationships between perinatal interventions, maternal-infant microbiomes, and neonatal outcomes. *Clin Perinatol.* 2018;45(2):339-355. doi:10.1016/j.clp.2018.01.008.
13. Santos S, Voerman E, Amiano P, et al. Impact of maternal body mass index and gestational weight gain on pregnancy complications: an individual participant data meta-analysis of European, North American, and Australian cohorts. *BJOG.* 2019;126(8):984-995. doi:10.1111/1471-0528.15661.
14. Middleton P, Gomersall JC, Gould JF, Shepherd E, Olsen SF, Makrides M. Omega-3 fatty acid addition during pregnancy. *Cochrane Database Syst Rev.* 2018;11:CD003402. doi:10.1002/14651858.CD003402.pub3.
15. Macpherson AJ, de Agüero MG, Ganal-Vonarburg SC. How nutrition and the maternal microbiota shape the neonatal immune system. *Nat Rev Immunol.* 2017;17(8):508-517. doi:10.1038/nri.2017.58.
16. Torow N, Hornef MW. The neonatal window of opportunity: setting the stage for life-long host-microbial interaction and immune homeostasis. *J Immunol.* 2017;198(2):557-563. doi:10.4049/jimmunol.1601253.
17. Willyard C. Could baby's first bacteria take root before birth? *Nature.* 2018;553(7688):264-266. doi:10.1038/d41586-018-00664-8.

18. Rackaityte E, Halkias J, Fukui EM, et al. Viable bacterial colonization is highly limited in the human intestine in utero. *Nat Med.* 2020;26(4):599-607. doi:10.1038/s41591-020-0761-3.

19. Parker EL, Silverstein RB, Mysorekar IU. Bacteria make T cell memories in utero. *Cell.* 2021;184(13):3356-3357. doi:10.1016/j.cell.2021.05.044.

20. Jain N. The early life education of the immune system: moms, microbes and (missed) opportunities. *Gut Microbes.* 2020;12(1):1824564. doi:10.1080/19490976.2020.1824564.

21. Socha-Banasiak A, Pawłowska M, Czkwianianc E, Pierzynowska K. From intrauterine to extrauterine life—the role of endogenous and exogenous factors in the regulation of the intestinal microbiota community and gut maturation in early life. *Front Nutr.* 2021;8:696966. doi:10.3389/fnut.2021.696966.

22. Koren O, Goodrich JK, Cullender TC, et al. Host remodeling of the gut microbiome and metabolic changes during pregnancy. *Cell.* 2012;150(3):470-480. doi:10.1016/j.cell.2012.07.008.

23. Zhang D, Huang Y, Ye D. Intestinal dysbiosis: an emerging cause of pregnancy complications? *Med Hypotheses.* 2015;84(3):223-226. doi:10.1016/j.mehy.2014.12.029.

24. Yang I, Corwin EJ, Brennan PA, Jordan S, Murphy JR, Dunlop A. The infant microbiome: implications for infant health and neurocognitive development. *Nurs Res.* 2016;65(1):76-88. doi:10.1097/nnr.0000000000000133.

25. Gronlund MM, Lehtonen OP, Eerola E, Kero P. Fecal microflora in healthy infants born by different methods of delivery: permanent changes in intestinal flora after cesarean delivery. *J Pediatr Gastroenterol Nutr.* 1999;28(1):19-25. doi:10.1097/00005176-199901000-00007.

26. Underwood MA, German JB, Lebrilla CB, Mills DA. Bifidobacterium longum subspecies infantis: champion colonizer of the infant gut. *Pediatr Res.* 2015;77(1-2):229-235. doi:10.1038/pr.2014.156.

27. Wampach L, Heintz-Buschart A, Fritz JV, et al. Birth mode is associated with earliest strain-conferred gut microbiome functions and immunostimulatory potential. *Nat Commun.* 2018;9(1):5091. doi:10.1038/s41467-018-07631-x.

28. Adeyeye TE, Yeung EH, McLain AC, Lin S, Lawrence DA, Bell EM. Wheeze and food allergies in children born via cesarean section—the Upstate KIDS Study. *Am J Epidemiol.* 2019;188(2):355-362. doi:10.1093/aje/kwy257.

29. Tamburini S, Shen N, Wu HC, Clemente JC. The microbiome in early life: implications for health outcomes. Review Article. *Nat Med.* 2016;22(7):713-722. doi:10.1038/nm.4142.

30. Keag OE, Norman JE, Stock SJ. Long-term risks and benefits associated with cesarean delivery for mother, baby, and subsequent pregnancies: systematic review and meta-analysis. *PLoS Med.* 2018;15(1):e1002494. doi:10.1371/journal.pmed.1002494.

31. Gibson MK, Crofts TS, Dantas G. Antibiotics and the developing infant gut microbiota and resistome. *Curr Opin Microbiol.* 2015;27:51-56. doi:10.1016/j.mib.2015.07.007.

32. Henderickx JGE, Zwittink RD, van Lingen RA, Knol J, Belzer C. The preterm gut microbiota: an inconspicuous challenge in nutritional neonatal care. *Front Cell Infect Microbiol.* 2019;9:85. doi:10.3389/fcimb.2019.00085.

33. Risnes KR, Belanger K, Murk W, Bracken MB. Antibiotic exposure by 6 months and asthma and allergy at 6 years: findings in a cohort of 1,401 US children. *Am J Epidemiol.* 2011;173(3):310-318. doi:10.1093/aje/kwq400.

34. Kronman MP, Zaoutis TE, Haynes K, Feng R, Coffin SE. Antibiotic exposure and IBD development among children: a population-based cohort study. *Pediatrics.* 2012;130(4):e794-e803. doi:10.1542/peds.2011-3886.

35. Torow N, Marsland BJ, Hornef MW, Gollwitzer ES. Neonatal mucosal immunology. *Mucosal Immunol.* 2017;10(1):5-17. doi:10.1038/mi.2016.81.

36. Drozdowski LA, Clandinin T, Thomson AB. Ontogeny, growth and development of the small intestine: understanding pediatric gastroenterology. *World J Gastroenterol.* 2010;16(7):787-799. doi:10.3748/wjg.v16.i7.787.

37. O'Hara AM, Shanahan F. The gut flora as a forgotten organ. *EMBO Rep.* 2006;7(7):688-693. doi:10.1038/sj.embor.7400731.

38. Niño DF, Sodhi CP, Hackam DJ. Necrotizing enterocolitis: new insights into pathogenesis and mechanisms. *Nat Rev Gastroenterol Hepatol.* 2016;13(10):590-600. doi:10.1038/nrgastro.2016.119.

39. Patel AL, Mutlu EA, Sun Y, et al. Longitudinal survey of microbiota in hospitalized preterm very-low-birth-weight infants. *J Pediatr Gastroenterol Nutr.* 2016;62(2):292-303. doi:10.1097/mpg.0000000000000913.

40. Carlisle EM, Morowitz MJ. The intestinal microbiome and necrotizing enterocolitis. *Curr Opin Pediatr.* 2013;25(3):382-387. doi:10.1097/MOP.0b013e3283600e91.

41. Cilieborg MS, Boye M, Sangild PT. Bacterial colonization and gut development in preterm neonates. *Early Hum Dev.* 2012; 88(suppl 1):S41-S49. doi:10.1016/j.earlhumdev.2011.12.027.

42. Wang Y, Hoenig JD, Malin KJ, et al. 16S rRNA gene-based analysis of fecal microbiota from preterm infants with and without necrotizing enterocolitis. *ISME J.* 2009;3(8):944-954. doi:10.1038/ismej.2009.37.

43. Chernikova DA, Madan JC, Housman ML, et al. The premature infant gut microbiome during the first 6 weeks of life differs based on gestational maturity at birth. *Pediatr Res.* 2018; 84(1):71-79. doi:10.1038/s41390-018-0022-z.

44. Biagi E, Aceti A, Quercia S, et al. Microbial community dynamics in mother's milk and infant's mouth and gut in moderately preterm infants. *Front Microbiol.* 2018;9:2512. doi:10.3389/fmicb.2018.02512.

45. Meyer-Hoffert U, Hornef MW, Henriques-Normark B, et al. Secreted enteric antimicrobial activity localises to the mucus surface layer. *Gut.* 2008;57(6):764-771. doi:10.1136/gut.2007.141481.

46. Oozeer R, van Limpt K, Ludwig T, et al. Intestinal microbiology in early life: specific prebiotics can have similar functionalities as human-milk oligosaccharides. *Am J Clin Nutr.* 2013;98(2):561s-571s. doi:10.3945/ajcn.112.038893.

47. Pourcyrous M, Nolan VG, Goodwin A, Davis SL, Buddington RK. Fecal short-chain fatty acids of very-low-birth-weight preterm infants fed expressed breast milk or formula. *J Pediatr Gastroenterol Nutr.* 2014;59(6):725-731. doi:10.1097/mpg.0000000000000515.

48. Hassiotou F, Hepworth AR, Metzger P, et al. Maternal and infant infections stimulate a rapid leukocyte response in breastmilk. *Clin Transl Immunology.* 2013;2(4):e3. doi:10.1038/cti.2013.1.

49. Moles JP, Tuaillon E, Kankasa C, et al. Breastmilk cell trafficking induces microchimerism-mediated immune system maturation in the infant. *Pediatr Allergy Immunol.* 2018;29(2):133-143. doi:10.1111/pai.12841.

50. McElroy SJ, Weitkamp JH. Innate immunity in the small intestine of the preterm infant. *Neoreviews.* 2011;12(9):e517-e526. doi:10.1542/neo.12-9-e517.

51. Lönnerdal B. Human milk microRNAs/exosomes: composition and biological effects. *Nestle Nutr Inst Workshop Ser.* 2019;90:83-92. doi:10.1159/000490297.

52. Urbaniak C, McMillan A, Angelini M, et al. Effect of chemotherapy on the microbiota and metabolome of human milk, a case report. *Microbiome.* 2014;2:24. doi:10.1186/2049-2618-2-24.

53. Morelli L. Postnatal development of intestinal microflora as influenced by infant nutrition. *J Nutr.* 2008;138(9):1791S-1795S. doi:10.1093/jn/138.9.1791S.

54. Kleinman RE, Walker WA. The enteromammary immune system: an important new concept in breast milk host defense. *Dig Dis Sci.* 1979;24(11):876-882. doi:10.1007/bf01324906.

55. Rautava S. Milk microbiome and neonatal colonization: overview. *Nestle Nutr Inst Workshop Ser.* 2020;94:65-74. doi:10.1159/000505030.

56. Rodríguez JM. The origin of human milk bacteria: is there a bacterial entero-mammary pathway during late pregnancy and lactation? *Adv Nutr.* 2014;5(6):779-784. doi:10.3945/an.114.007229.

57. Asbury MR, Butcher J, Copeland JK, et al. Mothers of preterm infants have individualized breast milk microbiota that changes temporally based on maternal characteristics. *Cell Host Microbe.* 2020;28(5):669-682.e4. doi:10.1016/j.chom.2020.08.001.

58. Cohen M, Steffen E, Axelrod R, et al. Availability of donor human milk decreases the incidence of necrotizing enterocolitis in VLBW infants. *Adv Neonatal Care.* 2021;21(5):341-348. doi:10.1097/anc.0000000000000804.

59. Picaud JC. Review highlights the importance of donor human milk being available for very low birth weight infants. *Acta Paediatr.* 2022;111(6):1127-1133. doi:10.1111/apa.16296.

60. Corpeleijn WE, de Waard M, Christmann V, et al. Effect of donor milk on severe infections and mortality in very low-birth-weight infants: the early nutrition study randomized clinical trial. *JAMA Pediatr.* 2016;170(7):654-661. doi:10.1001/jamapediatrics.2016.0183.

61. Ewaschuk JB, Unger S, Harvey S, O'Connor DL, Field CJ. Effect of pasteurization on immune components of milk: implications for feeding preterm infants. *Appl Physiol Nutr Metab.* 2011;36(2):175-182. doi:10.1139/h11-008.

62. O'Connor DL, Gibbins S, Kiss A, et al. Effect of supplemental donor human milk compared with preterm formula on neurodevelopment of very-low-birth-weight infants at 18 months: a randomized clinical trial. *JAMA.* 2016;316(18):1897-1905. doi:10.1001/jama.2016.16144.

63. Yu JC, Khodadadi H, Malik A, et al. Innate immunity of neonates and infants. *Front Immunol.* 2018;9:1759. doi:10.3389/fimmu.2018.01759.

64. Kollmann TR, Kampmann B, Mazmanian SK, Marchant A, Levy O. Protecting the newborn and young infant from infectious diseases: lessons from immune ontogeny. *Immunity.* 2017; 46(3):350-363. doi:10.1016/j.immuni.2017.03.009.

65. DiGiulio DB, Romero R, Kusanovic JP, et al. Prevalence and diversity of microbes in the amniotic fluid, the fetal inflammatory response, and pregnancy outcome in women with preterm pre-labor rupture of membranes. *Am J Reprod Immunol.* 2010;64(1):38-57. doi:10.1111/j.1600-0897.2010.00830.x.

66. Egan CE, Sodhi CP, Good M, et al. Toll-like receptor 4-mediated lymphocyte influx induces neonatal necrotizing enterocolitis. *J Clin Invest.* 2016;126(2):495-508. doi:10.1172/JCI83356.

67. Sharma AA, Jen R, Butler A, Lavoie PM. The developing human preterm neonatal immune system: a case for more research in this area. *Clin Immunol.* 2012;145(1):61-68. doi:10.1016/j.clim.2012.08.006.

68. Kollmann TR, Crabtree J, Rein-Weston A, et al. Neonatal innate TLR-mediated responses are distinct from those of adults. *J Immunol.* 2009;183(11):7150-7160. doi:10.4049/jimmunol.0901481.

69. Strunk T, Currie A, Richmond P, Simmer K, Burgner D. Innate immunity in human newborn infants: prematurity means more than immaturity. *J Matern Fetal Neonatal Med.* 2011;24(1):25-31. doi:10.3109/14767058.2010.482605.

70. Benkoe T, Baumann S, Weninger M, et al. Comprehensive evaluation of 11 cytokines in premature infants with surgical necrotizing enterocolitis. *PLoS One.* 2013;8(3):e58720. doi:10.1371/journal.pone.0058720.

71. Neish AS. Microbes in gastrointestinal health and disease. *Gastroenterology.* 2009;136(1):65-80. doi:10.1053/j.gastro.2008.10.080.

72. Ashayeri Ahmadabad R, Mirzaasgari Z, Gorji A, Khaleghi Ghadiri M. Toll-like receptor signaling pathways: novel therapeutic targets for cerebrovascular disorders. *Int J Mol Sci.* 2021;22(11):6153. doi:10.3390/ijms22116153.

73. Heel KA, McCauley RD, Papadimitriou JM, Hall JC. Review: Peyer's patches. *J Gastroenterol Hepatol.* 1997;12(2):122-136. doi:10.1111/j.1440-1746.1997.tb00395.x.

74. Maclennan KA. Reaction patterns of the lymph node. Part 1 cell types and functions. *J Clin Pathol.* 1991;44(12):1039.

75. Gleeson M, Cripps AW. Development of mucosal immunity in the first year of life and relationship to sudden infant death syndrome. *FEMS Immunol Med Microbiol.* 2004;42(1):21-33. doi:10.1016/j.femsim.2004.06.012.

76. Neu J. Necrotizing enterocolitis: the mystery goes on. *Neonatology.* 2014;106(4):289-295. doi:10.1159/000365130.

77. Wynn JL, Polin RA. Progress in the management of neonatal sepsis: the importance of a consensus definition. *Pediatr Res.* 2018;83(1-1):13-15. doi:10.1038/pr.2017.224.

78. Neu J, Modi N, Caplan M. Necrotizing enterocolitis comes in different forms: historical perspectives and defining the disease. *Semin Fetal Neonatal Med.* 2018;23(6):370-373. doi:10.1016/j.siny.2018.07.004.

79. Neu J, Walker WA. Necrotizing enterocolitis. *N Engl J Med.* 2011;364(3):255-264. doi:10.1056/NEJMra1005408.

80. Gonzalez-Rivera R, Culverhouse RC, Hamvas A, Tarr PI, Warner BB. The age of necrotizing enterocolitis onset: an application of Sartwell's incubation period model. *J Perinatol.* 2011;31(8):519-523. doi:10.1038/jp.2010.193.

81. Pitt J, Barlow B, Heird WC. Protection against experimental necrotizing enterocolitis by maternal milk. I. Role of milk leukocytes. *Pediatr Res.* 1977;11(8):906-909. doi:10.1203/00006450-197708000-00011.

82. Young CM, Kingma SD, Neu J. Ischemia-reperfusion and neonatal intestinal injury. *J Pediatr.* 2011;158(suppl 2):e25-e28. doi:10.1016/j.jpeds.2010.11.009.

83. Torrazza RM, Ukhanova M, Wang X, et al. Intestinal microbial ecology and environmental factors affecting necrotizing enterocolitis. *PLoS One.* 2013;8(12):e83304. doi:10.1371/journal.pone.0083304.

84. Mai V, Young CM, Ukhanova M, et al. Fecal microbiota in premature infants prior to necrotizing enterocolitis. *PLoS One.* 2011;6(6):e20647. doi:10.1371/journal.pone.0020647.

85. Pammi M, Cope J, Tarr PI, et al. Intestinal dysbiosis in preterm infants preceding necrotizing enterocolitis: a systematic review and meta-analysis. *Microbiome.* 2017;5(1):31. doi:10.1186/s40168-017-0248-8.

86. Lucas A, Cole TJ. Breast milk and neonatal necrotising enterocolitis. *Lancet*. 1990;336(8730):1519-1523. doi:10.1016/0140-6736(90)93304-8.

87. Raymond SL, Stortz JA, Mira JC, Larson SD, Wynn JL, Moldawer LL. Immunological defects in neonatal sepsis and potential therapeutic approaches. *Front Pediatr*. 2017;5:14. doi:10.3389/fped.2017.00014.

88. Madan JC, Salari RC, Saxena D, et al. Gut microbial colonisation in premature neonates predicts neonatal sepsis. *Arch Dis Child Fetal Neonatal Ed*. 2012;97(6):F456-F462. doi:10.1136/fetalneonatal-2011-301373.

89. Fasano A. Zonulin, regulation of tight junctions, and autoimmune diseases. *Ann N Y Acad Sci*. 2012;1258(1):25-33. doi:10.1111/j.1749-6632.2012.06538.x.

90. Anand RJ, Leaphart CL, Mollen KP, Hackam DJ. The role of the intestinal barrier in the pathogenesis of necrotizing enterocolitis. *Shock*. 2007;27(2):124-133. doi:10.1097/01.shk.0000239774.02904.65.

Chapter 3

Microbiome and Multiomics of the Developing Intestine: Nutritional and Environmental Perturbations

Mohan Pammi and Josef Neu

Chapter Outline

Key Points

1. Exposure of the intestine to certain microbes and/or their components and metabolites has implications for the future health of the individual as well as implications across generations via epigenetic mechanisms.
2. Responses of the host to the interactions of microbes, their antigens, and metabolic products need to be evaluated to better understand how they relate to the future health of the individual.
3. New developments in the field of artificial intelligence will synergize with multiomics and provide tools for precision nutrition and early diagnostics.

Antenatal Origins of the Perinatal Microbiome

The development of the neonatal microbiome, immunity, and metabolic homeostasis may be influenced by antenatal factors such as maternal modifiers or maternal determinants.[1,2] Maternal microbial colonization has been shown to affect neonatal microbial colonization and development of neonatal immunity.[3] Animal studies have demonstrated the effects of maternal microbiota on infants' transcription profiles, including those involved in innate immunity (antibacterial peptides), inflammation, and metabolism of microbial molecules.[3] Maternal Immunoglobulin A (IgA) in breast milk binds to infant intestinal bacteria (especially *Enterobacteriaceae*, a family of bacteria under the phylum *Proteobacteria*) and may play a protective role against necrotizing enterocolitis (NEC).[4] Maternal obesity and a high-fat diet during pregnancy may have an effect on the neonate's immune system, affect neonatal microbial colonization, and predispose the neonate to metabolic disease later in life.[1] The hypothesized mechanisms for this effect may be that the maternal metabolic derangement affects the infant's liver and other end organs through altered metabolite production, altered gut barrier integrity, and hematopoietic immune cells. Maternal programming of the fetal immune system may be effected by maternal antibodies, inflammatory mediators, micronutrients, microbial products, and maternal cells.[2]

Prior to birth, the maternal and fetal ecosystems may play a role in the timing of delivery. Specific microbiome communities or specific organisms that predispose to preterm births have not been identified. However, perturbations of the maternal microbiome, including the vaginal, gastrointestinal, amniotic fluid, and placental microbiomes, have been reported in preterm birth.[5–8] Inflammation and the presence of microbial DNA (or microbiome) in the amniotic fluid have been associated with preterm delivery.[9–11] The presence of a placental microbiome or intrauterine microbiome in normal pregnancies not complicated by chorioamnionitis or preterm rupture of membranes is a matter of debate. Aagaard and colleagues, in a population-based cohort of placental specimens collected under sterile conditions from 320 subjects, reported a unique placental microbiome niche composed of nonpathogenic commensal microbiota from the *Firmicutes*, *Tenericutes*, *Proteobacteria*, *Bacteroidetes*, and *Fusobacteria* phyla.[12] In aggregate, the placental microbiome profiles were most like the maternal oral microbiome. The placental microbiome was associated with a remote history of antenatal infection such as urinary tract infection in the first trimester, as well as with preterm birth. Other investigators have questioned the presence of the placental microbiome in normal pregnancies and attributed results to environmental contamination of samples.[13–15] Analyses of microbiota from first-pass meconium indicate the possibility of *in utero* colonization of the fetal gastrointestinal system.[5,16,17] Intrapartum antibiotic prophylaxis causes perturbations in the infant gut microbiome in both vaginal and caesarean section deliveries that may last up to a year, especially in those who are not breastfed.[18]

After Birth: Determinants of the Development of the Neonatal Microbiome

The neonatal microbiome undergoes a major transition during the birthing process: *in utero* the fetal skin is bathed in amniotic fluid, and after birth the neonate encounters a gaseous microbe-rich environment. The naïve neonatal microbiome matures and evolves rapidly into an adult-like microbiome during infancy and early childhood.[19–21] The composition of the developing neonatal microbiome is influenced at birth by mode of delivery (vaginal or cesarean) and later by feeding, antibiotic exposure, and the environment.[22–25] Mode of delivery has been reported to be a major variable in acquisition of the microbiome at birth and in the first weeks of life.[26] Investigators have reported that the differences in microbiome composition and diversity by mode of delivery may persist in the first few years of life and may be associated with allergic diseases in childhood.[27–31] However, Chu et al. found that by 6 weeks after delivery, the infant microbiota structure and function had substantially expanded and diversified, with the body site serving as the primary determinant of the composition of the bacterial community and its functional capacity and not the effect of mode of delivery.[32]

Composition of the gut microbiota in preterm infants shows a predominance of bacteria belonging to the phylum *Proteobacteria* in contrast to adults and older children where members of the *Firmicutes* predominate.[33,34] La Rosa et al. observed an orchestrated patterned progression of gut microbiota toward an abundance of *Clostridia* with increasing gestational age and predominance of *Proteobacteria*.[22] Antibiotics, feeding, or mode of delivery causes abrupt shifts in microbiota but may not change this seemingly predestined progression. Intestinal injury classified as NEC using a set of unclear diagnostic criteria is associated with a *Proteobacteria* bloom[35] and decreased abundances of anaerobic bacterial taxa (esp. *Negativicutes*).[36] Metagenomic evaluation of the intestinal microbiome in intestinal injury has also been shown to be associated uropathogenic *Escherichia coli* (a member of the class gamma-*Proteobacteria* and phylum *Proteobacteria*).[37]

During the neonatal period, microbial dysbiosis has been implicated in neonatal diseases such as NEC and bronchopulmonary dysplasia.[38,39] The intestinal microbiome (gut)–brain axis has been implicated in neurodevelopmental disorders such as autism.[40,41]

Infant feeding practices and antibiotic exposure are major determinants of the development of gut microbiota in the neonatal period and infancy.[42] Human milk contains proteins, fats, and carbohydrates in optimal concentrations and ratios for the well-being of the newborn infant and the preterm neonate. In addition, human milk has immune-protective factors, including immunoglobulins, lysozyme, lactoferrin, immunoregulatory cytokines (IL-10, TGF-β), and lymphocytes, among others.[43] Human milk may affect the development of the human gut microbiota by providing nutrients for bacterial proliferation, commensal bacteria, and immunoregulatory molecules. Human milk oligosaccharides (HMOs) are prebiotics that favor the growth of beneficial commensal bacteria such as *Bifidobacteria*.[44–46] These bacteria have the enzymatic machinery to digest the galacto-oligosaccharides in the milk, producing short-chain fatty acids (SCFAs) that have beneficial effects on preterm physiology. Breast milk is not sterile and has been known to have a microbiome with *Firmicutes* and *Lactobacilli*, which are beneficial for normal development of the gastrointestinal microbiome.[47,48] Fatty acids in breast milk and ratios of polyunsaturated fatty acids contribute to host health and immune development.[49] Formula-fed infants have enriched facultative and obligatory anaerobes such as clostridium and *Bacteroides* and increased *Proteobacteria*.[42,50] Pasteurized human donor milk partially restores the gut microbiome toward breast milk–fed infants compared to formula-fed infants.[51] After weaning to solid foods, the microbiome of both the breast-fed and formula-fed infants converges toward the mature adult microbiome.[52]

Antibiotic exposure early in life has profound effects on the normal development of the infant gut microbiota. Antibiotic exposure in early life skews gut microbiome development toward *Proteobacteria*, decreases microbial diversity, and leads to development of antibiotic-resistant bacteria.[53–56] Increased antibiotic exposure in early infancy is associated with increased risk of NEC in preterm infants.[57–59] The immediate environment of the preterm infant may also affect microbial exposure and colonization. Studies have shown the acquisition of gut microbiota including fungal colonization that may be related to the NICU environment.[60–62]

Mechanisms by Which the Neonatal/Perinatal Microbiome Influences Pathophysiology in Preterm Neonates: Immune Regulation, Inflammation, and Epigenetic Changes

The mechanisms of the altered perinatal microbiome on preterm pathophysiology have been studied in both animal models and *in vitro* studies. The preterm intestinal microbiome is closer to that of germ-free mice than that of adult mice. Germ-free mice lack normal immune regulation by commensal bacteria, and accumulation of invariant natural killer T cells (iNKT) in the colon and lung may result in mucosal pathology.[63] An interesting observation is that in neonatal germ-free mice (but not adult mice) exposed to conventional microbiota, decreased methylation of the Cxcl16 gene results in decreased expression and decreased accumulation of iNKT. This suggests that neonatal exposure to conventional microbiota is critical in immune regulation and may have long-lasting effects.[63]

IMMUNE REGULATION AND INFLAMMATION

Microbiota and metabolites drive innate immune responses and inflammation. Microbiota on human body surfaces and their metabolites act as environmental triggers that influence mammalian gene expression.[64,65] Recognition of commensal-derived pathogen-associated molecular patterns (PAMPs) such as lipopolysaccharides by intestinal epithelial cells (IECs) induces secretion of the antimicrobial peptide RegIIIγ, which mediates colonization resistance in the gut.[66] The microbiota-derived signals butyrate, propionate, and acetate (SCFAs) induce IL-18 production from the IEC through activation of nucleotide oligomerization domain (NOD)–like receptors (NLRs).[67] Acetate produced by *Bifidobacteria* promotes epithelial cell barrier function by inducing an antiapoptotic response in the IEC. Thus microbiota and their metabolites mediate immune response via the IEC and immune cells.[66,68]

EPIGENETIC CHANGES

Microbiota and metabolites influence the human epigenome and expression of genes associated with inflammation. Epigenetics involves the molecular processes that permit changes in gene expression without a change in the genetic code.[69] The most characterized epigenetic mechanisms are DNA methylation and histone modifications, which alter gene transcription in response to environmental triggers. Epigenomic modifications are maintained by the balancing activity of epigenomic modifying enzymes such as DNA methyltransferases, histone acetyltransferases, and histone methyltransferases.[64,65,69] Animal studies report repression of proinflammatory genes by microbiota; such repression is not seen in germ-free mice. Studies in germ-free mice have shown that DNA methylation of the TLR4 gene in the IECs was lower compared to conventional mice, indicating that TLR4 gene expression is repressed in wild-type mice.[70] Other experiments have shown that mononuclear phagocytes from conventionally housed mice compared to germ-free mice carried commensal bacteria with increased histone H3 methylation and decreased transcription of inflammatory genes.[71] Increased abundances of *Firmicutes* and *Bacteroidetes* are associated with obesity and cardiovascular risk, possibly due to their effects on glucose absorption, generation of fatty acids, hepatic lipogenesis, and tissue adipocyte deposition.[72,73]

Microbial metabolites (i.e., metabolites produced by microbiota) may induce changes in the epigenome. It is known that germ-free mice have lower levels of SCFAs compared to conventionally housed animals.[74,75] SCFAs inhibit histone deacetylase activity, which may be a potential target for epigenomic changes.[76,77] SCFAs also have been shown to stimulate histone acetylation of the forkhead box P3 (FOXP3) locus on naïve CD4+ T cells, increase FOXP3 expression, and promote differentiation of Tregs (antiinflammatory effects).[67,74,78] *Faecalibacterium prausnitzii* and *Eubacterium rectale/Roseburia* species (members of the phylum *Firmicutes*) are major contributors of butyrate, which regulates gene expression by histone modifications.[79] Lipopolysaccharides, an inflammatory marker for cardiovascular disease, may also have a role in epigenetic regulation of intestinal and immune cells.[80]

Leveraging Artificial Intelligence for Multiomics Investigation Into Health and Disease: the Need for Precision Medicine

The National Institutes of Health (NIH) defines *precision medicine* as "an innovative approach that takes into account individual differences in patients' genes, environments, and lifestyles." There is an urgent need to shift our current thinking on traditional symptom-based medicine to proactive precision medicine in which the trajectory toward health and disease can be predicted in advance so that interventions can be instituted to improve survival and decrease morbidity.

Recent advances in high-throughput technologies have provided access to multiomic biological data (including microbiomes, genomics, epigenomics, transcriptomics, proteomics, metabolomics, and immunomics) and provide a holistic view of pathophysiology in maternal and child health.[81] There is an ever-increasing need for integrative analysis of the human microbiome with information from the genome, the proteome, the metabolome, and the epigenome. Biological insights gained from multiomics should be integrated with clinical and social data and applied for the best possible clinical outcomes. Integration of these heterogeneous datasets using state-of-the-art artificial intelligence (AI) technology enables the development of biomarkers that can predict short- and long-term health trajectories and early timely interventions to improve outcomes. There are several forms of AI, including machine learning, neural networks, and deep learning, that yield reliable holistic models to predict mortality, morbidity, or other complications in pregnant women and preterm infants. The insights gained through integration of multiomic datasets with these different forms of AI are likely to lead to personalized healthcare decision-making (precision medicine) and biomarker discovery.

Summary

The developing intestinal microbiome in neonates and beyond has implications for health and disease. In preterm neonates, microbial dysbiosis has been implicated in NEC, bronchopulmonary dysplasia, and sepsis. The maternal microbiome and immunity may shape the immune development of the fetus and determine neonatal colonization during the process of delivery and immediately after. Postnatally infant nutrition with maternal milk and exposure to antibiotics appear to be major determinants for patterning the infant intestinal microbiome. It is imperative to integrate microbiome data with other multiomics to develop a holistic view of infant health and disease. Huge amount of data generated by multiomic investigations can be integrated by AI for predictive analytics and discovery of biomarkers which can facilitate the paradigm of Precision Medicine in Neonatology.

REFERENCES

1. Mulligan CM, Friedman JE. Maternal modifiers of the infant gut microbiota: metabolic consequences. *J Endocrinol*. 2017;235(1): R1-R12. doi:10.1530/joe-17-0303.
2. Jennewein MF, Abu-Raya B, Jiang Y, Alter G, Marchant A. Transfer of maternal immunity and programming of the newborn immune system. *Semin Immunopathol*. 2017;39(6):605-613. doi:10.1007/s00281-017-0653-x.
3. Gomez de Aguero M, Ganal-Vonarburg SC, Fuhrer T, et al. The maternal microbiota drives early postnatal innate immune development. *Science*. 2016;351(6279):1296-1302. doi:10.1126/science.aad2571.
4. Gopalakrishna KP, Macadangdang BR, Rogers MB, et al. Maternal IgA protects against the development of necrotizing enterocolitis in preterm infants. *Nat Med*. 2019;25(7):1110-1115. doi:10.1038/s41591-019-0480-9.
5. Ardissone AN, de la Cruz DM, Davis-Richardson AG, et al. Meconium microbiome analysis identifies bacteria correlated with premature birth. *PloS One*. 2014;9(3):e90784. doi:10.1371/journal.pone.0090784.
6. Cao B, Stout MJ, Lee I, Mysorekar IU. Placental microbiome and its role in preterm birth. *Neoreviews*. 2014;15(12): e537-e545. doi:10.1542/neo.15-12-e537.
7. Chu DM, Seferovic M, Pace RM, Aagaard KM. The microbiome in preterm birth. *Best Pract Res Clin Obstet Gynaecol*. 2018;52:103-113. doi:10.1016/j.bpobgyn.2018.03.006.
8. Prince AL, Ma J, Kannan PS, et al. The placental membrane microbiome is altered among subjects with spontaneous preterm birth with and without chorioamnionitis. *Am J Obstet Gynecol*. 2016;214(5):627.e1-627.e16. doi:10.1016/j.ajog.2016.01.193.
9. Urushiyama D, Suda W, Ohnishi E, et al. Microbiome profile of the amniotic fluid as a predictive biomarker of perinatal outcome. *Sci Rep*. 2017;7(1):12171. doi:10.1038/s41598-017-11699-8.
10. DiGiulio DB. Diversity of microbes in amniotic fluid. *Semin Fetal Neonatal Med*. 2012;17(1):2-11. doi:10.1016/j.siny.2011.10.001.
11. DiGiulio DB, Gervasi MT, Romero R, et al. Microbial invasion of the amniotic cavity in pregnancies with small-for-gestational-age fetuses. *J Perinat Med*. 2010;38(5):495-502. doi:10.1515/jpm.2010.076.
12. Aagaard K, Ma J, Antony KM, Ganu R, Petrosino J, Versalovic J. The placenta harbors a unique microbiome. *Sci Transl Med*. 2014;6(237):237ra65. doi:10.1126/scitranslmed.3008599.
13. Leiby JS, McCormick K, Sherrill-Mix S, et al. Lack of detection of a human placenta microbiome in samples from preterm and term deliveries. *Microbiome*. 2018;6(1):196. doi:10.1186/s40168-018-0575-4.
14. Perez-Munoz ME, Arrieta MC, Ramer-Tait AE, Walter J. A critical assessment of the "sterile womb" and "in utero colonization" hypotheses: implications for research on the pioneer infant microbiome. *Microbiome*. 2017;5(1):48. doi:10.1186/s40168-017-0268-4.
15. Theis KR, Romero R, Winters AD, et al. Does the human placenta delivered at term have a microbiota? Results of cultivation, quantitative real-time PCR, 16S rRNA gene sequencing, and metagenomics. *Am J Obstet Gynecol*. 2019;220(3):267.e1-267.e39. doi:10.1016/j.ajog.2018.10.018.
16. Rackaityte E, Halkias J, Fukui EM, et al. Viable bacterial colonization is highly limited in the human intestine in utero. *Nat Med*. 2020;26(4):599-607. doi:10.1038/s41591-020-0761-3.
17. Turunen J, Tejesvi MV, Paalanne N, et al. Presence of distinctive microbiome in the first-pass meconium of newborn infants. *Sci Rep*. 2021;11(1):19449. doi:10.1038/s41598-021-98951-4.
18. Azad MB, Konya T, Persaud RR, et al. Impact of maternal intrapartum antibiotics, method of birth and breastfeeding on gut microbiota during the first year of life: a prospective cohort study. *BJOG*. 2016;123(6):983-993. doi:10.1111/1471-0528.13601.
19. Kim CS, Claud EC. Necrotizing enterocolitis pathophysiology: how microbiome data alter our understanding. *Clin Perinatol*. 2019;46(1):29-38. doi:10.1016/j.clp.2018.10.003.
20. Baranowski JR, Claud EC. Necrotizing enterocolitis and the preterm infant microbiome. *Adv Exp Med Biol*. 2019;1125: 25-36. doi:10.1007/5584_2018_313.
21. Underwood MA, Sohn K. The microbiota of the extremely preterm infant. *Clin Perinatol*. 2017;44(2):407-427. doi:10.1016/j.clp.2017.01.005.
22. La Rosa PS, Warner BB, Zhou Y, et al. Patterned progression of bacterial populations in the premature infant gut. *Proc Natl Acad Sci U S A*. 2014;111(34):12522-12527. doi:10.1073/pnas.1409497111.
23. Stewart CJ, Embleton ND, Marrs ECL, et al. Longitudinal development of the gut microbiome and metabolome in preterm neonates with late onset sepsis and healthy controls. *Microbiome*. 2017;5(1):75. doi:10.1186/s40168-017-0295-1.
24. Stewart CJ, Embleton ND, Marrs EC, et al. Temporal bacterial and metabolic development of the preterm gut reveals specific signatures in health and disease. *Microbiome*. 2016;4(1):67. doi:10.1186/s40168-016-0216-8.
25. Shao Y, Forster SC, Tsaliki E, et al. Stunted microbiota and opportunistic pathogen colonization in caesarean-section birth. *Nature*. 2019;574(7776):117-121. doi:10.1038/s41586-019-1560-1.
26. Dominguez-Bello MG, Costello EK, Contreras M, et al. Delivery mode shapes the acquisition and structure of the initial microbiota across multiple body habitats in newborns. *Proc Natl Acad Sci U S A*. 2010;107(26):11971-11975. doi:10.1073/pnas.1002601107.
27. Ma J, Li Z, Zhang W, et al. Comparison of the gut microbiota in healthy infants with different delivery modes and feeding types: a cohort study. *Front Microbiol*. 2022;13:868227. doi:10.3389/fmicb.2022.868227.
28. Mueller NT, Differding MK, Østbye T, Hoyo C, Benjamin-Neelon SE. Association of birth mode of delivery with infant faecal microbiota, potential pathobionts, and short chain fatty acids: a longitudinal study over the first year of life. *BJOG*. 2021;128(8):1293-1303. doi:10.1111/1471-0528.16633.
29. Reyman M, van Houten MA, van Baarle D, et al. Impact of delivery mode-associated gut microbiota dynamics on health in the first year of life. *Nat Commun*. 2019;10(1):4997. doi:10.1038/s41467-019-13014-7.
30. Galazzo G, van Best N, Bervoets L, et al. Development of the microbiota and associations with birth mode, diet, and atopic disorders in a longitudinal analysis of stool samples, collected

from infancy through early childhood. *Gastroenterology*. 2020;158(6):1584-1596. doi:10.1053/j.gastro.2020.01.024.

31. Shaterian N, Abdi F, Ghavidel N, Alidost F. Role of cesarean section in the development of neonatal gut microbiota: a systematic review. *Open Med (Wars)*. 2021;16(1):624-639. doi:10.1515/med-2021-0270.

32. Chu DM, Ma J, Prince AL, Antony KM, Seferovic MD, Aagaard KM. Maturation of the infant microbiome community structure and function across multiple body sites and in relation to mode of delivery. *Nat Med*. 2017;23(3):314-326. doi:10.1038/nm.4272.

33. Zhang H, DiBaise JK, Zuccolo A, et al. Human gut microbiota in obesity and after gastric bypass. *Proc Natl Acad Sci U S A*. 2009;106(7):2365-2370. doi:10.1073/pnas.0812600106.

34. Saulnier DM, Riehle K, Mistretta TA, et al. Gastrointestinal microbiome signatures of pediatric patients with irritable bowel syndrome. *Gastroenterology*. 2011;141(5):1782-1791. doi:10.1053/j.gastro.2011.06.072.

35. Torrazza RM, Neu J. The altered gut microbiome and necrotizing enterocolitis. *Clin Perinatol*. 2013;40(1):93-108. doi:10.1016/j.clp.2012.12.009.

36. Warner BB, Deych E, Zhou Y, et al. Gut bacteria dysbiosis and necrotising enterocolitis in very low birthweight infants: a prospective case-control study. *Lancet*. 2016;387(10031):1928-1936. doi:10.1016/S0140-6736(16)00081-7.

37. Ward DV, Scholz M, Zolfo M, et al. Metagenomic sequencing with strain-level resolution implicates uropathogenic *E. coli* in necrotizing enterocolitis and mortality in preterm infants. *Cell Rep*. 2016;14(12):2912-2924. doi:10.1016/j.celrep.2016.03.015.

38. Pammi M, Lal CV, Wagner BD, et al. Airway microbiome and development of bronchopulmonary dysplasia in preterm infants: a systematic review. *J Pediatr*. 2019;204:126-133.e2. doi:10.1016/j.jpeds.2018.08.042.

39. Pammi M, Cope J, Tarr PI, et al. Intestinal dysbiosis in preterm infants preceding necrotizing enterocolitis: a systematic review and meta-analysis. *Microbiome*. 2017;5(1):31. doi:10.1186/s40168-017-0248-8.

40. Vuong HE, Hsiao EY. Emerging roles for the gut microbiome in autism spectrum disorder. *Biol Psychiatry*. 2017;81(5):411-423. doi:10.1016/j.biopsych.2016.08.024.

41. Luna RA, Oezguen N, Balderas M, et al. Distinct microbiome-neuroimmune signatures correlate with functional abdominal pain in children with autism spectrum disorder. *Cell Mol Gastroenterol Hepatol*. 2017;3(2):218-230. doi:10.1016/j.jcmgh.2016.11.008.

42. Chong CYL, Bloomfield FH, O'Sullivan JM. Factors affecting gastrointestinal microbiome development in neonates. *Nutrients*. 2018;10(3):274. doi:10.3390/nu10030274.

43. Sánchez C, Franco L, Regal P, Lamas A, Cepeda A, Fente C. Breast milk: a source of functional compounds with potential application in nutrition and therapy. *Nutrients*. 2021;13(3):1026. doi:10.3390/nu13031026.

44. Berger B, Porta N, Foata F, et al. Linking human milk oligosaccharides, infant fecal community types, and later risk to require antibiotics. *mBio*. 2020;11(2):e03196-e03119. doi:10.1128/mBio.03196-19.

45. Masi AC, Stewart CJ. Untangling human milk oligosaccharides and infant gut microbiome. *iScience*. 2022;25(1):103542. doi:10.1016/j.isci.2021.103542.

46. Singh RP, Niharika J, Kondepudi KK, Bishnoi M, Tingirikari JMR. Recent understanding of human milk oligosaccharides in establishing infant gut microbiome and roles in immune

system. *Food Res Int*. 2022;151:110884. doi:10.1016/j.foodres.2021.110884.

47. Pannaraj PS, Li F, Cerini C, et al. Association between breast milk bacterial communities and establishment and development of the infant gut microbiome. *JAMA Pediatr*. 2017;171(7):647-654. doi:10.1001/jamapediatrics.2017.0378.

48. Mantziari A, Rautava S. Factors influencing the microbial composition of human milk. *Semin Perinatol*. 2021;45(8):151507. doi:10.1016/j.semperi.2021.151507.

49. Kumar H, du Toit E, Kulkarni A, et al. Distinct patterns in human milk microbiota and fatty acid profiles across specific geographic locations. *Front Microbiol*. 2016;7:1619. doi:10.3389/fmicb.2016.01619.

50. Vandenplas Y, Carnielli VP, Ksiazyk J, et al. Factors affecting early-life intestinal microbiota development. *Nutrition*. 2020;78:110812. doi:10.1016/j.nut.2020.110812.

51. Gregory KE, Samuel BS, Houghteling P, et al. Influence of maternal breast milk ingestion on acquisition of the intestinal microbiome in preterm infants. *Microbiome*. 2016;4(1):68. doi:10.1186/s40168-016-0214-x.

52. Stewart CJ, Ajami NJ, O'Brien JL, et al. Temporal development of the gut microbiome in early childhood from the TEDDY study. *Nature*. 2018;562(7728):583-588. doi:10.1038/s41586-018-0617-x.

53. Greenwood C, Morrow AL, Lagomarcino AJ, et al. Early empiric antibiotic use in preterm infants is associated with lower bacterial diversity and higher relative abundance of Enterobacter. *J Pediatr*. 2014;165(1):23-29. doi:10.1016/j.jpeds.2014.01.010.

54. Moore AM, Ahmadi S, Patel S, et al. Gut resistome development in healthy twin pairs in the first year of life. *Microbiome*. 2015;3:27. doi:10.1186/s40168-015-0090-9.

55. Tanaka S, Kobayashi T, Songjinda P, et al. Influence of antibiotic exposure in the early postnatal period on the development of intestinal microbiota. *FEMS Immunol Med Microbiol*. 2009;56(1):80-87. doi:10.1111/j.1574-695X.2009.00553.x.

56. Fouhy F, Guinane CM, Hussey S, et al. High-throughput sequencing reveals the incomplete, short-term recovery of infant gut microbiota following parenteral antibiotic treatment with ampicillin and gentamicin. *Antimicrob Agents Chemother*. 2012;56(11):5811-5820. doi:10.1128/aac.00789-12.

57. Cotten CM, Taylor S, Stoll B, et al. Prolonged duration of initial empirical antibiotic treatment is associated with increased rates of necrotizing enterocolitis and death for extremely low birth weight infants. *Pediatrics*. 2009;123(1):58-66. doi:10.1542/peds.2007-3423.

58. Alexander VN, Northrup V, Bizzarro MJ. Antibiotic exposure in the newborn intensive care unit and the risk of necrotizing enterocolitis. *J Pediatr*. 2011;159(3):392-397. doi:10.1016/j.jpeds.2011.02.035.

59. Kuppala VS, Meinzen-Derr J, Morrow AL, Schibler KR. Prolonged initial empirical antibiotic treatment is associated with adverse outcomes in premature infants. *J Pediatr*. 2011;159(5):720-725. doi:10.1016/j.jpeds.2011.05.033.

60. Brooks B, Firek BA, Miller CS, et al. Microbes in the neonatal intensive care unit resemble those found in the gut of premature infants. *Microbiome*. 2014;2(1):1. doi:10.1186/2049-2618-2-1.

61. Brooks B, Olm MR, Firek BA, et al. Strain-resolved analysis of hospital rooms and infants reveals overlap between the human and room microbiome. *Nat Commun*. 2017;8(1):1814. doi:10.1038/s41467-017-02018-w.

62. Olm MR, West PT, Brooks B, et al. Genome-resolved metagenomics of eukaryotic populations during early colonization of premature infants and in hospital rooms. *Microbiome*. 2019;7(1):26. doi:10.1186/s40168-019-0638-1.

63. Olszak T, An D, Zeissig S, et al. Microbial exposure during early life has persistent effects on natural killer T cell function. *Science*. 2012;336(6080):489-493. doi:10.1126/science.1219328.

64. Alenghat T, Artis D. Epigenomic regulation of host-microbiota interactions. *Trends Immunol*. 2014;35(11):518-525. doi:10.1016/j.it.2014.09.007.

65. Alenghat T. Epigenomics and the microbiota. *Toxicol Pathol*. 2015;43(1):101-106. doi:10.1177/0192623314553805.

66. Kabat AM, Srinivasan N, Maloy KJ. Modulation of immune development and function by intestinal microbiota. *Trends Immunol*. 2014;35(11):507-517. doi:10.1016/j.it.2014.07.010.

67. Smith PM, Howitt MR, Panikov N, et al. The microbial metabolites, short-chain fatty acids, regulate colonic Treg cell homeostasis. *Science*. 2013;341(6145):569-573. doi:10.1126/science.1241165.

68. Deshmukh HS, Liu Y, Menkiti OR, et al. The microbiota regulates neutrophil homeostasis and host resistance to *Escherichia coli* K1 sepsis in neonatal mice. *Nat Med*. 2014;20(5):524-530. doi:10.1038/nm.3542.

69. Arrowsmith CH, Bountra C, Fish PV, Lee K, Schapira M. Epigenetic protein families: a new frontier for drug discovery. *Nat Rev Drug Discov*. 2012;11(5):384-400. doi:10.1038/nrd3674.

70. Takahashi K, Sugi Y, Nakano K, et al. Epigenetic control of the host gene by commensal bacteria in large intestinal epithelial cells. *J Biol Chem*. 2011;286(41):35755-35762. doi:10.1074/jbc.M111.271007.

71. Ganal SC, Sanos SL, Kallfass C, et al. Priming of natural killer cells by nonmucosal mononuclear phagocytes requires instructive signals from commensal microbiota. *Immunity*. 2012;37(1):171-186. doi:10.1016/j.immuni.2012.05.020.

72. Kumar H, Lund R, Laiho A, et al. Gut microbiota as an epigenetic regulator: pilot study based on whole-genome methylation analysis. *mBio*. 2014;5(6):e02113-e02114. doi:10.1128/mBio.02113-14.

73. Caesar R, Fåk F, Bäckhed F. Effects of gut microbiota on obesity and atherosclerosis via modulation of inflammation and lipid metabolism. *J Intern Med*. 2010;268(4):320-328. doi:10.1111/j.1365-2796.2010.02270.x.

74. Arpaia N, Campbell C, Fan X, et al. Metabolites produced by commensal bacteria promote peripheral regulatory T-cell generation. *Nature*. 2013;504(7480):451-455. doi:10.1038/nature12726.

75. Høverstad T, Midtvedt T. Short-chain fatty acids in germfree mice and rats. *J Nutr*. 1986;116(9):1772-1776. doi:10.1093/jn/116.9.1772.

76. Macfarlane S, Macfarlane GT. Regulation of short-chain fatty acid production. *Proc Nutr Soc*. 2003;62(1):67-72. doi:10.1079/PNS2002207.

77. Waldecker M, Kautenburger T, Daumann H, Busch C, Schrenk D. Inhibition of histone-deacetylase activity by short-chain fatty acids and some polyphenol metabolites formed in the colon. *J Nutr Biochem*. 2008;19(9):587-593. doi:10.1016/j.jnutbio.2007.08.002.

78. Furusawa Y, Obata Y, Fukuda S, et al. Commensal microbe-derived butyrate induces the differentiation of colonic regulatory T cells. *Nature*. 2013;504(7480):446-450. doi:10.1038/nature12721.

79. Canani RB, Costanzo MD, Leone L, Pedata M, Meli R, Calignano A. Potential beneficial effects of butyrate in intestinal and extraintestinal diseases. *World J Gastroenterol*. 2011;17(12):1519-1528. doi:10.3748/wjg.v17.i12.1519.

80. Angrisano T, Pero R, Peluso S, et al. LPS-induced IL-8 activation in human intestinal epithelial cells is accompanied by specific histone H3 acetylation and methylation changes. *BMC Microbiol*. 2010;10:172. doi:10.1186/1471-2180-10-172.

81. Neu J. Multiomics-based strategies for taming intestinal inflammation in the neonate. *Curr Opin Clin Nutr Metab Care*. 2019;22(3):217-222. doi:10.1097/mco.0000000000000559.

Chapter 4

The Brain-Gut-Microbiota Axis

Flavia Indrio and Josef Neu

Chapter Outline

Key Points

1. Bidirectional signaling occurs between the brain and intestine.
2. Microbes in the intestinal tract play a major role in the regulation of this signaling.
3. Disruption of these signaling processes can have a major effect on brain development and pathogenesis of neurobehavioral diseases such as depression, anxiety, and autism.

Introduction

The realization that gastrointestinal physiology is closely linked to the brain and vice versa is not new. Almost 2500 ago, Hippocrates, the "father of medicine," allegedly stated that "All disease begins in the gut." From direct observation, the brain has a direct effect on the stomach and intestine, where the very thought of eating can cause the release of intestinal digestive products before the food even arrives. On the other hand, distress in the gastrointestinal tract can send signals to the brain.

It is clear from human experience that various foods can affect mood. Some foods have a calming effect whereas others may cause excitement. Anxiety and excitement are often accompanied with changes in bowel habits. These are a few examples of bidirectional signaling between the gut and the brain, termed the *gut-brain axis*. Relationships suggesting bidirectional signaling between gut and brain have been described for several centuries.[1] Additional support for the gut-brain axis concept is emerging.[2–5] This includes the finding that there is a cooperation between intestinal bacteria and their animal hosts that regulates development and function of the immune system as well as the metabolic and nervous systems.[2] Nevertheless, many aspects of this cooperative triad remain unclear largely because their mechanisms remain to be elucidated.[6]

In this chapter we will provide an overview of several aspects of the gut-brain-microbiota axis. These include bidirectional signaling processes, how the components of this axis interact in disease, the evidence linking brain injury with the intestinal microbiota, immunology, inflammation as it pertains to the fetus and preterm infants, and the effects of antibiotics and other environmental perturbations on neurodevelopment via inflammatory processes and microbial metabolites.

It is important to note that much of the information currently available on the gut-brain-microbiota axis and its relation to health and disease in humans is based on single-omic technologies and is associative rather than causal. Although we have extrapolated considerable information from in vitro studies and studies in animals, how well they directly relate to the human remains unclear. We will briefly describe how integrated multiomics may help us better understand mechanisms and causality of central nervous system (CNS) diseases in humans and how they relate to the gut-brain axis.

Here we also present some of the information relating intestinal microbes to neurologic disorders, identify gaps in our current knowledge, and discuss future directions for research to clarify these relationships with the hope that this will lead to preventive and therapeutic strategies.

Overview of Brain-Gut-Microbial Signaling

BIDIRECTIONAL SIGNALING

The CNS plays a major role in various gut functions. Included among these are motility, secretion, blood flow, and gut-associated immune function in response to psychological and physical stressors.[7] This has been known for a long time but was amplified in the 1840s when William Beaumont, the father of gastrointestinal medicine, experimentally showed that emotional status affected the rate of digestion and thus that the brain affects the gut.[8] Beaumont's observations of Alexis St. Martin, a fur trader who incurred a gunshot wound that exposed his stomach, showed how various behaviors of the stomach related to mood, hunger, and other factors and thus

was one of the first direct observations of a brain-gut axis. This concept was subsequently recognized by numerous famous scientists including Darwin and Pavlov, but it took until the early to mid-20th century for accurate observations to be made that correlated gut physiology changes with changes in emotion.[8]

The gastrointestinal tract also sends signals to the brain via the gut-brain axis. The intestinal microbiota play an integral role in this signaling.[2] Components of the gut-brain axis include the CNS, neuroendocrine system, neuroimmune system, hypothalamic-pituitary-adrenal axis, autonomic nervous systems (both sympathetic and parasympathetic), enteric nervous system, vagus nerve, and intestinal microbiota.[9,10]

As seen in Fig. 4.1, the bidirectional communication is accomplished by neural, humoral, endocrine, and immune connections between the gastrointestinal tract and the CNS.[11] The microbes in the intestinal tract influence the brain via the release of cytokines, neurotransmitters, neuropeptides, endocrine messengers, and microbial metabolites.[3]

ENTERIC NERVOUS SYSTEM

The enteric nervous system (ENS) is one of the main divisions of the nervous system and consists of a mesh-like system of neurons that govern the function of the gastrointestinal system. The ENS utilizes numerous neurotransmitters, such as acetylcholine, dopamine, and serotonin. More than 90% of the body's serotonin and about 50% of the body's dopamine lie in the gut and are among several functions involved in regulation of motility.[12]

Development of Gut-Brain-Microbial Axis

FETUS

Despite a considerable number of studies suggesting live fetal placental and intestinal microbiota,[13,14] more recent studies indicate that the microbial signals detected in the fetal intestinal tract are likely the result of contamination during clinical procedures to obtain fetal samples or during DNA extraction and DNA sequencing.[15] This remains a matter of debate,[16] but whether a direct presence of microbes in the fetal intestinal tract is necessary for functional responses and development is not clear. Maternal microbes are still

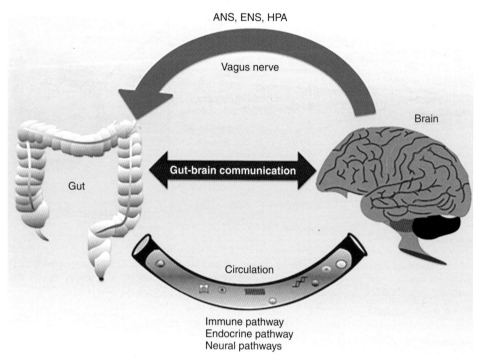

ANS, ENS, HPA

Vagus nerve

Brain

Gut-brain communication

Gut

Circulation

Immune pathway
Endocrine pathway
Neural pathways

Fig. 4.1 Bidirectional communication between the intestine and brain mediated by the intestinal microbiota. *ANS*, Autonomic nervous system; *ENS*, enteric nervous system; *HPA*, hypothalamus-pituitary-adrenal axis. From Suganya K, Koo BS. Gut–brain axis: role of gut microbiota on neurological disorders and how probiotics/prebiotics beneficially modulate microbial and immune pathways to improve brain functions. *Int J Mol Sci*. 2020;21(20):7551. doi:10.3390/ijms21207551.

likely to play a role in development of the fetal gut-brain axis. The mother–infant dyad is actually triangulated with a third component, the microbiota,[17] which in the maternal intestine release large quantities of metabolites that can be transported to the fetus and are known to be highly active (Fig. 4.2).[18]

Maternal diet, antibiotic usage, obesity, hypertension, and exposure to various environmental perturbations can affect this relationship with the fetus through the microbiota. The maternal intestinal microbiota undergo changes during different stages of pregnancy,[20] and several complications of pregnancy and subsequent outcomes in the offspring have been linked to perturbations of the microbiota,[18,19] especially those due to antibiotic use.[21]

As seen in Fig. 4.2, maternal intestinal microbial–derived metabolites are transmitted via the placenta to the fetus.[22] Some of the main end products of bacterial metabolism are the short-chain fatty acids (SCFAs) acetate, propionate, and butyrate. These have been

demonstrated to have beneficial effects during early fetal development, which includes their effects on control of insulin levels in the fetus; however, they have also been linked to the development of metabolic syndrome.[23] The presence of normally balanced intestinal microbiota and metabolites, which include SCFAs such as butyrate, is essential in maintenance of an intact blood–brain barrier.

Another putative function of SCFAs in the fetus is development of the nervous system.[23] Gut microbiota development occurring during the third trimester of pregnancy is associated with synaptogenesis, myelination, and development of specific brain areas.[24,25]

NEWBORN

During and after birth, the mode of delivery, gestational age, type of feeding (breast versus formula) used in the infant, and immediate neonatal perturbations such as being housed in a NICU versus being in a more sheltered home environment play a role in the

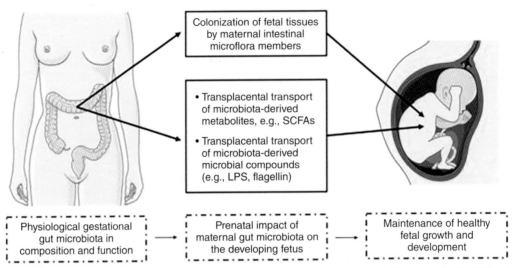

Fig. 4.2 Action of the maternal gut microbiota on the developing embryo and fetus during pregnancy. *LPS*, Lipopolysaccharide; *SCFAs*, short-chain fatty acids. From Miko E, Csaszar A, Bodis J, Kovacs K. The maternal-fetal gut microbiota axis: physiological changes, dietary influence, and modulation possibilities. *Life (Basel)*. 2022;12(3):424. doi:10.3390/life12030424.

colonization process. Areas where intensive research has been done include the blood–brain barrier, neurogenesis, myelination, and maturation of microglia.[26] Recent evidence describes how developmental processes in the brain can be facilitated by gut microbes and their interaction with the immune system as well as the production of metabolites.[27] In this descriptive model, dysbiosis of the gut microbiome in preterm infants predisposes the neonate to intestinal injury and sepsis, potentially leading to adverse neurologic outcomes later in life.[27] This suggests that optimizing the microbiota during early life is crucial for protecting infants from prematurity-related neurodevelopmental diseases and for developing preventive and therapeutic strategies. One of the most obvious interventions relates to promotion of a healthy microbiota, which has yet to be clearly defined.[28]

Early Life Disruptions of the Gut-Brain Axis

Several perturbations of the intestinal microbial environment in early life affect various aspects of intestinal development and the gut-brain axis during the lifespan of the individual.[29] These include maternal factors such as maternal diet, obesity, maternal antibiotic usage, mode of delivery, gestational age at birth, various stressors such as medication usage, type of diet such as being breastfed versus formula fed, and environmental pollutants.[30–32]

The specific mechanisms that cause these neurodevelopmental disorders often related to inflammatory conditions[33] remain poorly understood but are the targets of investigation. The inflammatory response initiated through the innate immune system triggers intracellular signaling pathways by activating toll-like receptors. These, in turn, signal for the expression of interferons, cytokines, and other immunologic mediators. These pathways may play an integral role in development of neurodevelopmental disorders (Fig. 4.3).[34]

There are also gut microbes that can counteract inflammation. These can act by inhibiting inflammation-induced microbes, producing SCFAs that strengthen the interepithelial junction barrier or interact directly with components of the innate immune system. These microbes induce this antiinflammatory response by increasing the ratio of interleukin (IL)-10 to IL-12.[35,36]

As mentioned, one highly relevant area related to microbes, inflammation, and the gut-brain axis is intestinal interepithelial junction integrity.[37] The concept of a "leaky gut" versus an intact barrier has been implicated in numerous pediatric clinical conditions.[38] Breakdown of the intestinal barrier can facilitate communication between the microbiota and key signaling pathways and may be the basis of chronic

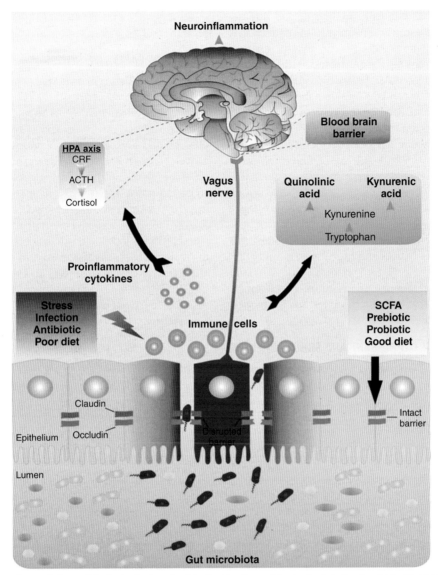

Fig. 4.3 Signaling pathways between intestinal microbes, the intestinal barrier, and the brain. A dysfunctional intestinal barrier or "leaky gut" permits a microbiota-driven proinflammatory state with implications for neuroinflammation. *ACTH*, Adrenocorticotropic hormone; *CRH*, corticotropin-releasing hormone; *HPA*, hypothalamus-pituitary-adrenal axis; *SCFA*, short-chain fatty acid. From Kelly JR, Kennedy PJ, Cryan JF, Dinan TG, Clarke G, Hyland NP. Breaking down the barriers: the gut microbiome, intestinal permeability and stress-related psychiatric disorders. *Front Cell Neurosci.* 2015;9:392. doi:10.3389/fncel.2015.00392.

low-grade inflammation observed in disorders such as depression.[39]

Functional Gastrointestinal Disorders

Recent data suggest a close link between gastrointestinal symptoms and gastroesophageal reflux (GER) and delayed relaxation of the lower esophageal sphincter triggered by gastric distension through activation of stretch receptors present in the stomach.[12]

COLIC

The brain-gut axis has important clinical implications and may relate to the pathophysiology of infant colic.

Colic is defined as frequent, prolonged, and intense crying or fussiness in a healthy infant. It is particularly frustrating for parents because the infant's distress seems to arise from no reason. Infants with colic are very difficult to console. Episodes usually peak at about 6 weeks of age and decline after about 4 months of age. Episodes of colic often occur in the evening when the parents are tired.

Treatment of colic has been very elusive.[13] Some studies suggest that the use of certain probiotics along with breast milk has been shown to reduce the crying time of colicky infants.[14] In fact, the action of the microbiota and its modulation by certain probiotics on upper gastrointestinal motility can be explained in several ways. Metabolites of intestinal bacteria such as SCFAs modify upper motility by inducing relaxation of the proximal stomach and lower esophageal sphincter and reduce gastric emptying through the action of gastrointestinal hormones such as polypeptide YY.[15]

AUTISM, ANXIETY, DEPRESSION, AND SCHIZOPHRENIA

Alterations in the bacterial composition of the intestine during early life are associated with various mental and behavioral consequences such as autism, anxiety, depression, and schizophrenia. The mechanisms of these relationships remain unclear, but in addition to alterations in barrier function as mentioned previously, the process of myelination has been related to health of the intestine.[40,41] At birth, whether born term or preterm, humans do not have well-developed myelination of their axons. This occurs rapidly in the first few years after birth, but any aberration in the process of myelination may have long-lasting effects. Intestinal dysbiosis such as that caused by antibiotic use and stress has been related to irregular myelination and has a harmful effect on social behavior.[42,43] The precise mechanisms are unclear, but SCFAs produced by commensal microbes play a role by modulating the impact of stress-induced regulation of the myelinization process, thus counteracting the effects of dysbiosis.[44] Furthermore, serotonin, a transmitter and signaling molecule, can also be synthesized by intestinal microbes into the gut lumen and is known to promote neurogenesis.[45] Deficiency of these microbes caused by stress or antibiotics is likely involved in the mechanism of action

of these pathologies by decreasing the microbes that produce SCFAs and/or serotonin.

EFFECTS OF EARLY LIFE STRESS

Early life stress such as maternal separation from the infant has been related to the development of neurobehavioral problems.[46] It is thought that neuroinflammatory mechanisms mediate this process,[47] but other studies suggest additional pathways are involved as well.[9] The interaction between the hypothalamus, pituitary gland, and adrenal gland in response to stress is known as the *hypothalamus-pituitary-adrenal axis (HPA)*. Corticotropin-releasing factor plays a central role in the stress response by initiating the release of glucocorticoids from the adrenal cortex. Commensal microbiota play a significant role in this interaction.[9] Studies done in germ-free (GF) and specific pathogen-free (SPF) mice are of interest in explaining the role of microbes in the interactions between corticosteroids and neurobehavior. SPF status indicates that the rodents have been tested and determined free of designated pathogens but not necessarily free of all pathogens or microbes. GF (or *gnotobiotic*) mice are obtained via C-section and raised in sterile isolators. Studies comparing GF and SPF animals showed that (1) the increase in plasma adrenocorticotropic hormone (ACTH) and corticosterone in response to restraint stress was substantially higher in GF mice than in SPF mice, suggesting an important role for intestinal microbiota in modulating stress; and (2) the enhanced HPA response of GF mice was partly corrected by reconstitution with SPF feces at an early stage but not by any reconstitution exerted at a later stage. The authors of these studies concluded that an early developmental stage is required for the HPA system to become fully susceptible to inhibitory neural regulation by microbes. In GF mice, a deficiency of dopamine appears to be one of the major causes of improper stress regulation and anxiety-like behavior. Certain microbial strains considered to be probiotics have been found to decrease the level of anxiety produced by various stressors. Recent evidence supports that microbes, their ligands, and metabolic products likely play a role in programming of the CNS and regulation of innate immunity.[48]

In Fig. 4.4, the brain-gut-microbiome axis regulates interactions between characteristics of infants such as gestational age, early life experiences, and how signaling occurs through the brain-gut axis.

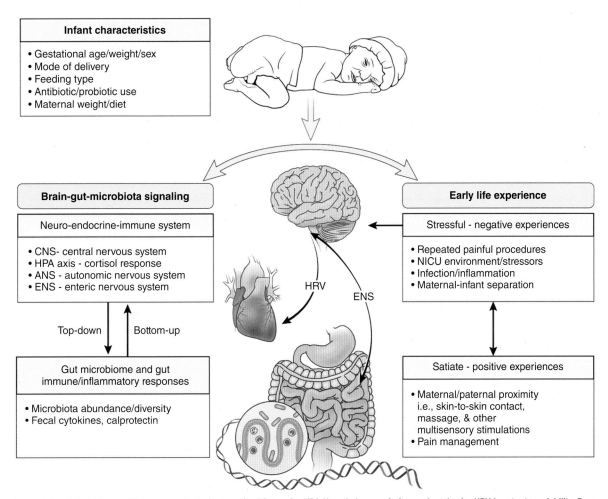

Fig. 4.4 Regulation of early life stress by the brain-gut-microbiota axis. *HPA*, Hypothalamus-pituitary-adrenal axis; *HRV*, heart rate variability. From Cong X, Henderson WA, Graf J, McGrath JM. Early life experience and gut microbiome: the brain-gut-microbiota signaling system. *Adv Neonatal Care*. 2015;15(5):314-323; quiz E1-E2. doi:10.1097/ANC.0000000000000191.

EFFECT OF ANTIBIOTICS

As mentioned, the use of antibiotics has a negative effect on gut microbiota and subsequent neurogenesis.[49] This effect is like that caused by early stress.[50] Most of the studies demonstrating this relationship have been in rodent models. However, a study of human preterm infants demonstrated a relationship between antibiotic use and several neurotransmitters and related them to the intestinal microbiome of these infants. Preterm infants (<33 weeks gestation) randomized to antibiotics or no antibiotics for the 48 hours after birth showed an association was discovered between lower *Veillonella*

and the neurotransmitter gamma-aminobutyric acid (GABA) in the antibiotics-treated group.[51] Significant differences were also seen in the fecal metabolomes in the antibiotics versus no antibiotics groups, including pathways related to vitamin biosynthesis, bile acids, amino acid metabolism, and neurotransmitters, with some of the most well-known of these, such as GABA, being lower in the antibiotics-treated group.[52]

AUTISM

A wide range of problems are associated with autism spectrum disorder (ASD).[53] ASD is a range of developmental neurobehavioral disorders characterized by impaired social interaction and communication. Some of these children show lack of interest and social involvement, avoid physical contact, have difficulty speaking, exhibit restrictive and repetitive behavior, and suffer from gastrointestinal symptoms.

Evidence has accumulated that there is an association between gut microbiota dysbiosis and ASDs.[54] Some of the microbes can synthesize metabolites that may play a role in the pathogenesis of ASDs. The SCFAs, especially butyrate, regulate the formation of the blood–brain barrier. Butyrate and propionate also exert strong epigenetic effects that regulate the expression of neurotransmitters as well as other molecules related to brain metabolism.

In children with ASDs, increased plasma concentrations of IL-8, tumor necrosis factor alpha (TNF)α, and IL-1β are observed. This suggests a proinflammatory condition.[55] Along with these, decreased levels of TGFβ have been reported and are thought to relate to the inflammation associated with ASDs.[55]

Autism is just one of the many disorders that have been associated with alterations in the developing microbiome in the gastrointestinal tract and the gut-brain axis. Others include attention deficit hyperactivity disorders, schizophrenia, and depression. Again, most of these are associations, and rigorous studies showing mechanistic causality are needed.

Maintaining a Healthy Gut-Brain Axis

Strategies to promote homeostasis should start in very early life. In fact, nutrition of the parents and health status prior to conception are crucial to development of the CNS. Certain nutrients, such as folate, have epigenetic potential and are well known to prevent infant neural tube defects and other congenital malformations. Certain drugs, such as antiepileptics, may decrease the availability of folate and thus risk CNS malformations. The father is not a totally innocent bystander in subsequent neurodevelopment of the infant; it has been shown that pathogenic infections of rodent fathers modulate offspring behavior via epigenetic regulation of the paternal reproductive cells and these effects could last for at least two generations.[56]

Maternal nutrition can have a major effect on microbial metabolites in the maternal intestines. Dietary fibers are fermented by maternal microbes, and this results in the subsequent release of SCFAs. SCFAs have been associated with altered microbial profiles in obese compared to normal-weight individuals. Furthermore, other studies have shown decreased abundance of bifidobacteria in babies born to overweight mothers compared to babies born to mothers with normal weight.

A vaginal delivery versus a caesarean section delivery is known to affect the subsequent development of microbiota in the neonate. Infants who are born via C-section have been shown to develop microbial signatures more like those of the maternal skin compared to those who are born vaginally, which shows a greater resemblance to vaginal and fecal microbiota. Whether these changes are completely due to the mode of delivery or to other variables such as more common exposure to antibiotics in C-section deliveries, longer hospital stays for infants delivered via C-section, or a delay in not being fed with maternal milk is not known.

Soon after birth, the gut microbiota are nurtured by the type of milk provided. In contrast to mother's own milk (fresh or frozen), those infants fed donor milk or formula are not provided with any live microbes, Furthermore, it appears that there is an enteromammary system that is highly dynamic and involves the maternal response to microbes in the environment or colonizing in the infant that may induce a response in the mother that results in specific immunity passed on through the milk to the infant.[57,58]

There are also numerous bioactive components in fresh maternal breast milk that are not present in formulas or may be inactivated by the pasteurization process that donor milk undergoes. Examples of these bioactive components include immunoglobulins, live cells, live microbes, enzymes such as lipase and alkaline phosphatase, and growth factors.

There has been considerable interest in pre-, pro-, and postbiotics that may alter the intestinal microbes of infants and their mothers to provide advantages. Although there are considerable theoretical considerations, the studies done in human infants in terms of protection against gut injury have mostly been small studies not adequately powered for various outcomes such as death, necrotizing enterocolitis (NEC), or feeding intolerance. Most randomized studies have been underpowered to test the effect of probiotics on the development of NEC, and the one that was adequately powered with over 1300 subjects did not demonstrate advantages.[59] The concern raised in the use of some of these agents and extremely low-birthweight infants necessitates the need for careful, adequately powered studies with agents that are pharmaceutical grade rather than food grade and that provide the most optimal protection against potential detrimental effects in these highly vulnerable infants.[60]

Summary

We have come a long way in our understanding of the brain-gut axis over the past couple of decades. It is now recognized that intestinal microbes play a major intermediary role in this axis, and thus we may consider that this is not a dyad but rather a triad. Despite considerable progress, much of the knowledge we have in this area related to the human remains associative rather than mechanistic and causal. In the future, researchers will need to utilize newly developing technologies such as artificial intelligence and multiomics to better understand mechanisms and causality and to provide the necessary information for developing early biomarkers that might be used to prevent disease as well as promote optimization of health in mothers and infants.

REFERENCES

1. Lewandowska-Pietruszka Z, Figlerowicz M, Mazur-Melewska K. The history of the intestinal microbiota and the gut-brain axis. *Pathogens*. 2022;11(12):1540. doi:10.3390/pathogens11121540.
2. Morais LH, Schreiber HL IV, Mazmanian SK. The gut microbiota-brain axis in behaviour and brain disorders. *Nat Rev Microbiol*. 2021;19(4):241-255. doi:10.1038/s41579-020-00460-0.
3. Cryan JF, O'Riordan KJ, Cowan CSM, et al. The microbiota-gut-brain axis. *Physiol Rev*. 2019;99(4):1877-2013. doi:10.1152/physrev.00018.2018.
4. Fasano A. All disease begins in the (leaky) gut: role of zonulin-mediated gut permeability in the pathogenesis of some chronic inflammatory diseases. *F1000Res*. 2020;9:F1000 Faculty Rev-69. doi:10.12688/f1000research.20510.1.
5. Lynch SV, Pedersen O. The human intestinal microbiome in health and disease. *N Engl J Med*. 2016;375(24):2369-2379. doi:10.1056/NEJMra1600266.
6. Lyon L. 'All disease begins in the gut': was Hippocrates right? *Brain*. 2018;141(3):e20. doi:10.1093/brain/awy017.
7. Mayer EA. The neurobiology of stress and gastrointestinal disease. *Gut*. 2000;47(6):861-869. doi:10.1136/gut.47.6.861.
8. Margolis KG, Cryan JF, Mayer EA. The microbiota-gut-brain axis: from motility to mood. *Gastroenterology*. 2021;160(5):1486-1501. doi:10.1053/j.gastro.2020.10.066.
9. Sudo N, Chida Y, Aiba Y, et al. Postnatal microbial colonization programs the hypothalamic-pituitary-adrenal system for stress response in mice. *J Physiol*. 2004;558(Pt 1):263-275. doi:10.1113/jphysiol.2004.063388.
10. Dinan TG, Cryan JF. The microbiome-gut-brain axis in health and disease. *Gastroenterol Clin North Am*. 2017;46(1):77-89. doi:10.1016/j.gtc.2016.09.007.
11. Carabotti M, Scirocco A, Maselli MA, Severi C. The gut-brain axis: interactions between enteric microbiota, central and enteric nervous systems. *Ann Gastroenterol*. 2015;28(2):203-209.
12. Martinucci I, Blandizzi C, de Bortoli N, et al. Genetics and pharmacogenetics of aminergic transmitter pathways in functional gastrointestinal disorders. *Pharmacogenomics*. 2015;16(5):523-539. doi:10.2217/pgs.15.12.
13. Aagaard K, Ma J, Antony KM, Ganu R, Petrosino J, Versalovic J. The placenta harbors a unique microbiome. *Sci Transl Med*. 2014;6(237):237ra65. doi:10.1126/scitranslmed.3008599.
14. Ardissone AN, Cruz DM, Davis-Richardson AG, et al. Meconium microbiome analysis identifies bacteria correlated with premature birth. *PLoS One*. 2014;9(3):e90784. doi:10.1371/journal.pone.0090784.
15. Kennedy KM, de Goffau MC, Perez-Muñoz ME, et al. Questioning the fetal microbiome illustrates pitfalls of low-biomass microbial studies. *Nature*. 2023;613(7945):639-649. doi:10.1038/s41586-022-05546-8.
16. Blaser MJ, Devkota S, McCoy KD, Relman DA, Yassour M, Young VB. Lessons learned from the prenatal microbiome controversy. *Microbiome*. 2021;9(1):8. doi:10.1186/s40168-020-00946-2.
17. Nuriel-Ohayon M, Neuman H, Koren O. Microbial changes during pregnancy, birth, and infancy. *Front Microbiol*. 2016;7:1031. doi:10.3389/fmicb.2016.01031.
18. Neuman H, Koren O. The pregnancy microbiome. *Nestle Nutr Inst Workshop Ser*. 2017;88:1-9. doi:10.1159/000455207.
19. Koren O, Goodrich JK, Cullender TC, et al. Host remodeling of the gut microbiome and metabolic changes during pregnancy. *Cell*. 2012;150(3):470-480. doi:10.1016/j.cell.2012.07.008.
20. Miko E, Csaszar A, Bodis J, Kovacs K. The maternal-fetal gut microbiota axis: physiological changes, dietary influence, and modulation possibilities. *Life (Basel)*. 2022;12(3):424. doi:10.3390/life12030424.
21. Kuperman AA, Koren O. Antibiotic use during pregnancy: how bad is it? *BMC Med*. 2016;14(1):91. doi:10.1186/s12916-016-0636-0.
22. Jašarević E, Bale TL. Prenatal and postnatal contributions of the maternal microbiome on offspring programming. *Front Neuroendocrinol*. 2019;55:100797. doi:10.1016/j.yfrne.2019.100797.
23. Kimura I, Miyamoto J, Ohue-Kitano R, et al. Maternal gut microbiota in pregnancy influences offspring metabolic phenotype in mice. *Science*. 2020;367(6481):eaaw8429. doi:10.1126/science.aaw8429.
24. Georgieff MK. Nutrition and the developing brain: nutrient priorities and measurement. *Am J Clin Nutr*. 2007;85(2):614s-620s. doi:10.1093/ajcn/85.2.614S.
25. Jašarević E, Howard CD, Morrison K, et al. The maternal vaginal microbiome partially mediates the effects of prenatal stress

on offspring gut and hypothalamus. *Nat Neurosci.* 2018;21(8): 1061-1071. doi:10.1038/s41593-018-0182-5.

26. Dash S, Syed YA, Khan MR. Understanding the role of the gut microbiome in brain development and its association with neurodevelopmental psychiatric disorders. *Front Cell Dev Biol.* 2022;10:880544. doi:10.3389/fcell.2022.880544.

27. Lu J, Claud EC. Connection between gut microbiome and brain development in preterm infants. *Dev Psychobiol.* 2019;61(5): 739-751. doi:10.1002/dev.21806.

28. Shanahan F, Ghosh TS, O'Toole PW. The healthy microbiome—what is the definition of a healthy gut microbiome? *Gastroenterology.* 2021;160(2):483-494. doi:10.1053/j.gastro.2020.09.057.

29. Indrio F, Neu J, Pettoello-Mantovani M, et al. Development of the gastrointestinal tract in newborns as a challenge for an appropriate nutrition: a narrative review. *Nutrients.* 2022;14(7): 1405. doi:10.3390/nu14071405.

30. Balaguer-Trias J, Deepika D, Schuhmacher M, Kumar V. Impact of contaminants on microbiota: linking the gut-brain axis with neurotoxicity. *Int J Environ Res Public Health.* 2022;19(3):1368. doi:10.3390/ijerph19031368.

31. Glinert A, Turjeman S, Elliott E, Koren O. Microbes, metabolites and (synaptic) malleability, oh my! The effect of the microbiome on synaptic plasticity. *Biol Rev Camb Philos Soc.* 2022; 97(2):582-599. doi:10.1111/brv.12812.

32. Tochitani S. Vertical transmission of gut microbiota: points of action of environmental factors influencing brain development. *Neurosci Res.* 2021;168:83-94. doi:10.1016/j.neures.2020.11.006.

33. Nutma E, Willison H, Martino G, Amor S. Neuroimmunology—the past, present and future. *Clin Exp Immunol.* 2019;197(3): 278-293. doi:10.1111/cei.13279.

34. Rutsch A, Kantsjö JB, Ronchi F. The gut-brain axis: how microbiota and host inflammasome influence brain physiology and pathology. *Front Immunol.* 2020;11:604179. doi:10.3389/fimmu.2020.604179.

35. Fung TC, Olson CA, Hsiao EY. Interactions between the microbiota, immune and nervous systems in health and disease. *Nat Neurosci.* 2017;20(2):145-155. doi:10.1038/nn.4476.

36. Bharwani A, Mian MF, Surette MG, Bienenstock J, Forsythe P. Oral treatment with Lactobacillus rhamnosus attenuates behavioural deficits and immune changes in chronic social stress. *BMC Med.* 2017;15(1):7. doi:10.1186/s12916-016-0771-7.

37. Kelly JR, Kennedy PJ, Cryan JF, Dinan TG, Clarke G, Hyland NP. Breaking down the barriers: the gut microbiome, intestinal permeability and stress-related psychiatric disorders. *Front Cell Neurosci.* 2015;9:392. doi:10.3389/fncel.2015.00392.

38. Liu L, Li N, Neu J. Tight junctions, leaky intestines, and pediatric diseases. *Acta Paediatr.* 2005;94(4):386-393. doi:10.1111/j.1651-2227.2005.tb01904.x.

39. Obrenovich MEM. Leaky gut, leaky brain? *Microorganisms.* 2018;6(4):107. doi:10.3390/microorganisms6040107.

40. Ahmed S, Travis SD, Díaz-Bahamonde FV, et al. Early influences of microbiota on white matter development in germ-free piglets. *Front Cell Neurosci.* 2021;15:807170. doi:10.3389/fncel.2021.807170.

41. Keogh CE, Kim DHJ, Pusceddu MM, et al. Myelin as a regulator of development of the microbiota-gut-brain axis. *Brain Behav Immun.* 2021;91:437-450. doi:10.1016/j.bbi.2020.11.001.

42. Rincel M, Aubert P, Chevalier J, et al. Multi-hit early life adversity affects gut microbiota, brain and behavior in a sex-dependent

manner. *Brain Behav Immun.* 2019;80:179-192. doi:10.1016/j.bbi.2019.03.006.

43. Leclercq S, Mian FM, Stanisz AM, et al. Low-dose penicillin in early life induces long-term changes in murine gut microbiota, brain cytokines and behavior. *Nat Commun.* 2017;8:15062. doi:10.1038/ncomms15062.

44. Panther EJ, Dodd W, Clark A, Lucke-Wold B. Gastrointestinal microbiome and neurologic injury. *Biomedicines.* 2022;10(2): 500. doi:10.3390/biomedicines10020500.

45. Gershon MD. The shaggy dog story of enteric signaling: serotonin, a molecular megillah. *Adv Exp Med Biol.* 2022;1383: 307-318. doi:10.1007/978-3-031-05843-1_28.

46. Halladay LR, Herron SM. Lasting impact of postnatal maternal separation on the developing BNST: lifelong socioemotional consequences. *Neuropharmacology.* 2023;225:109404. doi:10.1016/j.neuropharm.2022.109404.

47. Lumertz FS, Kestering-Ferreira E, Orso R, et al. Effects of early life stress on brain cytokines: a systematic review and meta-analysis of rodent studies. *Neurosci Biobehav Rev.* 2022;139: 104746. doi:10.1016/j.neubiorev.2022.104746.

48. Cong X, Henderson WA, Graf J, McGrath JM. Early life experience and gut microbiome: the brain-gut-microbiota signaling system. *Adv Neonatal Care.* 2015;15(5):314-323; quiz E1-E2. doi:10.1097/ANC.0000000000000191.

49. Vicentini FA, Keenan CM, Wallace LE, et al. Intestinal microbiota shapes gut physiology and regulates enteric neurons and glia. *Microbiome.* 2021;9(1):210. doi:10.1186/s40168-021-01165-z.

50. Ruiz-González R, Lajud N, Tejeda-Martínez AR, et al. Antibiotic-induced microbiota depletion in normally-reared adult rats mimics the neuroendocrine effects of early life stress. *Brain Res.* 2022;1793:148055. doi:10.1016/j.brainres.2022.148055.

51. Russell JT, Lauren Ruoss J, de la Cruz D, et al. Antibiotics and the developing intestinal microbiome, metabolome and inflammatory environment in a randomized trial of preterm infants. *Sci Rep.* 2021;11(1):1943. doi:10.1038/s41598-021-80982-6.

52. Patton L, Li N, Garrett TJ, et al. Antibiotics effects on the fecal metabolome in preterm infants. *Metabolites.* 2020;10(8):331. doi:10.3390/metabo10080331.

53. Talantseva OI, Romanova RS, Shurdova EM, et al. The global prevalence of autism spectrum disorder: a three-level meta-analysis. *Front Psychiatry.* 2023;14:1071181. doi:10.3389/fpsyt.2023.1071181.

54. Hsiao EY, McBride SW, Hsien S, et al. Microbiota modulate behavioral and physiological abnormalities associated with neurodevelopmental disorders. *Cell.* 2013;155(7):1451-1463. doi:10.1016/j.cell.2013.11.024.

55. Nour-Eldine W, Ltaief SM, Abdul Manaph NP, Al-Shammari AR. In search of immune cellular sources of abnormal cytokines in the blood in autism spectrum disorder: a systematic review of case-control studies. *Front Immunol.* 2022;13:950275. doi:10.3389/fimmu.2022.950275.

56. Tyebji S, Hannan AJ, Tonkin CJ. Pathogenic infection in male mice changes sperm small RNA profiles and transgenerationally alters offspring behavior. *Cell Rep.* 2020;31(4):107573. doi:10.1016/j.celrep.2020.107573.

57. Kleinman RE, Walker WA. The enteromammary immune system: an important new concept in breast milk host defense. *Dig Dis Sci.* 1979;24(11):876-882. doi:10.1007/BF01324906.

58. Wiggins JB, Trotman R, Perks PH, Swanson JR. Enteral nutrition: the intricacies of human milk from the immune system to the microbiome. *Clin Perinatol.* 2022;49(2):427-445. doi:10.1016/j.clp.2022.02.009.
59. Costeloe K, Bowler U, Brocklehurst P, et al. A randomised controlled trial of the probiotic Bifidobacterium breve BBG-001 in preterm babies to prevent sepsis, necrotising enterocolitis and death: the Probiotics in Preterm infantS (PiPS) trial. *Health Technol Assess Rep.* 2016;20(66):1-194. doi:10.3310/hta20660.
60. Poindexter B, Committee on Fetus and Newborn. Use of probiotics in preterm infants. *Pediatrics.* 2021;147(6):e2021051485. doi:10.1542/peds.2021-051485.

Chapter 5

Trophic Factors in the Neonatal Gastrointestinal Tract

Caitlin Elizabeth Vonderohe and Douglas G. Burrin

Chapter Outline

Key Points

1. The neonatal period is a highly dynamic period of gastrointestinal growth and functional development, and physiological changes during the fetal-neonatal period facilitate the transition from placental nutrient assimilation to oral ingestion via the gastrointestinal tract.

2. The cells within the fetal and neonatal gastrointestinal tract are influenced by extracellular signals from multiple sources, including (1) blood-borne factors in the circulation, such as hormones that act via endocrine mechanisms; (2) luminal factors derived from amniotic fluid, mammary secretions, or microbes; and (3) local factors secreted via autocrine or paracrine mechanisms from surrounding cells.

3. Several clinical studies have demonstrated that the practice of minimal enteral feeding or trophic feeding can enhance gastrointestinal motility and intestinal function and can improve feeding outcomes.

4. Cells within the gut can respond to extracellular concentrations of nutrients directly via intracellular signaling pathways, including mammalian target of rapamycin, that mediate downstream cellular function, such as cell proliferation, protein synthesis, and apoptosis.

5. Several specific nutrients have trophic actions when supplemented to a complete diet. Among them are glutamine, arginine, and long-chain polyunsaturated fatty acids.

6. Some of the gut hormones that have been implicated in the stimulation of trophic functional response to enteral nutrition include glucagon-like peptide 2, gastrin, cholecystokinin, peptide YY, and neurotensin.

7. Glucagon-like peptide 2 has significant trophic effects on the neonatal small intestine that are mediated by increased cell proliferation, protein synthesis, blood flow, and glucose transport.

8. Vascular endothelial growth factor, hepatocyte growth factor, and keratinocyte growth factor are expressed in the cells located within the intestinal mucosal layer and may play a role in mucosal angiogenesis, growth, and repair.

9. The gut is also a major producer of serotonin, which is involved in modulating and initiating intestinal motility, gastrointestinal secretions, vasodilation, and activation of afferent nerves. Serotonin also promotes growth and survival of enterochromaffin cells and other enteric nerves.

Introduction

Gastrointestinal growth and function are significant facets of neonatal development that are highly regulated by both intrinsic and extrinsic factors. The development and function of gastrointestinal organs during the neonatal period have been extensively examined using novel molecular biological and genetic approaches, including the use of *in vitro* enteroids and organoids cultivated from fetal and neonatal tissues. This has revealed microenvironments within intestinal crypts and villi, allowing stem cell proliferation in crypts while simultaneously regulating cellular differentiation, function, and eventual quiescence at the villus tip. Extrinsic factors, such as nutrients and hormones, are also important determinants that prepare the fetus and neonate gut for birth and weaning. Enteral nutrition is the most significant stimulus for gastrointestinal growth and protein synthesis. Select nutrients, such as glutamine, arginine, threonine, and leucine; nucleotides; and short-chain fatty acids (SCFAs) and long-chain fatty acids (LCFAs) also have trophic effects. The gut is also a significant endocrine organ secreting hormones such as glucagon-like peptide 2 that have profound effects on gastrointestinal growth. Other hormones, such as glucocorticoids, are important in triggering fetal intestinal maturation before birth. Additionally, local and endocrine growth factors such as serotonin and the epidermal growth factor and insulin-like growth factor (IGF) families play significant roles in the regulation of gastrointestinal

function and proliferation. There is a highly coordinated balance between cellular proliferation and function in the gastrointestinal tract that is imperative for neonatal health and survival.

The Nature of Gut Growth

The neonatal period is a highly dynamic period of gastrointestinal growth and functional development. In the case of the intestine, this includes the development of swallowing and mature motility patterns,[1] tissue vascular hemodynamics,[2] and nutrient transporters.[3] Together, these physiologic changes during the fetal-neonatal period facilitate the transition from placental nutrient assimilation to oral ingestion via the gastrointestinal tract. Intestinal epithelial growth at the tissue and cellular levels is characterized by increased cell numbers (i.e., *hyperplasia*) and increased cellular size (i.e., *hypertrophy*). Intestinal growth also involves expansion of the number and size of crypt and villus units.[4] An important aspect of growth in the gut is the continual proliferation, migration, and loss of epithelial cells along the mucosal surface. In the intestine, this process involves multiple cell lineages (absorptive enterocyte, goblet, Paneth, endocrine, tuft) that differentiate from pluripotent stem cells located in the crypt.[5] Growth is also characterized by structural and functional changes in innervation and vascularization within the gut. Gastrointestinal growth involves the proliferation, growth, and development of cells and structures, including blood vessels, endothelial cells, smooth muscle cells, submucosal nerves, and myenteric nerves. The normal growth and development of the gastrointestinal tract is critical to normal development of the neonate, as the gut is a central organ for nutrient digestion and absorption and is a major environmental interface for innate immune function, nutrient sensing, and neuroendocrine crosstalk between the gut and brain. The timing and characteristics of neonatal gastrointestinal growth are exquisitely coordinated with the events of birth and weaning to ensure survival of the organism. The regulation of neonatal gastrointestinal growth is complex and involves multiple and often redundant factors. Among these factors are intrinsic cell programs or signals arising from gene expression, as well as extracellular signals such as peptide growth factors, hormones, nutrients, and microbes, which originate from surrounding cells, the blood, and the gut lumen.

In the past decade, the development of *in vitro* models of fetal and neonatal gastrointestinal physiology in the form of intestinal enteroids and organoids has provided new insights about the role of stem cells and growth factors in the proliferation and maintenance of the intestinal epithelium.[6] Intestinal organoids are specifically representative of fetal tissue and have been used to examine signaling pathways that determine the eventual developmental fate (endoderm, mesoderm, or ectoderm) of pluripotent stem cells, from gastrulation onward. Growth factors such as TGF-β initiate gastrulation in early fetal life, but other factors such as Wnt, fibroblast growth factors

(FGFs), retinoic acid, and bone morphogenetic protein (BMP) pathways are essential for the development and subsequent differentiation of the intestinal epithelium (Fig. 5.1). Enteroids are cultured from stem cells present in the base of intestinal crypts and represent the physiology of the tissue the cells were isolated from.[7] For example, if stem cells are harvested from diseased or aging tissue, they will differentiate into enteroids that reflect the ratio of epithelial cell lineages observed in the original tissue. In enteroid culture, Wnt signaling is amplified by R-spondin to maximize enteroid proliferation and survivability, while epidermal growth factor (EGF) has a similar, profound mitogenic effect on stem cells. In intestinal tissue, BMP signaling is greatest at the villus tip and lowest

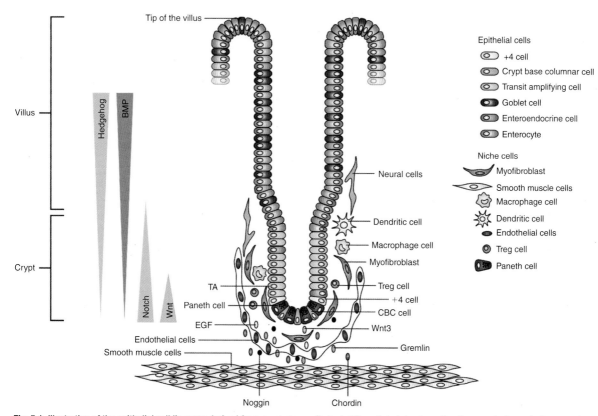

Fig. 5.1 Illustration of the epithelial cell lineages derived from crypt stem cells that differentiate into absorptive lineages (enterocytes) or secretory lineages (enteroendocrine cells, goblet cells, tuft cells, and Paneth cells). The niche consists of multiple components and cell types, including the extracellular matrix, fibroblasts, myofibroblasts, smooth muscle cells, neural cells, endothelial cells, lymphocytes, and macrophages, along with secreted factors (Wnt3, epidermal growth factor). *BMP*, Basic metabolic panel; *CBC*, complete blood count; *EGF*, epidermal growth factor; *TA*, transit-amplifying. Adapted with permission from Sailaja BS, He XC, Li L. The regulatory niche of intestinal stem cells. *J Physiol*. 2016;594(17):4829. doi:10.1113/JP271931.

at the crypt base, driving terminal differentiation.[8] Additionally, R-spondin has been shown to promote the expansion of the stem cell niche in intestinal tissue.[9] Other growth factors used in organoid and enteroid culture are still under investigation for their clinical significance in nonneoplastic and neonatal gut tissue.

Gut Adaptation in the Perinatal Period

Normal gastrointestinal growth and development during fetal life are critical to facilitate successful adaptation from nutritional support via umbilical circulation to oral ingestion of breast milk. An increase in circulating fetal glucocorticoid concentration just prior to and during vaginal birth is an important trigger of gut functional development.[10,11] In the neonatal period, growth of the gastrointestinal tract is influenced by multiple physiologic factors that serve to prepare the developing neonate for separation from maternal nutritional support (i.e., weaning). In addition, several important environmental cues signal adaptive changes in gastrointestinal function to facilitate postweaning survival. For example, the microbial colonization of the gut may serve to prime intestinal lymphoid cell development for normal innate and adaptive immune function.[12,13] During these processes, extracellular signals such as peptide growth factors are believed to be important trophic factors that influence growth. However, the term *trophic* also pertains to nutrition, and in the case of the gut, nutrients present in amniotic fluid and breast milk are a major trophic influence. Thus there are numerous extracellular trophic signals including foods, nutrients, peptide growth factors, gut peptide hormones, steroid and thyroid hormones, microbes, and neural inputs. The cells within the fetal and neonatal gastrointestinal tract are influenced by extracellular signals from multiple sources, including (1) blood-borne factors in the circulation such as hormones that act via endocrine mechanisms; (2) luminal factors derived from amniotic fluid, mammary secretions, or microbes; and (3) local factors secreted via autocrine or paracrine mechanisms from surrounding cells. Additionally, intrinsic intracellular signals such as transcription factors interact with these extracellular signals to affect mucosal hyperplasia and hypertrophy.

Preterm birth creates major problems for newborn infants' adaptation to normal oral feeding and enteral nutrition. These problems are often manifested clinically as feeding intolerance, sepsis, and necrotizing enterocolitis (NEC). These problems are linked with immature gastroduodenal motor function, hemodynamic regulation, nutrient malabsorption, a dysfunctional mucosal immune system, and microbial dysbiosis. Thus the challenge for clinicians caring for preterm infants is to provide the appropriate combination of clinical support, nutritional or otherwise, to stimulate the normal growth and development of these organ systems and physiologic functions.

How Soon and How Much to Feed Enterally

Enteral nutrition is the most potent trophic stimulus of gastrointestinal tract growth. Enteral feeding acts directly by supplying nutrients for growth and oxidative metabolism of the mucosal epithelial cells. However, it also acts indirectly by triggering the release of local growth factors and gut hormones and activating neural pathways (Fig. 5.2). Neonatal starvation and total parenteral nutrition (TPN) reduce gut tissue mass and mucosal surface area, increase catabolism, and decrease protein synthesis.[14,15] Evidence from numerous animal studies and some human studies shows that enteral nutrition is critical to maintain normal intestinal growth and development. The enteral nutrient stimulation of gut growth begins in the late-gestation fetus with the onset of amniotic fluid swallowing. Studies in fetal sheep and pigs have shown that preventing amniotic fluid swallowing by esophageal ligation suppresses intestinal growth.[10,16]

In most infants, enteral feeding of human milk or formula after birth stimulates the growth and adaptive development of the gastrointestinal tract. However, in the immediate postnatal period premature infants normally receive most of their nutrition parenterally due to poor feeding tolerance. Studies in neonatal pigs show that TPN leads to significantly reduced growth and to atrophy of the intestinal mucosa marked by reduced cell proliferation, villus height, and protein synthesis as well as increased apoptosis.[17] Additional studies with neonatal animals and human infants suggest that lack of enteral nutrition is also associated with reduced secretion of many gut peptide hormones

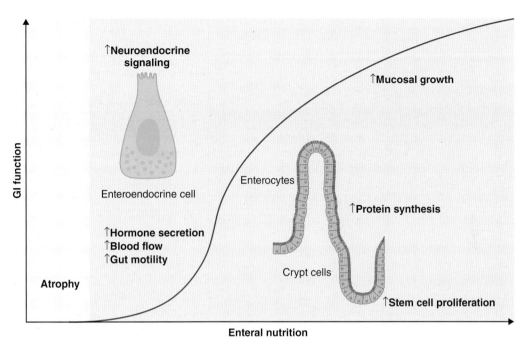

Fig. 5.2 Illustration showing the relationship between enteral nutrition and gastrointestinal function.

and growth factors as well as dysbiotic intestinal microbiota colonization, all of which may be linked to reduced gut functional development during TPN.[18–20]

Therefore, in premature infants, the question is how soon and how much to feed enterally. Several clinical studies have demonstrated that the practice of minimal enteral feeding or trophic feeding can enhance gastrointestinal motility and intestinal function and improve feeding outcomes[21] (Fig. 5.1). The introduction of minimal enteral nutrition usually starts at birth at a daily intake of ~24–25 mL/kg, an amount that is insufficient for the total nutrient needs of the infant.[22] Meta-analyses have shown that while minimal enteral nutrition reduces time to full feeding and length of hospital stay, the impact on overall health and disease risk for premature infants is yet to be established.[23,24] However, recent clinical trials suggest that advancement of enteral feeding by 20–30 mL/kg/d may be safe and may not increase the risk of NEC.[21,22,25–27] Clinical studies in premature infants have indicated that enteral feeding is positively linked to intestinal mucosal growth but that lactose digestion is more closely correlated to lactase activity and gestational age than feeding

status.[28,29] Studies in piglets suggest that enteral nutrition is critical to maintain normal lactose digestion and glucose absorption.[30] Studies in neonatal piglets also suggest that an enteral intake of at least 40% of total nutrient intake is necessary to maintain normal growth, which would imply that minimal enteral nutrition may not be trophic to gut mucosa.[11] An additional consideration is whether to provide enteral nutrition intragastrically, intraduodenally, as a bolus, or continuously. Evidence from clinical studies is equivocal as to clinical outcome.[31,32] Studies in piglets suggest that, in comparison with continuous feeding, bolus feeding resulted in increased gut growth and improvement in trophic insulin response in skeletal muscle in term pigs[33,34] but was not linked to secretion of trophic gut peptides or improvements in insulin response to feeding in preterm pigs.[35,36]

The Trophic Role of Breast Milk Versus Formula

The relative significance of milk-borne trophic factors has been an intensely studied area of pediatric nutrition and gastroenterology.[37–40] Several trophic peptide growth factors are present in mother's own breast milk but not in infant formulas and have been implicated in the beneficial outcomes of breast-fed infants, particularly in the reduced incidence of NEC and sepsis. However, the stability of these growth factors in donor human milk that has been pasteurized has not been well established. Studies conducted in neonatal animals have shown evidence that breast milk has a greater trophic effect on the gastrointestinal tract than formula, as measured by typical indices of structural and cellular growth. However, the most significant advantage of breast milk on the neonatal intestine, especially of preterm infants, may be related not to growth but to mucosal barrier and immune function. There is considerable evidence showing that immunoprotective factors in breast milk (e.g., secretory IgA, lactoferrin, oligosaccharides) act to modulate mucosal immune function and bacterial colonization, thereby limiting the incidence of infection, sepsis, and NEC.[41–44] Other novel human milk, plasma, and bovine colostrum–derived bioactive ingredients are being explored for their utility to reduce bacteria-mucosal interaction and therefore improve mucosal growth by reducing inflammation.[45] Many of the trophic factors in milk are polypeptides that survive digestion, retain their biological activity, and interact with specific receptors present on the mucosal epithelium of neonates. Several studies have shown that these milk-borne growth factors stimulate neonatal intestinal growth when given in purified and recombinant forms either orally or systemically.[46] Moreover, in preterm neonates the presence of increased intestinal permeability could facilitate the intestinal absorption of milk-borne peptide growth factors; however, there are limited instances where this process has been found to be physiologically significant.

Another important stimulus of intestinal growth associated with feeding is the secretion of bile acids from the liver. Historically, bile acids were solely considered as detergent molecules that emulsify lipids and function in fat digestion and absorption. In the past two decades, the scope of bile acid biology has greatly expanded, with studies showing that luminal bile acids act as signaling molecules that regulate gastrointestinal functions by binding to a host of membrane and nuclear receptors present on epithelial cells as well as other cell types located within the small intestine and colon. Secondary bile acids present in the colon can directly stimulate epithelial proliferation by activating epithelial growth factor receptor pathways.[47] Studies in neonatal piglets have shown that enterally administering chenodeoxycholic acid was able to prevent TPN-induced small intestinal atrophy and restore normal glucagon-like peptide 2 (GLP-2) secretion.[48,49] In the distal ileum, bile acids act as ligands for farnesoid X receptor (FXR), triggering the production of fibroblast growth factor 19 (FGF19). FGF19 has multiple systemic effects, but the primary target is to reduce bile acid synthesis in the liver by reducing the expression of CYP7a1. Additionally, FGF19 has been shown to have an insulin-like effect on hepatic protein synthesis and gluconeogenesis, along with a proliferative effect on hepatocytes via the receptors FGFR4 and βklotho.[50] However, the direct effect of FGF19 on intestinal epithelial function remains to be determined.

Key Nutrients to Provide Enterally

Despite the important functional effect of growth factors and immunologic factors in human milk, the dominant trophic stimulus on the neonatal intestine can be attributed to macronutrient content. The chemical form and nutrient composition also influence the impact of enteral nutrition on gastrointestinal growth and function.[15,18] Some studies indicate that enteral nutrition in a complex, polymeric form is more trophic to the small intestine than in a simpler, elemental form, yet results in piglets refute this idea.[51] Dietary restriction of protein and energy generally suppresses gut growth and mucosal immune function. The enteral infusion of individual nutrients, by themselves, can have a trophic stimulus on the gut if administered in a sufficiently large amount. Cells within the gut can respond to extracellular concentrations of nutrients directly via intracellular signaling pathways, including mammalian target of rapamycin (mTOR), that mediate downstream cellular functions such as cell proliferation, protein synthesis, and apoptosis (Fig. 5.3). However, there are several specific nutrients that have trophic actions when supplemented to a complete diet; among those are glutamine, arginine, and long-chain polyunsaturated fatty acids (LC-PUFAs). In the past, evidence of the metabolic and

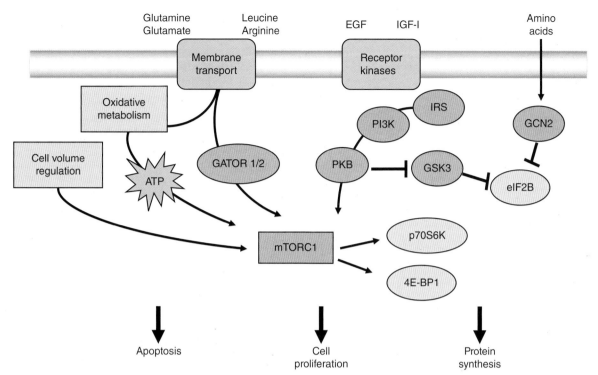

Fig. 5.3 The role of extracellular signals, including amino acids and growth factors, on cellular signaling pathways that mediate cellular growth. *ATP,* Adenosine triphosphate; *EGF,* Epidermal growth factor; *GCN2,* general control nonderepressible 2; *GSK3,* glycogen synthase kinase 3; *IGF-1,* insulin-like growth factor-1; *IRS,* insulin receptor substrate; *mTORC1,* mammalian target of rapamycin complex 1; *PI3K,* phosphoinositide 3-kinase; *PKB,* protein kinase B.

cellular effects of glutamine and arginine has prompted numerous studies aimed at evaluating the efficacy of their supplementation in clinical situations to act as antiinflammatory and trophic factors. This has spawned the concept of immunonutrition and the commercial introduction of enteral diets that target immune cell functions with nutrients, including arginine, glutamine, SCFAs, and n-3 LCFAs. Numerous clinical trials and meta-analyses of immune-enhancing diets with largely adult critical care patients have shown reduced infectious complications, yet the relative role of specific immunonutrients remains to be established.

GLUTAMINE

Glutamine is a key intestinal oxidative fuel that is extensively metabolized and oxidized to CO_2 by intestinal tissues when fed either enterally or parenterally[18,52,53] (Fig. 5.3). However, several studies have shown that enteral and parenteral glutamine also stimulates intestinal growth and enhances function in healthy and diseased conditions.[54–56] Evidence from clinical studies with premature infants has also suggested that enteral glutamine may reduce infectious morbidity.[57,58] Further studies are warranted to determine whether enteral glutamine enhances gut immune function and whether this translates to reduced infectious morbidity. Clinical studies show that parenteral glutamine does not reduce mortality or the incidence of sepsis in hospitalized infants.[59,60] Studies in rodents indicate that enteral glutamine stimulates intestinal blood flow, yet a recent clinical study found no effect of glutamine on superior mesenteric arterial flow.[61,62] Studies in cultured intestinal epithelial cells indicate that glutamine, but not other nonessential amino acids, specifically stimulates cell proliferation, activates mitogenic intracellular signaling pathways, and may be a critical precursor for glucosamine, pyrimidine, and arginine synthesis.[63–70]

ARGININE

Arginine is an essential amino acid for neonates and may be an especially important substrate for maintenance of intestinal nitric oxide synthesis, blood flow, and immune function. L-arginine is a precursor for the synthesis of nitric oxide, and nitric oxide plays a key role in regulating intestinal blood flow.[71] A recent study in pigs demonstrates that arginine administered enterally or parenterally increases NO production in the gastrointestinal tract.[72] Arginine has also been shown to affect the molecular mechanisms of cell metabolism and growth. These include the downstream targets of mTOR, an amino acid–responsive serine/threonine kinase that affects cell growth. Specifically, arginine was shown to affect the phosphorylation of p70S6 kinase and 4E-BP1, important components in the regulation of cell growth.[73] Despite these findings, it is uncertain whether arginine can affect intestinal epithelial proliferation directly, but arginine has been shown to stimulate intestinal cell migration.[74–76] Another study showed that arginine was able to re-epithelialize porcine ileal mucosa via inducible nitric oxide synthase (iNOS) but only in the presence of serum.[77]

A major cause of mortality and morbidity in preterm infants is NEC. The etiology of NEC has not been firmly established but is associated with prematurity, enteral formula feeding, and small-bowel bacterial colonization. Additional contributing factors thought to play a role in NEC are intestinal ischemia, proinflammatory stimulation, and an immature mucosal immune barrier function. Arginine supplementation has been considered as a particularly attractive strategy to prevent the incidence of neonatal NEC because it is the immediate precursor for nitric oxide, which acts as a major vasodilator and participates in the inflammatory response, and because arginine also augments B- and T-lymphocyte function. Some studies have shown that enteral arginine supplementation can reduce the incidence of NEC in neonatal infants and piglets.[78,79] The benefits of enteral arginine in preterm NEC also may stem from an underlying deficiency in endogenous gut arginine synthesis shown in preterm piglets.[80] A systematic review of limited clinical studies demonstrated that arginine supplementation may prevent NEC, but more studies are needed.[81] Commercially available enteral formulas

designed to enhance immune function in critically ill and surgical patients contain arginine, yet the safety and efficacy of these diets in infants is untested. Further studies are needed to characterize the impact of enteral arginine on intestinal blood flow, NO production, mucosal growth, and immune function in neonatal infants and animal models.

Other nonessential amino acids, including glutamate, proline, and citrulline, may have stimulatory actions on the gut because they are precursors for glutamine and arginine synthesis.[52,82] This may be especially important in infants after small-bowel resection, since studies in rodents indicate that arginine is conditionally essential under these conditions due to the loss of intestinal citrulline production.[83,84] Threonine is also a key nutrient for the intestinal synthesis of threonine-rich mucins by goblet cells. Studies in piglets have shown that the gut extracts ~80% of enteral threonine for intestinal mucosal protein synthesis.[85] The sulfur-containing amino acids methionine and cysteine also have important metabolic roles in maintaining antioxidant function since methionine is metabolized via transsulfuration to cysteine, which is a precursor of glutathione, a critical antioxidant in the gut. Studies in neonatal piglets indicate that intestinal metabolism accounts for ~30% of the daily methionine requirement,[86] and diets deficient in sulfur amino acids specifically limit intestinal growth.[87,88]

SHORT-CHAIN FATTY ACIDS

SCFAs, largely in the form of acetate, propionate, and butyrate, are produced by microbial fermentation of carbohydrates in the large bowel.[89,90] Colonic epithelial cells derive most (60% to 70%) of their energy from SCFAs, and butyrate is the preferred oxidative fuel compared with glucose, glutamine, or ketone bodies. The diet of the human neonate is largely devoid of fiber, yet the production of SCFAs from large-bowel microbial fermentation increases with the degree of microbial colonization and postnatal age. Normal substrates for colonic SCFA production in neonates include endogenous secretions and small-intestinal malabsorption of dietary carbohydrates, such as lactose or maltodextrins. Colonic SCFAs are also produced through bacterial metabolism of oligosaccharides, which are the second most abundant carbohydrate in human milk, but infant formulas are substantially devoid of these compounds.[91] There is considerable evidence for the specific intestinal trophic effects of SCFAs. Intraluminal and systemic infusions of SCFAs have a stimulatory effect on intestinal mucosal proliferation, gene expression, blood flow, and gut hormone secretion; yet, studies with cultured colonic tumor cell lines indicate that butyrate induces differentiation and apoptosis, thereby suppressing neoplasia.[92]

N-3 PUFAS

As with SCFAs, there is considerable interest in dietary LCFAs because breast milk generally contains higher concentrations of n-3 LC-PUFAs than infant formulas; many infant formulas are now formulated with these fatty acids. Interest in the n-3 LC-PUFAs or omega-3 fatty acids, particularly docosahexaenoic acid (DHA), eicosapentaenoic acid (EPA), and arachidonic acid (ARA), stems from studies showing that dietary supplementation can lower the incidence and inflammatory effects of NEC in neonatal infants and rats.[93] Omega-3 fatty acids have been shown to attenuate inflammatory proteins in the small intestine of a preterm rat pup

model of NEC.[94] There is limited information regarding the intestinal trophic effects of either n-3 LC-PUFA or other LCFAs in developing animals. However, studies have demonstrated that n-3 LC-PUFAs enhance intestinal adaptation after small-bowel resection, and their effects were greater than those of less saturated oils; they also found that medium-chain triglycerides are less trophic than long-chain triglycerides.[18] In contrast, studies with neonatal piglets indicated that the LCFA oleic acid can cause significant mucosal injury and increased permeability and that this effect is more severe in newborn piglets than in 1-month-old piglets.[95]

Key Gut Hormone and Growth Factors

GUT HORMONES

The gut is one of the largest endocrine organs in the body and secretes numerous peptide hormones from specialized endocrine cells acting as chemical sensors that respond to the composition and amount of luminal nutrients[96] (Fig. 5.4). In many cases these hormones function as neuroendocrine factors that activate extrinsic and intrinsic nerves, which mediate

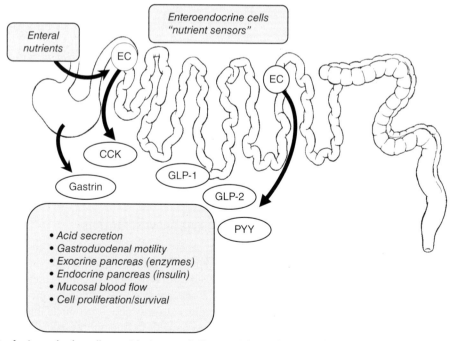

Fig. 5.4 The role of enteroendocrine cells as nutrient sensors in the neonatal gastrointestinal tract and secretion of key hormones that regulate intestinal functions. *CCK*, Cholecystokinin; *EC*, enteroendocrine cell; *GLP-1*, glucagon-like peptide 1; *PYY*, peptide YY.

secretory and motor reflexes in the gastrointestinal tract. Some of the gut hormones that have been implicated in the stimulation of trophic functional response to minimal enteral nutrition include gastrin, cholecystokinin (CCK), peptide YY (PYY), and neurotensin.[19]

Gastrin is secreted from G cells within the antrum of the stomach and acts primarily to stimulate proliferation of parietal and enterochromaffin-like cells within the gastric mucosa.[97] Studies have shown that hypogastrinemia, produced by antrectomy and targeted disruption of the gastrin gene, leads to atrophy of the gastric mucosal cells and that dysregulation of gastrin secretion can lead to neoplasia.[98] The neonate exhibits hypergastrinemia and comparatively high gastric pH, yet gastrin secretion is induced by feeding.[19] The trophic effects of gastrin are most evident in the stomach and are mediated by increased ornithine decarboxylase activity and cell proliferation.[99] The development of pentagastrin-responsive gastric acid secretion occurs within 1 week in neonatal piglets and can be prematurely induced with glucocorticoids, consistent with upregulation of gastrin receptor expression with age.[100] The trophic effects of gastrin are most evident in the stomach and are mediated by increased ornithine decarboxylase activity and cell proliferation.

CCK is expressed in endocrine cells of the gut and in neurons within the gut and brain, while its primary target tissues are the pancreas and gallbladder. CCK stimulates pancreatic growth and cell proliferation, and these trophic effects have been attributed exclusively to interaction via the CCK-A receptor. Genetic knockout of this receptor in rodent models results in hypoplasia of gastric mucosa.[101] PYY is secreted from enteroendocrine L cells and stimulates gut growth in developing rats.[18] Studies using PYY knockout and overexpression models demonstrate that PYY plays a significant role in regulation of metabolism and satiety.[102] Studies also indicate that PYY stimulates gut growth in some but not all cases and does not stimulate proliferation of cultured epithelial cells. Neurotensin is a 13–amino acid peptide secreted from the enteroendocrine N cells located exclusively in the gut within the distal small intestine.[103] Neurotensin expression is markedly increased during the neonatal period, and secretion is

stimulated specifically by ingestion of fat. Administration of neurotensin stimulates gut growth in animals after small-bowel resection, even in the absence of enteral nutrients. Apart from the effects on gastrointestinal tissue growth, CCK and PYY may be more important in the maturation and development of gastroduodenal motor and secretory function, which is critical for premature infants. CCK is a key hormone involved in pancreatic and biliary section and has been examined as possible treatment for TPN-induced cholestasis; however, a recent clinical study suggests that CCK was ineffective.[104,105] Other work in rodent models suggests limited efficacy of CCK as a trophic factor in TPN-fed rats.[106]

GLP-2 is a gut peptide that has gained considerable attention as an intestinal trophic factor.[107] GLP-2, like PYY, is secreted by enteroendocrine L cells in response to enteral nutrition, and secretion appears to be developmentally upregulated in late gestation.[108] GLP-2 has significant trophic effects on the neonatal small intestine that are mediated by increased cell proliferation, protein synthesis, blood flow, and glucose transport.[109,110] Moreover, GLP-2 increased superior mesenteric artery (SMA) blood flow without increasing systemic blood pressure or affecting brain blood flow in neonatal piglets, suggesting that its effects occur locally.[111,112] GLP-2 treatment also has been shown to reduce proinflammatory cytokines and restore intestinal structure in animal models of GLP-2 inflammatory bowel disease and enteritis.[107] Studies have shown that treatment with native GLP-2 and the long-acting GLP-2 analogs, including teduglutide, promote intestinal adaptation in neonatal piglets with short bowel syndrome (SBS).[113,114] Teduglutide was recently US Food and Drug Administration (FDA) approved for pediatric patients with SBS over the age of 1 year who require parenteral nutrition or fluid support[115–117] (Fig. 5.5).

TISSUE GROWTH FACTORS

Another class of molecules that may be key growth factors for the neonatal gut can be generally categorized as polypeptides that are secreted locally and act via the paracrine or autocrine mechanism to affect cellular growth and function (Table 5.1). Several of these growth factors are present in the blood, gastrointestinal secretions, and amniotic fluid and thus may act via endocrine mechanism (e.g., insulin-like growth

Postsurgical adaptation
- Longer villi and crypts
- Increased crypt cell proliferation
- Increased GLP-2 secretion by endocrine cells
- Increased angiogenesis

Total parenteral nutrition
- Shorter villi and crypts
- More goblet cells
- Increased inflammation and immune cells (e.g., macrophages and lymphocytes)
- Increased intercellular permeability
- Reduced blood flow

Healthy enteral fed

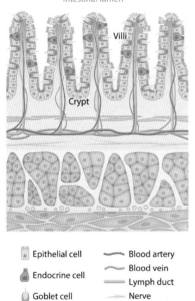

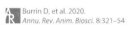

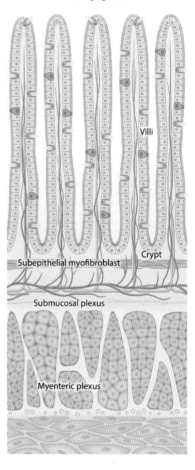

Fig. 5.5 Intestinal mucosal adaptation to TPN and intestinal resection. Illustrated is the influence of TPN, a common clinical practice in hospitalized preterm infants that deprives the gut lumen of enteral nutrition and results in mucosal villus atrophy, deterioration of intestinal barrier function, and infiltration of immune cells. Also shown is the influence of surgical resection of the intestine, which occurs due to congenital and acquired gastrointestinal diseases, that results in activation of adaptive processes promoting mucosal growth, such as increased GLP-2 secretion, crypt cell proliferation, and blood flow. GLP-2 is a key gut hormone that functions to activate mucosal enteric neuron release of NO and VIP as well as subepithelial fibroblast release of EGF and IGF-1. *EGF*, Epidermal growth factor; *GLP-2*, glucagon-like peptide 2; *GLP-2R*, glucagon-like peptide 2 receptor; *IGF-1*, insulin-like growth factor 1; *NO*, nitric oxide; *TPN*, total parenteral nutrition; *VIP*, vasoactive intestinal peptide. Adapted with permission from Burrin D, Sangild PT, Stoll B, et al. Translational advances in pediatric nutrition and gastroenterology: new insights from pig models. *Annu Rev Anim Biosci.* 2020;8:326. doi:10.1146/annurev-animal-020518-115142.

> ### TABLE 5.1 **Tissue Growth Factors Present in Breast Milk and Produced Locally in Intestinal Mucosal Tissue**
>
> - EGF
>   Intestinal cell growth
>   Stimulation of brush border enzymes
>   Stimulation of angiogenesis
>   Prevention of NEC
> - HB-EGF
>   Increased crypt cell proliferation
>   Inhibits epithelial cell apoptosis
>   Stimulation of brush border enzymes
>   Stimulation of angiogenesis
>   Prevention of NEC
> - IGF-1
>   Epithelial cell growth
>   Submucosal tissue growth
>   Intestinal smooth muscle growth
>   Increased lactase activity and glucose transport
> - VEGF
>   Vascular development and angiogenesis
>   Host defense/monocyte migration
> - KGF
>   Epithelial cell growth/proliferation
>   Inhibition epithelial cell apoptosis
>   Goblet cell hyperplasia
>   Increased glucose transport

EGF, Epidermal growth factor; *HB-EGF,* heparin-binding epidermal growth factor; *IGF-1,* insulin-like growth factor-1; *KGF,* keratinocyte growth factor; *NEC,* necrotizing enterocolitis; *VEGF,* vascular endothelial growth factor.

factor-1 [IGF-1]). More importantly, however, many of these growth factors are present in breast milk and are thought to influence neonatal gut growth.[18,39,118,119] Among the most well-known of these is EGF, a member of a family of peptides that includes transforming growth factor-α, heparin-binding EGF (HB-EGF), amphiregulin, epiregulin, betacellulin, and neuregulin.[120] Most of the EGF family of peptides are trophic to the gut, stimulating cell proliferation and suppressing apoptosis; however, they also modulate a number of other physiologic functions including enhanced tooth eruption, decreased gastric acid secretion, increased mucus secretion and gastric blood flow, reduced gastric emptying, and increased sodium and glucose transport.[121–124] EGF also has been found to increase mucosal growth and functional adaptation following intestinal resection, when infused during administration of TPN and to prevent the incidence of NEC.[125–130] Recent reports in premature infants suggest that EGF concentrations in saliva, serum, and urine are lower in infants that have NEC than in healthy infants.[128,131] Another EGF family member, HB-EGF, has been shown to reduce the incidence of NEC in neonatal rats and intestinal injury resulting from ischemia/ reperfusion injury in adult rats.[119,132] The mechanism whereby these two growth factors protect against NEC seems to involve their ability to induce cell proliferation and epithelial cell restitution and inhibit apoptosis. Enteral nutrition stimulates gastrointestinal secretion, resulting in the release of salivary and pancreatic EGF into the gut lumen where it is postulated to play a protective role. Many neonatal animal studies have shown that oral EGF administration augments gut growth and functional development.[18] These findings, combined with recent evidence from transgenic mice, support the idea that both local expression and milk- borne ingestion of EGF play a physiologic role in neonatal gut growth and development.

The IGF family of peptides includes insulin, IGF-1, and IGF-2.[18,37,133] Although insulin secretion is largely confined to the pancreas, both IGF-1 and IGF-2 are expressed throughout the body, including the gut. However, within the intestinal mucosa, expression of both IGF-1 and IGF-2 appears to be localized to subepithelial myofibroblast cells, although epithelial cells may also produce IGF-2. IGF-1 is also involved in growth of the submucosal and muscularis layers of the intestine.[134] The expression of IGF-1 and IGF-2 in the gut is highest in the fetal and neonatal periods and declines with age. The insulin and type 1 IGF receptors are present in epithelial cells; they are more abundant on the basolateral than apical membrane and more abundant in proliferating crypt cells than in differentiated enterocytes. IGF-1 appears to stimulate intestinal smooth muscle cell growth, and IGF-1 knockout mice exhibit thinning of the submucosa, identical to that in mice treated with dexamethasone.[135,136] Studies in enteroids and irradiated mice showed that IGF-1 enhances stem cell proliferation *in vivo* and *in vitro*.[137] Diminishment of IGF-1 expression may play a role in spontaneous ileal perforation seen in low-birth-weight infants treated with dexamethasone.[135] Numerous studies have shown that either administering IGF systemically or increasing its expression locally (as in transgenic mice) stimulates intestinal growth and function in normal animals receiving TPN, and following gut resection, dexamethasone treatment, sepsis, and radiation therapy. Some studies with fetal and neonatal animals given pharmacologic oral doses of insulin and IGF-1 have demonstrated a stimulation of gut growth, disaccharidase activity, and glucose transport.[18,138] Yet, others have shown only limited effects of oral IGF on the neonatal gut, suggesting that the IGFs may not have a physiologic role in the neonate.[113] Vascular endothelial growth factor (VEGF), hepatocyte growth factor (HGF), and keratinocyte growth factor (KGF) are expressed in the gut tissues and may play a role in mucosal angiogenesis, growth, and repair.[18] VEGF is expressed in the small intestine in the vascular endothelium and mast cells.[18] The receptor (flt-1) for the VEGF 165 amino acid isoform is present in intestinal epithelial cells; however, VEGF did not stimulate proliferation of these cells. The VEGF receptor has also been found on human colonic vascular endothelial cells. VEGF is found in human milk, decreasing in concentration as lactation progresses.[139,140] The role of VEGF in the intestine remains uncertain, but unpublished work by Andersson et al. showed that labeled VEGF was not absorbed by the intestine into systemic circulation, suggesting local action on the intestine. VEGF has also been shown to enhance monocyte migration, highlighting a possible role in intestinal host defense.[141] A recent report demonstrated that VEGF reduces the rate of crypt cell apoptosis in mice following total body irradiation treatment. VEGF has been implicated in angiogenesis during intestinal repair.[142]

HGF is expressed by mesenchymal but not epithelial cells, whereas the HGF receptor (c-met) is found in epithelial cells; the c-met receptor is localized on the basolateral membrane. Studies with cultured intestinal epithelial cells demonstrate that HGF stimulates cell proliferation and wound closure proliferation.[143,144] HGF is found in human milk mononuclear cells and partially accounts for the stimulatory effect of human milk on intestinal cell proliferation. Studies in rats have shown that HGF, given either systemically or orally, increased gut growth and nutrient transport after massive small-bowel resection. Increased local expression of KGF has been found in patients with inflammatory bowel disease (IBD), and administration of KGF enhanced mucosal healing in rats following induction of colitis.[145] Studies in mice demonstrate that systemic KGF administration prevents intestinal apoptosis in TPN-fed mice and augments intestinal adaptation after massive small-bowel resection.[146–150]

GLUCOCORTICOIDS

The role of glucocorticoids in neonatal intestinal development has been studied extensively, especially in rodents.[151,152] The impact of glucocorticoids, particularly dexamethasone, on human intestinal growth and development has received considerable attention in the past because of their use in treatment of pulmonary function in premature infants.[153] Studies in fetal rodents and pigs suggest that increased endogenous glucocorticoid levels are critical signals that stimulate gastrointestinal tract development and growth.[154] The prenatal cortisol surge is an important signal for intestinal development of the neonate, and premature birth precludes exposure to this key maturational signal. This idea is supported by studies in infants and piglets showing that premature birth results in insufficient intestinal maturation of intestinal lactase and lactose digestive capacity.[155] Numerous studies demonstrate how glucocorticoids stimulate neonatal intestinal development and maturation, especially regarding disaccharidase expression. However, their effects on neonatal mucosal growth, per se, as indicated by cell proliferation, cell cycle, protein turnover, and apoptosis, are not completely understood.

GROWTH HORMONE

Growth hormone (GH) has a major influence on IGF-1 expression during postnatal growth, and studies in postweaning rodents indicate that hypophysectomy results in gut atrophy, whereas transgenic overexpression of GH in mice increases gut growth.[156,157] However, the significance of GH in neonatal gut and liver growth may be limited by the abundance and responsiveness of the GH receptor. Studies with hypophysectomized neonatal rats suggest some degree of pituitary-dependent intestinal growth and development. Other studies in rats demonstrate that GH treatment does not prevent TPN-induced intestinal atrophy but may augment intestinal growth after massive small-bowel resection. Like EGF, IGF-1 has been shown to mediate the local action of GLP-2.[158]

SEROTONIN

Serotonin (5-HT) is a neurotransmitter primarily produced by enterochromaffin cells using the rate-limiting enzyme tryptophan hydroxylase (TPH2) in the small intestine with local and systemic effects. Epithelial cells present in the mucosal layer of the small intestine express serotonin reuptake transporter (SERT), which controls 5-HT levels by removing 5-HT molecules from the interstitial space in the submucosa. 5-HT that diffuses into small-intestine capillaries is taken up by platelets for later release. Dysregulation and dysfunction of SERT–5-HT uptake has been associated with multiple gastrointestinal pathologies, such as diverticulitis and celiac disease.[159] Development of SERT-knockout (SERTKO) and TPH2-knockout rodent models has also indicated the significance of 5-HT production and regulation in modulating and initiating intestinal motility, gastrointestinal secretions, vasodilation, and activation of afferent nerves. 5-HT also promotes growth and survival of enterochromaffin cells and other enteric nerves.[159] Other investigators have implicated 5-HT and SERT as factors affecting mucosal wound healing in ulcerative colitis.[160] Additionally, SERTKO mice have taller villi, deeper crypts, greater mucosal surface area, and increased nutrient absorption compared to wild-type mice, indicating that 5-HT may play a part in regulating mucosal proliferation and absorption.[160–162]

Summary

The growth and development of the fetal and neonatal gastrointestinal tract is more dynamic than any other time during the life cycle and is stimulated by a host of multiple factors, including intrinsic cellular and extracellular signaling pathways. Many of these signals, such as transcription factors, peptide growth factors, and hormones, are triggered by environmental cues, such as nutrients and microbes. Many of the cellular receptors that sense and transmit these extracellular growth signals, such as nutrients, are now emerging from non-targeted mining of the genome to reveal families of G protein–coupled receptors. The nutritional support of gastrointestinal growth and function is a key consideration in the clinical care of neonatal infants, especially those born preterm. In most healthy infants, the provision of either breast milk or formula appears to support normal intestinal mucosal growth. The most significant advantages of breast milk may be for host defense or gut barrier–related functions that are involved in reducing microbial-induced inflammation and infection. However, enteral feeding is the most potent stimulus for intestinal growth and in infants given parenteral nutrition, future studies are needed to determine the minimal amounts and composition of specific nutrients and growth factors necessary to maintain specific intestinal functions. Some specific nutrients have trophic actions when fed enterally including glutamine, arginine, and long-chain polyunsaturated fatty acids. Moreover, the use of metabolomic and metagenomic approaches is identifying new metabolites and small molecules derived from specific gut microbes that induce trophic and functional effects on the gastrointestinal tract. New tools and experimental approaches have emerged to elucidate the existing and new trophic factors that regulate gastrointestinal tract growth, such as tissue organoids, stem cells and the clustered regularly interspaced short palindromic repeat (CRISPR)/Cas system for gene editing of cells and animals. New growth factors continue to be discovered, and some of those, such as R-spondins, have potent effects on stem cell growth and function in the gastrointestinal tract. These new approaches should provide important new advancements in the coming years in our understanding of the biology of gastrointestinal tract growth during early development.

Acknowledgments

This work is a publication of the USDA/ARS Children's Nutrition Research Center, Department of Pediatrics, Baylor College of Medicine and Texas Children's Hospital, Houston, Texas. The work was supported in part by federal funds from the US Department of Agriculture Agricultural Research Service, Cooperative Agreement 3092-51000-060-01, and grants from the National Institutes of Health Grant DK-094616 (D.G.B). Caitlin Vonderohe was supported by T32 DK007664.

REFERENCES

1. Bruhin-Feichter S, Meier-Ruge W, Martucciello G, Bruder E. Connective tissue in gut development: a key player in motility and in intestinal desmosis. *Eur J Pediatr Surg.* 2012;22(6):445-459. doi:10.1055/s-0032-1322544.

2. Nankervis CA, Reber KM, Nowicki PT. Age-dependent changes in the postnatal intestinal microcirculation. *Microcirculation.* 2001;8(6):377-387. doi:10.1038/sj/mn/7800110.

3. Buddington RK, Elnif J, Puchal-Gardiner AA, Sangild PT. Intestinal apical amino acid absorption during development of the pig. *Am J Physiol Regul Integr Comp Physiol.* 2001;280(1):R241-R247. doi:10.1152/ajpregu.2001.280.1.R241.

4. Cheng H, Bjerknes M. Whole population cell kinetics and postnatal development of the mouse intestinal epithelium. *Anat Rec.* 1985;211(4):420-426. doi:10.1002/ar.1092110408.

5. Haber AL, Biton M, Rogel N, et al. A single-cell survey of the small intestinal epithelium. *Nature.* 2017;551(7680):333-339. doi:10.1038/nature24489.

6. In JG, Foulke-Abel J, Estes MK, Zachos NC, Kovbasnjuk O, Donowitz M. Human mini-guts: new insights into intestinal physiology and host-pathogen interactions. *Nat Rev Gastroenterol Hepatol.* 2016;13(11):633-642. doi:10.1038/nrgastro.2016.142.

7. Sato T, van Es JH, Snippert HJ, et al. Paneth cells constitute the niche for Lgr5 stem cells in intestinal crypts. *Nature.* 2011;469(7330):415-418. doi:10.1038/nature09637.

8. Sato T, Clevers H. Growing self-organizing mini-guts from a single intestinal stem cell: mechanism and applications. *Science.* 2013;340(6137):1190-1194. doi:10.1126/science.1234852.

9. Hilkens J, Timmer NC, Boer M, et al. RSPO3 expands intestinal stem cell and niche compartments and drives tumorigenesis. *Gut.* 2017;66(6):1095-1105. doi:10.1136/gutjnl-2016-311606.

10. Sangild PT, Fowden AL, Trahair JF. How does the foetal gastrointestinal tract develop in preparation for enteral nutrition after birth? *Livest Prod Sci.* 2000;66(2):141-150. doi:10.1016/S0301-6226(00)00221-9.

11. Nanthakumar NN, Young C, Ko JS, et al. Glucocorticoid responsiveness in developing human intestine: possible role in prevention of necrotizing enterocolitis. *Am J Physiol Gastrointest Liver Physiol.* 2005;288(1):G85-G92. doi:10.1152/ajpgi.00169.2004.

12. Mackie RI, Sghir A, Gaskins HR. Developmental microbial ecology of the neonatal gastrointestinal tract. *Am J Clin Nutr.* 1999;69(5):1035s-1045s. doi:10.1093/ajcn/69.5.1035s.

13. Brandtzaeg PE. Current understanding of gastrointestinal immunoregulation and its relation to food allergy. *Ann N Y Acad Sci.* 2002;964:13-45. doi:10.1111/j.1749-6632.2002.tb04131.x.

14. Raul F, Schleiffer R. Intestinal adaptation to nutritional stress. *Proc Nutr Soc.* 1996;55(1b):279-289. doi:10.1079/pns19960029.

15. Jenkins AP, Thompson RP. Mechanisms of small intestinal adaptation. *Dig Dis.* 1994;12(1):15-27. doi:10.1159/000171433.

16. Trahair JF, Sangild PT. Systemic and luminal influences on the perinatal development of the gut. *Equine Vet J Suppl.* 1997;(24):40-50. doi:10.1111/j.2042-3306.1997.tb05077.x.

17. Burrin DG, Stoll B, Jiang R, et al. Minimal enteral nutrient requirements for intestinal growth in neonatal piglets: how much is enough? *Am J Clin Nutr.* 2000;71(6):1603-1610. doi:10.1093/ajcn/71.6.1603.

18. Burrin DG, Stoll B. Key nutrients and growth factors for the neonatal gastrointestinal tract. *Clin Perinatol.* 2002;29(1):65-96. doi:10.1016/s0095-5108(03)00065-4.

19. Berseth CL. Minimal enteral feedings. *Clin Perinatol.* 1995;22(1):195-205. doi:Not available.

20. Lavallee CM, MacPherson JAR, Zhou M, et al. Lipid emulsion formulation of parenteral nutrition affects intestinal microbiota and host responses in neonatal piglets. *JPEN J Parenter Enteral Nutr.* 2017;41(8):1301-1309. doi:10.1177/0148607116662972.

21. Salas AA, Li P, Parks K, Lal CV, Martin CR, Carlo WA. Early progressive feeding in extremely preterm infants: a randomized trial. *Am J Clin Nutr.* 2018;107(3):365-370. doi:10.1093/ajcn/nqy012.

22. Kwok TC, Dorling J, Gale C. Early enteral feeding in preterm infants. *Semin Perinatol.* 2019;43(7):151159. doi:10.1053/j.semperi.2019.06.007.

23. Tyson JE, Kennedy KA. Trophic feedings for parenterally fed infants. *Cochrane Database Syst Rev.* 2005;(3):CD000504. doi:10.1002/14651858.CD000504.pub2.

24. Morgan J, Bombell S, McGuire W. Early trophic feeding versus enteral fasting for very preterm or very low birth weight infants. *Cochrane Database Syst Rev.* 2013;(3):CD000504. doi:10.1002/14651858.CD000504.pub4.

25. Kennedy KA, Tyson JE, Chamnanvanakij S. Rapid versus slow rate of advancement of feedings for promoting growth and preventing necrotizing enterocolitis in parenterally fed low-birth-weight infants. *Cochrane Database Syst Rev.* 2000;(2):CD001241. doi:10.1002/14651858.CD001241.

26. Dorling J, Abbott J, Berrington J, et al. Controlled trial of two incremental milk-feeding rates in preterm infants. *N Engl J Med.* 2019;381(15):1434-1443. doi:10.1056/NEJMoa1816654.

27. Walsh V, Brown JVE, Copperthwaite BR, Oddie SJ, McGuire W. Early full enteral feeding for preterm or low birth weight infants. *Cochrane Database Syst Rev.* 2020;12(12):CD013542. doi:10.1002/14651858.CD013542.pub2.

28. Shulman RJ, Wong WW, Smith EO. Influence of changes in lactase activity and small-intestinal mucosal growth on lactose digestion and absorption in preterm infants. *Am J Clin Nutr.* 2005;81(2):472-479. doi:10.1093/ajcn.81.2.472.

29. Shulman RJ, Schanler RJ, Lau C, Heitkemper M, Ou CN, Smith EO. Early feeding, feeding tolerance, and lactase activity in preterm infants. *J Pediatr.* 1998;133(5):645-649. doi:10.1016/s0022-3476(98)70105-2.

30. Burrin DG, Stoll B, Chang X, et al. Parenteral nutrition results in impaired lactose digestion and hexose absorption when enteral feeding is initiated in infant pigs. *Am J Clin Nutr.* 2003;78(3):461-470. doi:10.1093/ajcn/78.3.461.

31. Schanler RJ, Shulman RJ, Lau C, Smith EO, Heitkemper MM. Feeding strategies for premature infants: randomized trial of gastrointestinal priming and tube-feeding method. *Pediatrics.* 1999;103(2):434-439. doi:10.1542/peds.103.2.434.

32. Premji S, Chessell L. Continuous nasogastric milk feeding versus intermittent bolus milk feeding for premature infants less than 1500 grams. *Cochrane Database Syst Rev.* 2003;(1):CD001819. doi:10.1002/14651858.CD001819.

33. El-Kadi SW, Boutry-Regard C, Suryawan A, et al. Intermittent bolus feeding promotes greater lean growth than continuous feeding in a neonatal piglet model. *Am J Clin Nutr.* 2018;108(4):nzaa170. doi:10.1093/ajcn/nqy133.

34. Shulman RJ, Redel CA, Stathos TH. Bolus versus continuous feedings stimulate small-intestinal growth and development in the newborn pig. *J Pediatr Gastroenterol Nutr.* 1994;18(3):350-354. doi:10.1097/00005176-199404000-00017.

35. van Goudoever JB, Stoll B, Hartmann B, Holst JJ, Reeds PJ, Burrin DG. Secretion of trophic gut peptides is not different in bolus- and continuously fed piglets. *J Nutr.* 2001;131(3):729-732. doi:10.1093/jn/131.3.729.

36. Rudar M, Naberhuis JK, Suryawan A, et al. Intermittent bolus feeding does not enhance protein synthesis, myonuclear accretion, or lean growth more than continuous feeding in a premature piglet model. *Am J Physiol Endocrinol Metab.* 2021; 321(6):E737-E752. doi:10.1152/ajpendo.00236.2021.

37. Donovan SM, Odle J. Growth factors in milk as mediators of infant development. *Annu Rev Nutr.* 1994;14:147-167. doi:10.1146/annurev.nu.14.070194.001051.

38. Grosvenor CE, Picciano MF, Baumrucker CR. Hormones and growth factors in milk. *Endocr Rev.* 1993;14(6):710-728. doi:10.1210/edrv-14-6-710.

39. Koldovský O. Hormonally active peptides in human milk. *Acta Paediatr Suppl.* 1994;402:89-93. doi:10.1111/j.1651-2227.1994.tb13368.x.

40. Hamosh M. Bioactive factors in human milk. *Pediatr Clin North Am.* 2001;48(1):69-86. doi:10.1016/s0031-3955(05)70286-8.

41. Bernt KM, Walker WA. Human milk as a carrier of biochemical messages. *Acta Paediatr Suppl.* 1999;88(430):27-41. doi:10.1111/j.1651-2227.1999.tb01298.x.

42. Claud EC, Walker WA. Hypothesis: inappropriate colonization of the premature intestine can cause neonatal necrotizing enterocolitis. *FASEB J.* 2001;15(8):1398-1403. doi:10.1096/fj.00-0833hyp.

43. Walker WA. The dynamic effects of breastfeeding on intestinal development and host defense. *Adv Exp Med Biol.* 2004;554:155-170. doi:10.1007/978-1-4757-4242-8_15.

44. Forchielli ML, Walker WA. The role of gut-associated lymphoid tissues and mucosal defence. *Br J Nutr.* 2005;93(suppl 1):S41-S48. doi:10.1079/bjn20041356.

45. Sangild PT, Vonderohe C, Melendez Hebib V, Burrin DG. Potential benefits of bovine colostrum in pediatric nutrition and health. *Nutrients.* 2021;13(8):2551. doi:10.3390/nu13082551.

46. Lönnerdal B, Erdmann P, Thakkar SK, Sauser J, Destaillats F. Longitudinal evolution of true protein, amino acids and bioactive proteins in breast milk: a developmental perspective. *J Nutr Biochem.* 2017;41:1-11. doi:10.1016/j.jnutbio.2016.06.001.

47. Ajouz H, Mukherji D, Shamseddine A. Secondary bile acids: an underrecognized cause of colon cancer. *World J Surg Oncol.* 2014;12:164. doi:10.1186/1477-7819-12-164.

48. Jain AK, Stoll B, Burrin DG, Holst JJ, Moore DD. Enteral bile acid treatment improves parenteral nutrition-related liver disease and intestinal mucosal atrophy in neonatal pigs. *Am J Physiol Gastrointest Liver Physiol.* 2012;302(2):G218-G224. doi:10.1152/ajpgi.00280.2011.

49. Villalona G, Price A, Blomenkamp K, et al. No gut no gain! Enteral bile acid treatment preserves gut growth but not parenteral nutrition-associated liver injury in a novel extensive short bowel animal model. *JPEN J Parenter Enteral Nutr.* 2018; 42(8):1238-1251. doi:10.1002/jpen.1167.

50. Markan KR, Potthoff MJ. Metabolic fibroblast growth factors (FGFs): mediators of energy homeostasis. *Semin Cell Dev Biol.* 2016;53:85-93. doi:10.1016/j.semcdb.2015.09.021.

51. Stoll B, Price PT, Reeds PJ, et al. Feeding an elemental diet vs a milk-based formula does not decrease intestinal mucosal growth in infant pigs. *JPEN J Parenter Enteral Nutr.* 2006;30(1):32-39. doi:10.1177/014860710603000132.

52. Stoll B, Burrin DG, Henry J, Yu H, Jahoor F, Reeds PJ. Substrate oxidation by the portal drained viscera of fed piglets. *Am J Physiol.* 1999;277(1):E168-E175. doi:10.1152/ajpendo.1999.277.1.E168.

53. Reeds PJ, Burrin DG. Glutamine and the bowel. *J Nutr.* 2001;131(suppl 9):2505S-2508S; discussion 2523S-2524S. doi:10.1093/jn/131.9.2505S.

54. Neu J. Glutamine in the fetus and critically ill low birth weight neonate: metabolism and mechanism of action. *J Nutr.* 2001; 131(suppl 9):2585S-2589S; discussion 2590S. doi:10.1093/jn/131.9.2585S.

55. Neu J, DeMarco V, Li N. Glutamine: clinical applications and mechanisms of action. *Curr Opin Clin Nutr Metab Care.* 2002;5(1):69-75. doi:10.1097/00075197-200201000-00013.

56. Ziegler TR, Bazargan N, Leader LM, Martindale RG. Glutamine and the gastrointestinal tract. *Curr Opin Clin Nutr Metab Care.* 2000;3(5):355-362. doi:10.1097/00075197-200009000-00005.

57. Neu J, Roig JC, Meetze WH, et al. Enteral glutamine supplementation for very low birth weight infants decreases morbidity. *J Pediatr.* 1997;131(5):691-699. doi:10.1016/s0022-3476(97)70095-7.

58. Vaughn P, Thomas P, Clark R, Neu J. Enteral glutamine supplementation and morbidity in low birth weight infants. *J Pediatr.* 2003;142(6):662-668. doi:10.1067/mpd.2003.208.

59. Ong EG, Eaton S, Wade AM, et al. Randomized clinical trial of glutamine-supplemented versus standard parenteral nutrition in infants with surgical gastrointestinal disease. *Br J Surg.* 2012;99(7):929-938. doi:10.1002/bjs.8750.

60. Poindexter BB, Ehrenkranz RA, Stoll BJ, et al. Parenteral glutamine supplementation does not reduce the risk of mortality or late-onset sepsis in extremely low birth weight infants. *Pediatrics.* 2004;113(5):1209-1215. doi:10.1542/peds.113.5.1209.

61. Houdijk AP, Van Leeuwen PA, Boermeester MA, et al. Glutamine-enriched enteral diet increases splanchnic blood flow in the rat. *Am J Physiol.* 1994;267(6 Pt 1):G1035-G1040. doi:10.1152/ajpgi.1994.267.6.G1035.

62. Mercier A, Eurin D, Poulet-Young V, Marret S, Dechelotte P. Effect of enteral supplementation with glutamine on mesenteric blood flow in premature neonates. *Clin Nutr.* 2003;22(2):133-137. doi:10.1054/clnu.2002.0621.

63. Rhoads M. Glutamine signaling in intestinal cells. *JPEN J Parenter Enteral Nutr.* 1999;23(suppl 5):S38-S40. doi:10.1177/014860719902300510.

64. Wu G, Meininger CJ, Knabe DA, Bazer FW, Rhoads JM. Arginine nutrition in development, health and disease. *Curr Opin Clin Nutr Metab Care.* 2000;3(1):59-66. doi:10.1097/00075197-200001000-00010.

65. Evans ME, Tian J, Gu LH, Jones DP, Ziegler TR. Dietary supplementation with orotate and uracil increases adaptive growth of jejunal mucosa after massive small bowel resection in rats. *JPEN J Parenter Enteral Nutr.* 2005;29(5):315-320; discussion 320-321. doi:10.1177/0148607105029005315.

66. Evans ME, Jones DP, Ziegler TR. Glutamine prevents cytokine-induced apoptosis in human colonic epithelial cells. *J Nutr.* 2003;133(10):3065-3071. doi:10.1093/jn/133.10.3065.

67. Nakajo T, Yamatsuji T, Ban H, et al. Glutamine is a key regulator for amino acid-controlled cell growth through the mTOR signaling pathway in rat intestinal epithelial cells. *Biochem Biophys Res Commun.* 2005;326(1):174-180. doi:10.1016/j.bbrc.2004.11.015.

68. Zhu Y, Lin G, Dai Z, et al. L-Glutamine deprivation induces autophagy and alters the mTOR and MAPK signaling pathways in porcine intestinal epithelial cells. *Amino Acids.* 2015;47(10):2185-2197. doi:10.1007/s00726-014-1785-0.

69. Moore SR, Guedes MM, Costa TB, et al. Glutamine and alanyl-glutamine promote crypt expansion and mTOR signaling in murine enteroids. *Am J Physiol Gastrointest Liver Physiol.* 2015;308(10):G831-G839. doi:10.1152/ajpgi.00422.2014.

70. Sampson LL, Davis AK, Grogg MW, Zheng Y. mTOR disruption causes intestinal epithelial cell defects and intestinal atrophy

postinjury in mice. *FASEB J.* 2016;30(3):1263-1275. doi:10.1096/fj.15-278606.

71. Hansen MB, Dresner LS, Wait RB. Profile of neurohumoral agents on mesenteric and intestinal blood flow in health and disease. *Physiol Res.* 1998;47(5):307-327. doi:Not available.

72. Bruins MJ, Luiking YC, Soeters PB, Lamers WM, Akkermans LMA, Deutz NEP. Effects of long-term intravenous and intragastric L-arginine intervention on jejunal motility and visceral nitric oxide production in the hyperdynamic compensated endotoxaemic pig. *Neurogastroenterol Motil.* 2004;16(6): 819-828. doi:10.1111/j.1365-2982.2004.00579.x.

73. Ban H, Shigemitsu K, Yamatsuji T, et al. Arginine and leucine regulate p70 S6 kinase and 4E-BP1 in intestinal epithelial cells. *Int J Mol Med.* 2004;13(4):537-543. doi:Not available.

74. Rhoads JM, Chen W, Gookin J, et al. Arginine stimulates intestinal cell migration through a focal adhesion kinase dependent mechanism. *Gut.* 2004;53(4):514-522. doi:10.1136/gut.2003. 027540.

75. Hou Q, Dong Y, Yu Q, et al. Regulation of the Paneth cell niche by exogenous L-arginine couples the intestinal stem cell function. *FASEB J.* 2020;34(8):10299-10315. doi:10.1096/fj.201902573RR.

76. Bauchart-Thevret C, Cui L, Wu G, Burrin DG. Arginine-induced stimulation of protein synthesis and survival in IPEC-J2 cells is mediated by mTOR but not nitric oxide. *Am J Physiol Endocrinol Metab.* 2010;299(6):E899-E909. doi:10.1152/ajpendo.00068.2010.

77. Gookin JL, Rhoads JM, Argenzio RA. Inducible nitric oxide synthase mediates early epithelial repair of porcine ileum. *Am J Physiol Gastrointest Liver Physiol.* 2002;283(1):G157-G168. doi:10.1152/ajpgi.00005.2001.

78. Di Lorenzo M, Bass J, Krantis A. Use of L-arginine in the treatment of experimental necrotizing enterocolitis. *J Pediatr Surg.* 1995;30(2):235-240; discussion 240-241. doi:10.1016/0022-3468(95)90567-7.

79. Amin HJ, Zamora SA, McMillan DD, et al. Arginine supplementation prevents necrotizing enterocolitis in the premature infant. *J Pediatr.* 2002;140(4):425-431. doi:10.1067/mpd.2002.123289.

80. Robinson JL, Smith VA, Stoll B, et al. Prematurity reduces citrulline-arginine-nitric oxide production and precedes the onset of necrotizing enterocolitis in piglets. *Am J Physiol Gastrointest Liver Physiol.* 2018;315(4):G638-G649. doi:10.1152/ajpgi.00198.2018.

81. Shah PS, Shah VS, Kelly LE. Arginine supplementation for prevention of necrotising enterocolitis in preterm infants. *Cochrane Database Syst Rev.* 2017;4(4):CD004339. doi:10.1002/14651858. CD004339.pub4.

82. Bertolo RF, Brunton JA, Pencharz PB, Ball RO. Arginine, ornithine, and proline interconversion is dependent on small intestinal metabolism in neonatal pigs. *Am J Physiol Endocrinol Metab.* 2003;284(5):E915-E922. doi:10.1152/ajpendo.00269.2002.

83. Dumas F, De Bandt JP, Colomb V, et al. Enteral ornithine alpha-ketoglutarate enhances intestinal adaptation to massive resection in rats. *Metabolism.* 1998;47(11):1366-1371. doi:10.1016/s0026-0495(98)90306-7.

84. Wakabayashi Y, Yamada E, Yoshida T, Takahashi H. Arginine becomes an essential amino acid after massive resection of rat small intestine. *J Biol Chem.* 1994;269(51):32667-32671. doi:Not available.

85. Schaart MW, Schierbeek H, van der Schoor SRD, et al. Threonine utilization is high in the intestine of piglets. *J Nutr.* 2005;135(4):765-770. doi:10.1093/jn/135.4.765.

86. Shoveller AK, Stoll B, Ball RO, Burrin DG. Nutritional and functional importance of intestinal sulfur amino acid metabolism. *J Nutr.* 2005;135(7):1609-1612. doi:10.1093/jn/135.7.1609.

87. Bauchart-Thevret C, Stoll B, Chacko S, Burrin DG. Sulfur amino acid deficiency upregulates intestinal methionine cycle activity and suppresses epithelial growth in neonatal pigs. *Am J Physiol Endocrinol Metab.* 2009;296(6):E1239-E1250. doi:10.1152/ajpendo.91021.2008.

88. Saito Y, Iwatsuki K, Hanyu H, et al. Effect of essential amino acids on enteroids: methionine deprivation suppresses proliferation and affects differentiation in enteroid stem cells. *Biochem Biophys Res Commun.* 2017;488(1):171-176. doi:10.1016/j. bbrc.2017.05.029.

89. Forchielli ML, Walker WA. The role of gut-associated lymphoid tissues and mucosal defence. *Br J Nutr.* 2005;93(suppl 1):S41-S48. doi:10.1079/bjn20041356.

90. Forchielli ML, Walker WA. The effect of protective nutrients on mucosal defense in the immature intestine. *Acta Paediatr Suppl.* 2005;94(449):74-83. doi:10.1111/j.1651-2227.2005.tb02159.x.

91. Smilowitz JT, Lebrilla CB, Mills DA, German JB, Freeman SL. Breast milk oligosaccharides: structure-function relationships in the neonate. *Annu Rev Nutr.* 2014;34:143-169. doi:10.1146/ annurev-nutr-071813-105721.

92. Roy CC, Kien CL, Bouthillier L, Levy E. Short-chain fatty acids: ready for prime time? *Nutr Clin Pract.* 2006;21(4): 351-366. doi:10.1177/0115426506021004351.

93. Caplan MS, Jilling T. The role of polyunsaturated fatty acid supplementation in intestinal inflammation and neonatal necrotizing enterocolitis. *Lipids.* 2001;36(9):1053-1057. doi:10.1007/ s11745-001-0816-3.

94. Ohtsuka Y, Okada K, Yamakawa Y, et al. ω-3 fatty acids attenuate mucosal inflammation in premature rat pups. *J Pediatr Surg.* 2011;46(3):489-495. doi:10.1016/j.jpedsurg.2010.07.032.

95. Crissinger KD, Burney DL, Velasquez OR, Gonzalez E. An animal model of necrotizing enterocolitis induced by infant formula and ischemia in developing piglets. *Gastroenterology.* 1994;106(5):1215-1222. doi:10.1016/0016-5085(94)90012-4.

96. Raybould HE, Cooke HJ, Christofi FL. Sensory mechanisms: transmitters, modulators and reflexes. *Neurogastroenterol Motil.* 2004;16(suppl 1):60-63. doi:10.1111/j.1743-3150.2004.00477.x.

97. Schubert ML. Gastric secretion. *Curr Opin Gastroenterol.* 2008;24(6):659-664. doi:10.1097/MOG.0b013e328311a65f.

98. Smith JP, Nadella S, Osborne N. Gastrin and gastric cancer. *Cell Mol Gastroenterol Hepatol.* 2017;4(1):75-83. doi:10.1016/ j.jcmgh.2017.03.004.

99. Walsh JH. Role of gastrin as a trophic hormone. *Digestion.* 1990;47(suppl 1):11-16; discussion 49-52. doi:10.1159/ 000200509.

100. Trahair JF, Sangild PT. Systemic and luminal influences on the perinatal development of the gut. *Equine Vet J Suppl.* 1997;(24):40-50. doi:10.1111/j.2042-3306.1997.tb05077.x.

101. Chen D, Zhao CM, Håkanson R, Rehfeld JF. Gastric phenotypic abnormality in cholecystokinin 2 receptor null mice. *Pharmacol Toxicol.* 2002;91(6):375-381. doi:10.1034/j. 1600-0773.2002.910616.x.

102. Kirchner H, Tong J, Tschöp MH, Pfluger PT. Ghrelin and PYY in the regulation of energy balance and metabolism: lessons from mouse mutants. *Am J Physiol Endocrinol Metab.* 2010;298(5):E909-E919. doi:10.1152/ajpendo.00191.2009.

103. Gomez GA, Englander EW, Greeley Jr GH. Postpyloric gastrointestinal peptides. In: Johnson LR, Kaunitz JD, Merchant JL, et al., eds. *Physiology of the Gastrointestinal Tract.* 5th ed. Waltham, MA: Elsevier Academic Press; 2012:155-198.

104. Teitelbaum DH, Tracy Jr TF, Aouthmany MM, et al. Use of cholecystokinin-octapeptide for the prevention of parenteral

nutrition-associated cholestasis. *Pediatrics.* 2005;115(5):1332-1340. doi:10.1542/peds.2004-1014.

105. Tsai S, Strouse PJ, Drongowski RA, Islam S, Teitelbaum DH. Failure of cholecystokinin-octapeptide to prevent TPN-associated gallstone disease. *J Pediatr Surg.* 2005;40(1):263-267. doi:10.1016/j.jpedsurg.2004.09.036.

106. Wu XM, Liao YW, Ji KQ, Li GF, Zang B. The trophic effect of cholecystokinin on the pancreas declines in rats on total parenteral nutrition. *J Anim Physiol Anim Nutr (Berl).* 2012;96(2):214-219.doi:10.1111/j.1439-0396.2011.01140.x.

107. Estall JL, Drucker DJ. Glucagon-like peptide-2. *Annu Rev Nutr.* 2006;26:391-411. doi:10.1146/annurev.nutr.26.061505.111223.

108. Burrin D, Guan X, Stoll B, Petersen YM, Sangild PT. Glucagon-like peptide 2: a key link between nutrition and intestinal adaptation in neonates? *J Nutr.* 2003;133(11):3712-3716. doi:10.1093/jn/133.11.3712.

109. Cottrell JJ, Stoll B, Buddington RK, et al. Glucagon-like peptide-2 protects against TPN-induced intestinal hexose malabsorption in enterally refed piglets. *Am J Physiol Gastrointest Liver Physiol.* 2006;290(2):G293-G300. doi:10.1152/ajpgi.00275.2005.

110. Guan X, Karpen HE, Stephens J, et al. GLP-2 receptor localizes to enteric neurons and endocrine cells expressing vasoactive peptides and mediates increased blood flow. *Gastroenterology.* 2006;130(1):150-164. doi:10.1053/j.gastro.2005.11.005.

111. Stephens J, Stoll B, Cottrell J, Chang X, Helmrath M, Burrin DG. Glucagon-like peptide-2 acutely increases proximal small intestinal blood flow in TPN-fed neonatal piglets. *Am J Physiol Regul Integr Comp Physiol.* 2006;290(2):R283-R289. doi:10.1152/ajpregu.00588.2005.

112. Burrin D, Sangild PT, Stoll B, et al. Translational advances in pediatric nutrition and gastroenterology: new insights from pig models. *Annu Rev Anim Biosci.* 2020;8:321-354. doi:10.1146/annurev-animal-020518-115142.

113. Sangild PT, Ney DM, Sigalet DL, Vegge A, Burrin D. Animal models of gastrointestinal and liver diseases. Animal models of infant short bowel syndrome: translational relevance and challenges. *Am J Physiol Gastrointest Liver Physiol.* 2014;307(12):G1147-G1168. doi:10.1152/ajpgi.00088.2014.

114. Slim GM, Lansing M, Wizzard P, et al. Novel long-acting GLP-2 analogue, FE 203799 (apraglutide), enhances adaptation and linear intestinal growth in a neonatal piglet model of short bowel syndrome with total resection of the ileum. *JPEN J Parenter Enteral Nutr.* 2019;43(7):891-898. doi:10.1002/jpen.1500.

115. Jeppesen PB, Hartmann B, Thulesen J, et al. Glucagon-like peptide 2 improves nutrient absorption and nutritional status in short-bowel patients with no colon. *Gastroenterology.* 2001;120(4):806-815. doi:10.1053/gast.2001.22555.

116. Jeppesen PB, Sanguinetti EL, Buchman A, et al. Teduglutide (ALX-0600), a dipeptidyl peptidase IV resistant glucagon-like peptide 2 analogue, improves intestinal function in short bowel syndrome patients. *Gut.* 2005;54(9):1224-1231. doi:10.1136/gut.2004.061440.

117. Rosete BE, Wendel D, Horslen SP. Teduglutide for pediatric short bowel syndrome patients. *Expert Rev Gastroenterol Hepatol.* 2021;15(7):727-733. doi:10.1080/17474124.2021.1913052.

118. Dvorak B. Milk epidermal growth factor and gut protection. *J Pediatr.* 2010;156(suppl 2):S31-S35. doi:10.1016/j.jpeds.2009.11.018.

119. Feng J, El-Assal ON, Besner GE. Heparin-binding EGF-like growth factor (HB-EGF) and necrotizing enterocolitis. *Semin Pediatr Surg.* 2005;14(3):167-174. doi:10.1053/j.sempedsurg.2005.05.005.

120. Barnard JA, Beauchamp RD, Russell WE, Dubois RN, Coffey RJ. Epidermal growth factor-related peptides and their relevance to gastrointestinal pathophysiology. *Gastroenterology.* 1995;108(2):564-580. doi:10.1016/0016-5085(95)90087-x.

121. Seare NJ, Playford RJ. Growth factors and gut function. *Proc Nutr Soc.* 1998;57(3):403-408. doi:10.1079/pns19980057.

122. Thompson JS. Epidermal growth factor and the short bowel syndrome. *JPEN J Parenter Enteral Nutr.* 1999;23(suppl 5):S113-S116. doi:10.1177/014860719902300528.

123. Uribe JM, Barrett KE. Nonmitogenic actions of growth factors: an integrated view of their role in intestinal physiology and pathophysiology. *Gastroenterology.* 1997;112(1):255-268. doi:Not available.

124. Wong WM, Wright NA. Epidermal growth factor, epidermal growth factor receptors, intestinal growth, and adaptation. *JPEN J Parenter Enteral Nutr.* 1999;23(suppl 5):S83-S88. doi:10.1177/014860719902300521.

125. Erwin CR, Helmrath MA, Shin CE, Falcone Jr RA, Stern LE, Warner BW. Intestinal overexpression of EGF in transgenic mice enhances adaptation after small bowel resection. *Am J Physiol.* 1999;277(3):G533-G540. doi:10.1152/ajpgi.1999.277.3.G533.

126. Helmrath MA, Shin CE, Fox JW, Erwin CR, Warner BW. Adaptation after small bowel resection is attenuated by sialoadenectomy: the role for endogenous epidermal growth factor. *Surgery.* 1998;124(5):848-854. doi:Not available.

127. Helmrath MA, Erwin CR, Warner BW. A defective EGF-receptor in waved-2 mice attenuates intestinal adaptation. *J Surg Res.* 1997;69(1):76-80. doi:10.1006/jsre.1997.5033.

128. Warner BW, Warner BB. Role of epidermal growth factor in the pathogenesis of neonatal necrotizing enterocolitis. *Semin Pediatr Surg.* 2005;14(3):175-180. doi:10.1053/j.sempedsurg.2005.05.006.

129. Clark JA, Lane RH, Maclennan NK, et al. Epidermal growth factor reduces intestinal apoptosis in an experimental model of necrotizing enterocolitis. *Am J Physiol Gastrointest Liver Physiol.* 2005;288(4):G755-G762. doi:10.1152/ajpgi.00172.2004.

130. Dvorak B, Halpern MD, Holubec H, et al. Epidermal growth factor reduces the development of necrotizing enterocolitis in a neonatal rat model. *Am J Physiol Gastrointest Liver Physiol.* 2002;282(1):G156-G164. doi:10.1152/ajpgi.00196.2001.

131. Shin CE, Falcone Jr RA, Stuart L, Erwin CR, Warner BW. Diminished epidermal growth factor levels in infants with necrotizing enterocolitis. *J Pediatr Surg.* 2000;35(2):173-176; discussion 177. doi:10.1016/s0022-3468(00)90005-8.

132. Pillai SB, Hinman CE, Luquette MH, Nowicki PT, Besner GE. Heparin-binding epidermal growth factor-like growth factor protects rat intestine from ischemia/reperfusion injury. *J Surg Res.* 1999;87(2):225-231. doi:10.1006/jsre.1999.5764.

133. MacDonald RS. The role of insulin-like growth factors in small intestinal cell growth and development. *Horm Metab Res.* 1999;31(2-3):103-113. doi:10.1055/s-2007-978706.

134. Zheng Y, Song Y, Han Q, et al. Intestinal epithelial cell-specific IGF1 promotes the expansion of intestinal stem cells during epithelial regeneration and functions on the intestinal immune homeostasis. *Am J Physiol Endocrinol Metab.* 2018;315(4):E638-E649. doi:10.1152/ajpendo.00022.2018.

135. Herman AC, Carlisle EM, Paxton JB, Gordon PV. Insulin-like growth factor-I governs submucosal growth and thickness in the newborn mouse ileum. *Pediatr Res.* 2004;55(3):507-513. doi:10.1203/01.PDR.0000110525.30786.50.

136. Rowland KJ, Trivedi S, Lee D, et al. Loss of glucagon-like peptide-2-induced proliferation following intestinal epithelial insulin-like growth factor-1-receptor deletion. *Gastroenterology.* 2011;141(6):2166-2175.e7. doi:10.1053/j.gastro.2011.09.014.

137. Van Landeghem L, Santoro MA, Mah AT, et al. IGF1 stimulates crypt expansion via differential activation of 2 intestinal stem cell populations. *FASEB J.* 2015;29(7):2828-2842. doi:10.1096/fj.14-264010.

138. Fesler Z, Mitova E, Brubaker PL. GLP-2, EGF, and the intestinal epithelial IGF-1 receptor interactions in the regulation of crypt cell proliferation. *Endocrinology.* 2020;161(4):bqaa040. doi:10.1210/endocr/bqaa040.

139. Siafakas CG, Anatolitou F, Fusunyan RD, Walker WA, Sanderson IR. Vascular endothelial growth factor (VEGF) is present in human breast milk and its receptor is present on intestinal epithelial cells. *Pediatr Res.* 1999;45(5 Pt 1):652-657. doi:10.1203/00006450-199905010-00007.

140. Vuorela P, Andersson S, Carpén O, Ylikorkala O, Halmesmäki E. Unbound vascular endothelial growth factor and its receptors in breast, human milk, and newborn intestine. *Am J Clin Nutr.* 2000;72(5):1196-1201. doi:10.1093/ajcn/72.5.1196.

141. Clauss M, Gerlach M, Gerlach H, et al. Vascular permeability factor: a tumor-derived polypeptide that induces endothelial cell and monocyte procoagulant activity, and promotes monocyte migration. *J Exp Med.* 1990;172(6):1535-1545. doi:10.1084/jem.172.6.1535.

142. Jones MK, Tomikawa M, Mohajer B, Tarnawski AS. Gastrointestinal mucosal regeneration: role of growth factors. *Front Biosci.* 1999;4:D303-D309. doi:10.2741/a428.

143. Göke M, Kanai M, Podolsky DK. Intestinal fibroblasts regulate intestinal epithelial cell proliferation via hepatocyte growth factor. *Am J Physiol.* 1998;274(5):G809-G818. doi:10.1152/ajpgi.1998.274.5.G809.

144. Nusrat A, Parkos CA, Bacarra AE, et al. Hepatocyte growth factor/scatter factor effects on epithelia. Regulation of intercellular junctions in transformed and nontransformed cell lines, basolateral polarization of c-met receptor in transformed and natural intestinal epithelia, and induction of rapid wound repair in a transformed model epithelium. *J Clin Invest.* 1994;93(5):2056-2065. doi:10.1172/JCI117200.

145. Farrell CL, Rex KL, Chen JN, et al. The effects of keratinocyte growth factor in preclinical models of mucositis. *Cell Prolif.* 2002;35(suppl 1):78-85. doi:10.1046/j.1365-2184.35.s1.8.x.

146. Wildhaber BE, Yang H, Teitelbaum DH. Total parenteral nutrition-induced apoptosis in mouse intestinal epithelium: modulation by keratinocyte growth factor. *J Surg Res.* 2003;112(2):144-151. doi:10.1016/s0022-4804(03)00160-4.

147. Wildhaber BE, Yang H, Teitelbaum DH. Keratinocyte growth factor decreases total parenteral nutrition-induced apoptosis in mouse intestinal epithelium via Bcl-2. *J Pediatr Surg.* 2003;38(1):92-96; discussion 92-96. doi:10.1053/jpsu.2003.50018.

148. Yang H, Antony PA, Wildhaber BE, Teitelbaum DH. Intestinal intraepithelial lymphocyte gamma delta-T cell-derived keratinocyte growth factor modulates epithelial growth in the mouse. *J Immunol.* 2004;172(7):4151-4158. doi:10.4049/jimmunol.172.7.4151.

149. Yang H, Wildhaber BE, Teitelbaum DH. 2003 Harry M. Vars Research Award. Keratinocyte growth factor improves epithelial function after massive small bowel resection. *JPEN J Parenter Enteral Nutr.* 2003;27(3):198-206; discussion 206-207. doi:10.1177/0148607103027003198.

150. Yang H, Wildhaber B, Tazuke Y, Teitelbaum DH. 2002 Harry M. Vars Research Award. Keratinocyte growth factor stimulates the recovery of epithelial structure and function in a mouse model of total parenteral nutrition. *JPEN J Parenter Enteral Nutr.* 2002;26(6):333-340; discussion 340-341. doi:10.1177/0148607102026006333.

151. Henning SJ, Rubin DC, Shulman RJ. Ontogeny of the intestinal mucosa. In: Johnson LR, Alpers DH, Christensen J, Jacobson E, eds. *Physiology of the Gastrointestinal Tract.* 3rd ed. New York: Raven; Press; 1994:576-610.

152. Drozdowski L, Thomson ABR. Intestinal hormones and growth factors: effects on the small intestine. *World J Gastroenterol.* 2009;15(4):385. doi:10.3748/wjg.15.385.

153. Yeung MY, Smyth JP. Hormonal factors in the morbidities associated with extreme prematurity and the potential benefits of hormonal supplement. *Biol Neonate.* 2002;81(1):1-15. doi:10.1159/000047178.

154. Rønnestad I, Akiba Y, Kaji I, Kaunitz JD. Duodenal luminal nutrient sensing. *Curr Opin Pharmacol.* 2014;19:67-75. doi:10.1016/j.coph.2014.07.010.

155. Sangild PT. Gut responses to enteral nutrition in preterm infants and animals. *Exp Biol Med.* 2006;231(11):1695-1711. doi:10.1177/153537020623101106.

156. Burrin DG, Stoll B. Key nutrients and growth factors for the neonatal gastrointestinal tract. *Clin Perinatol.* 2002;29(1):65-96. doi:10.1016/s0095-5108(03)00065-4.

157. Bortvedt SF, Lund PK. Insulin-like growth factor 1: common mediator of multiple enterotrophic hormones and growth factors. *Curr Opin Gastroenterol.* 2012;28(2):89-98. doi:10.1097/MOG.0b013e32835004c6.

158. Hellmich MR, Evers BM. Regulation of gastrointestinal normal cell growth. In: Johnson LR, Barrett KE, Ghishan FK, Merchant JL, Said HM, Wood JD, eds. *Physiology of the Gastrointestinal Tract.* 4th ed. Burlington, MA: Elsevier Academic Press; 2006:435-458.

159. Mawe GM, Hoffman JM. Serotonin signalling in the gut—functions, dysfunctions and therapeutic targets. *Nat Rev Gastroenterol Hepatol.* 2013;10(8):473-486. doi:10.1038/nrgastro.2013.105.

160. Tada Y, Ishihara S, Kawashima K, et al. Downregulation of serotonin reuptake transporter gene expression in healing colonic mucosa in presence of remaining low-grade inflammation in ulcerative colitis. *J Gastroenterol Hepatol.* 2016; 31(8):1443-1452. doi:10.1111/jgh.13268.

161. Park CJ, Armenia SJ, Shaughnessy MP, Greig CJ, Cowles RA. Potentiation of serotonin signaling leads to increased carbohydrate and lipid absorption in the murine small intestine. *J Pediatr Surg.* 2019;54(6):1245-1249. doi:10.1016/j.jpedsurg.2019.02.027.

162. Gross ER, Gershon MD, Margolis KG, Gertsberg ZV, Li Z, Cowles RA. Neuronal serotonin regulates growth of the intestinal mucosa in mice. *Gastroenterology.* 2012;143(2):408-417.e2. doi:10.1053/j.gastro.2012.05.007.

Chapter 6

The Liver and Cholestasis (Treatment and Prevention)

Daniel T. Robinson and Kara L. Calkins

Key Points

1. Parenteral nutrition (PN) and intravenous lipid emulsions (ILEs) play an important role in nutrition for premature infants and infants with intestinal failure.
2. Infants with intestinal failure require prolonged PN and are at high risk for intestinal failure–associated liver disease (IFALD), which is histologically hallmarked by cholestasis.
3. Various ILEs are available and their oil source varies.
4. Pure soybean oil (SO ILE) has a long-standing association with IFALD.
5. SO ILE's high concentration of hepatoxic phytosterols and proinflammatory omega-6 fatty acids along with its insufficient antioxidant protection in the form of vitamin E contribute to the development and severity of IFALD.
6. Pure fish oil (FO ILE) is used to manage pediatric IFALD and can prevent liver failure.
7. FO ILE contains antiinflammatory omega-3 fatty acids and vitamin E and is devoid of phytosterols.
8. Multi-oil ILEs replace soybean oil with medium-chain triglycerides, olive oil–derived monounsaturated fatty acids, and eicosapentaenoic acid and docosahexaenoic acid–rich fish oil.
9. It remains unclear as to whether an ILE type offers any specific advantages for preterm infants without intestinal failure who require short PN courses.
10. When prescribing ILEs to infants with intestinal failure and preterm infants, clinicians should be mindful of the dose and fatty acid, phytosterol, and vitamin E composition.

Neonatal Cholestasis and Parenteral Nutrition

Cholestasis affects 1 in every 2500 newborns worldwide.[1] Because of impaired bile acid flux and bilirubin elimination, bilirubin and bile acids are retained in the liver, causing hepatocyte injury and apoptosis. The sine qua non of cholestasis in infants is a rise in serum conjugated bilirubin (CB) and bile acids. Traditionally, cholestasis has been diagnosed by an increase in serum direct bilirubin or CB, not an increase in circulating bile acids. While there is no universally agreed-upon definition for cholestasis, an arbitrary cutoff of >2 mg/dL is often used. Other commonly used diagnostic thresholds include a CB >1 mg/dL (if the total serum bilirubin is <5 mg/dL) or a CB >15% to 20% of the total serum

bilirubin (if the total serum bilirubin is >5 mg/dL). Some data suggest that a lower cutoff should be used, particularly in the first two weeks of life (i.e., >0.8 mg/dL in the first 5 days or >0.5 mg/dL in the first 14 days).[2,3]

Fig. 6.1 illustrates the hepatocellular transport and excretion of bile acids and bilirubin. Bile acids are transported into and out of the hepatocyte by organic solute transporter subunit (OST)-α and -β, organic anion-transporter polypeptide 1 (OATP1), and sodium taurocholate cotransporter peptide (NTCP). CYP7A1 is a critical, rate-limiting enzyme that endogenously synthesizes bile acids from cholesterol. The nuclear receptors farnesoid X receptor (FXR) and liver X receptor (LXR) act as intracellular sensors for bile acids and sterols. When activated by bile acids, FXR represses CYP7A1 and NTCP via the small heterodimer partner

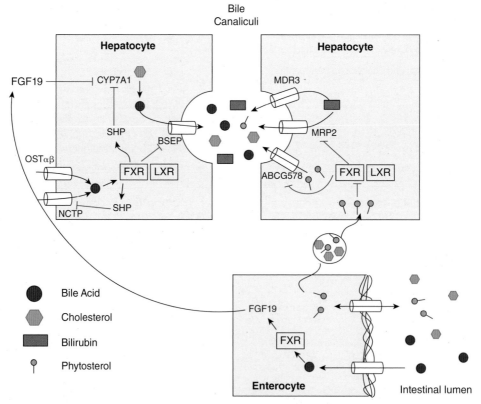

Fig. 6.1 Bilirubin, bile acid, and phytosterol metabolism. *ASBPT*, Apical sodium–bile acid transporter; *BSEP*, bile salt exporter; *FGF19*, fibroblast growth factor 19; *FXR*, farnesoid X receptor; *LXR*, liver X receptor; *MDR3*, multidrug resistance protein 3; *MRP2*, multidrug resistance–associated protein 2; *NTCP*, sodium taurocholate co-transporter peptide; *OST*, organic solute transporter subunit; *SHP*, small heterodimer partner.

(SHP) and upregulates the bile salt exporter (BSEP, *ABCB11*), an ATP-dependent efflux transporter. BSEP excretes bile acids into the bile canaliculi, and the multidrug resistance–associated protein 2 (MRP2) and multidrug resistance protein 3 (MDR3) excrete bilirubin into the bile canaliculi. At the intestinal level, bile acids are absorbed into the enterocyte via the apical sodium–bile acid transporter (ASBPT) and bind to FXR, which activates the expression of fibroblast growth factor 19 (FGF19), a hormone that travels to the liver via the portal circulation and inhibits CYP7A1, thereby downregulating bile acid synthesis.

A common cause of cholestasis in infants cared for in the NICU is parenteral nutrition (PN)–related cholestasis. PN, specifically intravenous lipid emulsions (ILEs), has a long-standing association with cholestasis.[4-15] Studies have demonstrated that phytosterols derived from ILEs with 100% soybean oil (SO ILEs) interfere with bilirubin and bile acid metabolism.[8,9] Infants at risk of PN- and ILE-induced liver injury include preterm infants and infants with underlying gastrointestinal pathology. Commonly encountered acquired and congenital gastrointestinal diseases in the NICU include necrotizing enterocolitis (NEC), intestinal perforation, gastroschisis, small bowel atresias, volvulus, meconium ileus, and Hirschsprung's disease. Infants with intestinal failure (IF) are at the highest risk for PN- and ILE-induced liver disease.[16] IF is defined as a reduction of gut function hallmarked by water, electrolyte, and nutrient malabsorption that leads to PN dependence.[17]

While the terms *parenteral nutrition–associated cholestasis* (PNAC) and *intestinal failure–associated liver disease* (IFALD) are often used interchangeably, they are distinctly different. PNAC generally refers to CB >2 mg/dL in the absence of other liver diseases and >14 days of PN. In uncomplicated scenarios, PNAC is transient without long-term sequelae. On the other hand, IFALD refers to hepatobiliary dysfunction secondary to the toxicities associated with the long-standing use of PN and ILE and underlying intestinal anatomic abnormalities. It remains unclear whether IFALD should be defined by clinical, laboratory, or histologic criteria. IFALD is initially characterized by cholestasis and hepatitis. Advanced IFALD is heralded by thrombocytopenia, coagulopathy, and portal hypertension. If IFALD cannot be stabilized or reversed by intestinal rehabilitation, it can progress to end-stage liver disease requiring a multivisceral, liver-inclusive transplant. While the prevalence of IFALD among children with IF is not well studied, approximately 20% to 30% of children with IF develop IFALD and 4% develop liver failure.[16] When appropriate, the term *IFALD* should be used in place of *PNAC* since it more accurately reflects this disease's complexity and multifactorial nature.

Well-known risk factors for PNAC and IFALD include prematurity, low birth weight, fetal growth restriction, small for gestational age, intestinal surgeries, hepatic injury secondary to infections, ischemia, medications, bacterial overgrowth, genetics, and specific PN micro- and macronutrients, including ILE.[16] The prevalence of PNAC and IFALD varies by population and report, given the absence of standardized definitions for cholestasis, PNAC, and IFALD. In a meta-analysis of studies, the incidence of PNAC in very-low-birthweight (birth weight <1.5 kg) and extremely low-birthweight infants (birth weight <1 kg) ranged from 0% to 67%. In the same meta-analysis, the incidence of IFALD in infants and children with short bowel syndrome (SBS) or who required intestinal surgery was 23% to 63%.[16] The incidence of PNAC or IFALD is directly proportional to PN duration. For example, infants who receive <14 to 30 days of PN have a reported incidence of 0% to 37%, while those who receive >60 days have a reported incidence of 36% to 100%.[16]

Neonatal Cholestasis and Intravenous Lipid Emulsions

ILEs are a standard companion to parenteral amino acids and carbohydrates when providing PN. ILEs provide nonprotein calories and fatty acids and help ensure appropriate growth and development when achieving sufficient enteral nutrition is not possible. While ILE duration and dose are associated with liver injury, specific ILE constituents, namely omega-6 fatty acids, phytosterols, and vitamin E, play a role in liver injury.[7-10,16,18-20] An ILE's fatty acid, phytosterol, and vitamin E content is determined by the ILE's oil source (Table 6.1). The first-generation ILE, which was first introduced in 1961 and approved for use in the United States in 1972, is composed of pure soybean

TABLE 6.1 **Intravenous Lipid Emulsions**					
	SO ILE	**SO,MCT ILE**	**SO,OO ILE**	**SO,MCT,OO, FO ILE**	**FO ILE**
Oil Source (%)					
Soybean oil	100	50	20	30	0
MCT	0	50	0	30	0
Olive oil	0	0	80	20	0
Fish oil	0	0	0	15	100
Fatty Acid (% by weight, mean value, or range)					
Medium Chain					
Caprylic	0%	28.5%	0%	$17 \pm 0.2\%$	0%
Capric	0%	20%	0%	$12 \pm 0.2\%$	0%
Long Chain					
Linoleic acid (18:2n–6)	44–62%	27%	13.8–22%	14–25%	1.5%
α-Linolenic acid (18:3n–3)	4–11%	4%	0.5–4.2%	1.5–3.5%	1.1%
Arachidonic acid (20:4n–6)	0%	0.2%	ND	0.5%	0.2–2%
Docosahexaenoic acid (22:6n–3)	0%	0%	0%	1–3.5%	14–27%
Eicosapentaenoic acid (20:5n–3)	0%	0%	0%	1–3.5%	13–26%
Oleic acid (18:1n–9)	19–30%	11%	44–80%	23–35%	4–11%
Omega-6 to omega-3 ratio	7:1	7:1	9:1	2.5:1	1:8
Phytosterols (mcg/mL)					
β-Sitosterol	243.26 ± 4.10	191.6	197.86 ± 5.38	131.58 ± 7.11	ND
Campesterol	37.19 ± 0.54	30.9	11.41 ± 0.33	20.45 ± 1.04	0.95 ± 0.08
Stigmasterol	49.57 ± 0.62	46	11.01 ± 0.54	18.51 ± 0.81	1.37 ± 0.35
Vitamin E (mg/L)					
α-Tocopherol	ND	169–171	32	163–225	150–300

FO, Fish oil; *ILE*, intravenous lipid emulsion; *MCT*, medium chain triglyceride; *ND*, not determined; *OO*, olive oil; *SO*, soybean oil.

oil (SO ILE, Intralipid Fresenius Kabi, Uppsala, Sweden). SO ILE has a skewed omega-6 to omega-3 ratio (7:1) and contains hepatotoxic phytosterols. SO ILE is also a rich source of long-chain triglycerides (LCTs) and the omega-6 polyunsaturated fatty acid (PUFA) linoleic acid (LA), which is prone to lipid peroxidation, which causes cellular injury. LA and α-linolenic acid (ALA) are considered to be essential fatty acids and are metabolized to downstream fatty acids (Fig. 6.2) and bioactive eicosanoids (Fig. 6.3). The eicosanoids generated from the LA pathway are considered to be proinflammatory, while the eicosanoids generated from the ALA pathway are considered to be less inflammatory and help promote the resolution of inflammation (Fig. 6.3).

To reduce the provision of phytosterols, LCTs, and LA while simultaneously lowering the omega-6 to omega-3

ratio, soybean oil can be replaced by other oils (coconut, olive, and fish oils). Several ILEs are now available globally, although approval for use in the pediatric population varies by country and indication (Table 6.1). Worldwide, many NICUs have transitioned from SO ILE to other ILE products. In 1984, a second-generation ILE, a 50:50 blend of soybean oil and medium-chain triglycerides (MCTs) (Lipofundin, B-Braun, Melsungen, Germany), was introduced. MCTs are derived from coconut oil. In contrast to LCTs, which are packaged into chylomicrons, MCTs are directly absorbed from the intestine into the portal circulation and transported to the liver for oxidation. MCT-based ILEs have some potential advantages when compared to LCT-based ILEs. In contrast to LCTs, MCTs are hydrolyzed more quickly and do not generate proinflammatory eicosanoids. Hence they are considered to be "immune neutral."

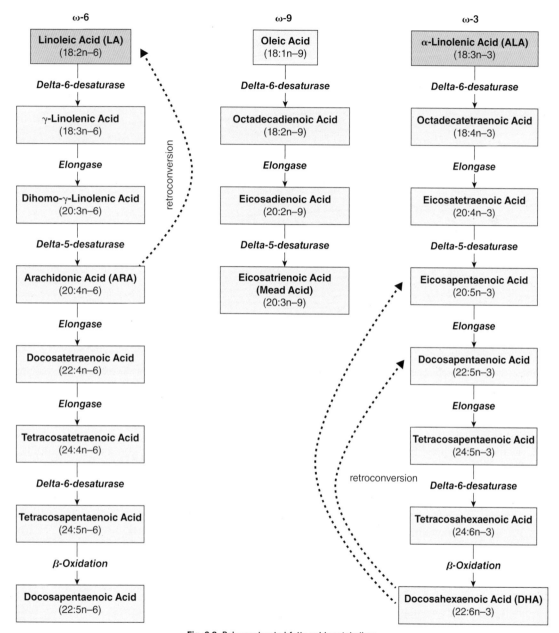

Fig. 6.2 Polyunsaturated fatty acid metabolism.

In the 1990s, a third-generation ILE blend of 80% olive oil with 20% soybean oil (ClinOleic, Baxter, Deerfield, IL) became available. Olive oil is enriched with the omega-9 monounsaturated fatty acid oleic acid, which, like MCTs, is considered to be "immune neutral." Monounsaturated fatty acids are less prone to lipid peroxidation than PUFAs. Free radicals attack double bonds, generating malondialdehyde and 4-hydroxy-2-nonenal, which are carcinogenic, mutagenic, and toxic. Furthermore, olive oil is a source of

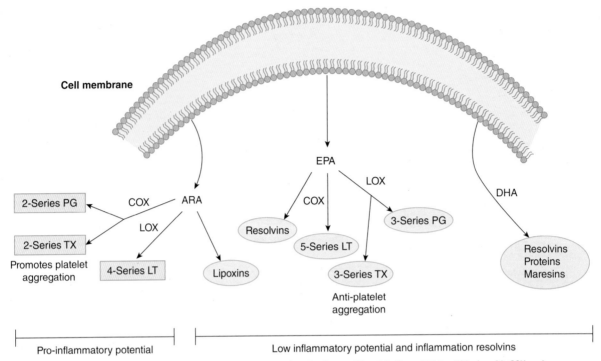

Fig. 6.3 Arachidonic acid, eicosapentaenoic acid, and docosahexaenoic acid eicosanoid metabolism. *ARA*, Arachidonic acid; *COX*, cyclooxygenase; *DHA*, docosahexaenoic acid; *EPA*, eicosapentaenoic acid; *LOX*, lipoxygenase; *LT*, leukotrienes; *PG*, prostaglandins; *TX*, thromboxanes.

α-tocopherol, a fat-soluble antioxidant that protects against lipid peroxidation.

Lastly, in the early 2000s, fish oil–containing ILEs were marketed. Fish oil supplies the antiinflammatory omega-3 fatty acids eicosapentaenoic acid (EPA) and docosahexaenoic acid (DHA). Fish oil also contains a negligible amount of phytosterols since it is not plant based. A 100% fish oil monotherapy (FO ILE, Omegaven, Fresenius Kabi, Bad Homburg, Germany) was US Food and Drug Administration (FDA) approved for use in the United States in 2018 to manage pediatric PNAC. In addition, a composite ILE (SMOF, Fresenius Kabi, Bad Homburg, Germany) combines 30% soybean oil with 30% coconut oil, 25% olive oil, and 15% fish oil (SO,MCT,OO,FO ILE). This composite ILE provides a more balanced omega-6 to omega-3 ratio (2.5:1) and is a source of DHA, EPA, and MCTs. Because fish oil–based ILEs contain PUFAs, they are supplemented with α-tocopherol.

FATTY ACIDS AND CHOLESTASIS

ILEs contain artificial chylomicrons consisting of a triglyceride core with a surrounding phospholipid bilayer. Triglycerides are tri-esters composed of a glycerol backbone with three fatty acids. Phospholipids, the ILE's emulsifier, contain a hydrophilic head with a phosphate group and a hydrophobic tail consisting of two fatty acids. Fatty acids are carbon-hydrogen chains with carboxylic acid and methyl ends. Fatty acids are classified by their carbon chain length (short [≤5 carbons], medium [6–12 carbons], long [13–21 carbons], and very long [>21 carbons]), the presence (unsaturated) or absence of a double bond (saturated), the number of double bonds (mono- or poly-), and double bond location. Omega-3, omega-6, or omega-9 indicates the location of the first double bond from the methyl end of the carbon chain (Fig. 6.4).

Fatty acids serve several critical functions in addition to providing and storing energy. Fatty acids affect cell membrane structure, fluidity, permeability, and cell-signaling pathways. LA and ALA are considered to be essential fatty acids because they cannot be synthesized de novo since mammals lack the enzymes (delta 12 and 15 desaturases) that are responsible for inserting a *cis* double bond past the ninth carbon.

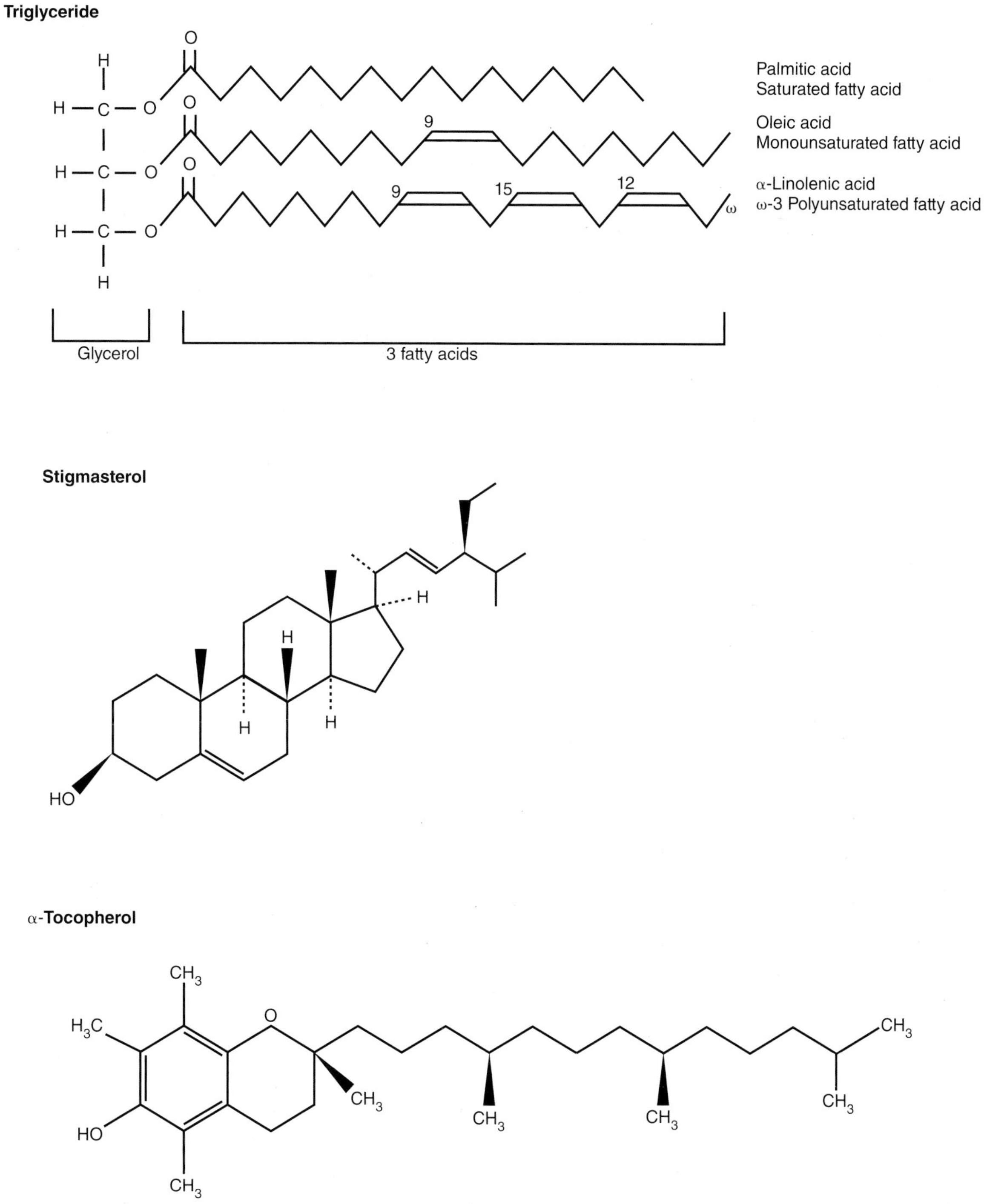

Triglyceride

Palmitic acid
Saturated fatty acid

Oleic acid
Monounsaturated fatty acid

α-Linolenic acid
ω-3 Polyunsaturated fatty acid

Glycerol

3 fatty acids

Stigmasterol

α-Tocopherol

Fig. 6.4 Fatty acids, phytosterols, and vitamin E.

Experiments by George Burr in the 1920s and 1930s demonstrated that rats fed a fat-free diet grew poorly, developed dry, scaly skin, were infertile, and eventually died. It is now well known that LA is a vital component of ceramides, which help maintain the epidermal barrier function and prevent transdermal water loss. When the rat's fat-free diet was supplemented with the LA-rich linseed, corn, and poppy seed oils, clinical manifestations associated with an essential fatty acid deficiency (EFAD) were prevented and reversed. While an ALA-supplemented fat-free diet in rats minimized EFAD symptomology, it was not as effective as an LA-supplemented fat-free diet.[21]

In the 1950s and 1960s, a series of experiments confirmed that LA was converted to arachidonic acid (ARA) and ALA was converted to EPA and DHA (Fig. 6.2). These experiments also demonstrated that ARA was more effective at curing an EFAD.[21] While the downstream fatty acids ARA, EPA, and DHA can be synthesized de novo from their upstream parent essential fatty acids, their "essentiality" was also confirmed. ARA, EPA, and DHA generate eicosanoids, important for cell signaling and various cellular functions, such as platelet aggregation, chemotaxis, and growth. The eicosanoid family includes leukotrienes, prostaglandins, thromboxanes, prostacyclins, lipoxins, and hydroperoxy fatty acids (Fig. 6.3). ARA-derived eicosanoids are potent inducers of inflammation, vasoconstriction, and coagulation. An excess of ARA-derived eicosanoids is associated with various disease states, including PNAC and IFALD.[20,22,23] In contrast, EPA-derived eicosanoids are less potent inducers of inflammation, vasoconstriction, and coagulation. ARA, EPA, and DHA give rise to specialized proresolving mediators; ARA gives rise to lipoxins, and DHA and EPA give rise to resolvins, protectins, and maresins. These mediators "turn off" inflammation. Increased provisions of DHA and EPA via FO ILE have been associated with the resolution of IFALD.[20,22,23]

While DHA and EPA may play a role in the cholestasis in PN-dependent neonates, ARA and DHA play a critical role in fetal and infant retinal and brain development, which may be equally if not more important. The placenta preferentially transfers DHA and ARA to the fetus.[24] In the third trimester of pregnancy, fetal accretion rates are 142 to 212 mg/kg/d and 43 mg/kg/d for ARA and DHA, respectively.[24] This process is known as *biomagnification*. Postnatally, breast milk and standard preterm and term formulas provide ARA and DHA. However, because very preterm infants are born prior to the transplacental biomagnification of ARA and DHA, lack sufficient adipose stores, and inefficiently convert LA and ALA into downstream metabolites, they quickly develop ARA and DHA deficiencies shortly after birth.[25] These deficiencies are further exacerbated by SO ILE that lacks exogenous ARA and DHA. Specific preterm comorbidities, including IFALD, retinopathy of prematurity, sepsis, chronic lung disease, and neurocognitive impairments, have been linked to poor ARA and DHA status.[7,26]

An EFAD has traditionally been defined by varying thresholds of the triene to tetraene ratio (Mead acid:ARA). When LA and ALA concentrations are low, the omega-9 fatty acid oleic acid is converted to Mead acid. Traditionally, a triene to tetraene ratio >0.2 was considered diagnostic of an EFAD. However, lower thresholds have been employed for infants.[27] Biochemical EFADs precede symptoms associated with an EFAD. These symptoms include poor growth; dry, scaly skin; thrombocytopenia; hepatitis; hypertriglyceridemia; and an increased risk for infections, bleeding, and poor wound healing. It is important to remember that an EFAD can develop within a few days in preterm and critically ill neonates if ILEs are withheld. To treat an EFAD in PN-dependent neonates, two potential approaches have been described. One approach is to increase the provision of the essential fatty acids LA and ALA by providing SO ILE or increasing the SO ILE dose.[28] The second approach is to provide the downstream fatty acids ARA, EPA, and DHA. This can be accomplished by providing FO ILE.[29]

When FO ILE was first introduced, many theorized that infants with IFALD who were treated with an ILE containing only fish oil would develop an EFAD. However, triene to tetraene ratios measured in infants receiving FO ILE did not identify an EFAD.[4,30] There are case reports of infants with IFALD whose EFAD and IFALD were reversed by FO ILE.[29] FO ILE is not associated with an EFAD because FO ILE's provision of EPA, DHA, and ARA is sufficient to generate the downstream bioactive lipid-signaling molecules that are necessary for cellular health. Moreover, ARA can be retroconverted into LA and DHA can be retroconverted into upstream PUFAs (Fig. 6.2).

PHYTOSTEROLS AND CHOLESTASIS

Phytosterols, which are cholesterol analogs, collectively include plant-derived sterols and stanols. Phytosterols have a fused polycyclic structure and are differentiated from one another by their carbon side chain and the presence of a double bond. Sterols lack a double bond while stanols do not. Sterols exist in three main forms (β-sitosterol, campesterol, and stigmasterol) and stanols exist in two forms (sitostanol and campestanol) (Fig. 6.4). Circulating phytosterol concentrations are 100 times lower than cholesterol concentrations. Less than 5% and <0.5% of sterols and stanols, respectively, enter the systemic circulation. When phytosterols are absorbed into the enterocyte, the *ABCG5/8* efflux transporter readily excretes the sterol back into the intestinal lumen. The small amount of phytosterols that are incorporated into chylomicrons travel to the liver and are readily excreted by the *ABCG5/8* efflux transporter into the biliary system for elimination in the stool (Fig. 6.1).

When high concentrations of phytosterols are infused intravenously, the *ABCG5/8* transporter, which protects against phytosterolemia, is bypassed. As a result, circulating phytosterol concentrations can rapidly increase in preterm infants and infants with IFALD who are receiving SO ILE.[31,32] In healthy newborns, phytosterol concentrations are usually <100 μmol, but in PN-fed infants, concentrations exceed 1000 μmol.[32,33] Studies have demonstrated a positive correlation between phytosterol and CB concentrations and inflammatory and fibrotic changes on liver biopsy in PN-dependent infants and children.[7,33,34] Compared to infants and young children with IFALD who receive SO ILE, those who receive FO ILE for IFALD treatment have substantially lower phytosterol concentrations, and an early decrease in stigmasterol is correlated with a later decrease in CB.[7]

Phytosterols contribute to IFALD in specific ways. Stigmasterol inhibits FXR, LXR, and CYP7A1. As a result, bilirubin, bile acids, and phytosterols accumulate in the liver, causing cholestasis and fibrosis. When mice were infused with SO ILE or FO ILE supplemented with stigmasterol, FXR- and LXR-dependent genes (BSEP, MRP2, *ABCG5/8*) were downregulated, and hepatic macrophages and Kupffer cells were activated by an increase in interleukin-6. As a result, these mice developed cholestasis and hepatitis, indicated by a rise in serum liver function tests, bile acids, and total serum bilirubin. In contrast, mice infused with FO ILE did not demonstrate any evidence of liver disease.[8,9] Other studies have highlighted the importance of FGF19. In PN-fed piglets, biliary stasis decreased FGF19, which inhibits CYP7A1. As a result, hepatic bile acid production was increased, causing liver injury.[35]

In other *in vitro* and *in vivo* experiments, the combination of PN and intestinal injury or a lipopolysaccharide infusion induces liver injury via the suppression of FXR and LXR. Animals that received PN alone or were subjected to intestinal injury without PN were free of liver disease.[36] This suggests that increased intestinal permeability facilitates bacterial translocation and that cytokine release from Kupffer cells acts synergistically with phytosterols to disrupt bile acid, bilirubin, and cholesterol homeostasis, causing IFALD.[8,9,36]

VITAMIN E AND CHOLESTASIS

Vitamin E protects PUFAs against lipid peroxidation. Naturally occurring vitamin E is a fat-soluble antioxidant that exists as four different tocopherols (α, β, γ, and δ) and four different tocotrienols (α, β, γ, and δ), each with different levels of biological activity (Fig. 6.4). Gamma-tocopherol sources include oils rich in PUFAs, like SO ILE. On the other hand, olive oil and coconut oil contain α-tocopherol, the most abundant form of vitamin E in the human body. In the liver, α-tocopherol is bound to the α-tocopherol transfer protein and then incorporated into lipoproteins to be delivered to various tissues and organs. In cell membranes, α-tocopherol neutralizes free radicals, preventing lipid peroxidation and cellular damage. Gamma-tocopherol is quite effective at scavenging peroxyl radicals and reactive nitrogen species. However, α-tocopherol is preferentially retained in the liver, while γ-tocopherol is readily excreted by the kidneys. In addition, when attached to lipoproteins, α-tocopherol protects these particles from oxidation.

SO ILE contains γ-tocopherol and is not supplemented with α-tocopherol. In contrast, MCT-based and olive oil–based ILEs contain α-tocopherol, and SO,MCT,OO,FO ILE and FO ILE are supplemented with α-tocopherol because of their high PUFA content. It is important to note that the tocopherols present in ILEs are included for product stability and are not specifically intended to impact clinical outcomes. In a piglet study, adding α-tocopherol to PN/SO ILE-fed piglets prevented cholestasis and preserved bile flow. In contrast, piglets fed PN/SO ILE, PN/FO ILE, or PN/FO ILE-supplemented phytosterols developed cholestasis.[8] It remains unclear which ILE constituent is the primary driver of IFALD. However, when the evidence is taken as a whole, it appears that a high concentration of phytosterols, LCTs, LA-derived eicosanoids, and PUFAs without sufficient α-tocopherol protection are responsible for ILE-induced liver injury.

Clinical Studies: IV Lipid Emulsions and Cholestasis

Efforts to evaluate associations between ILE dose and composition and cholestasis risk in infants differ on key aspects. The populations studied are not always comparable. As a result, their underlying risk for cholestasis and IF varies. Some studies exclusively include preterm infants who may or may not develop acquired bowel pathology such as NEC. Other studies exclusively include infants with acquired or congenital gastrointestinal disorders. Regardless of the underlying etiology of the intestinal disorder, infants with intestinal disease are at high risk for SBS, IF, and IFALD. In contrast, most preterm infants generally wean from PN and transition to full enteral nutrition without complications within the first couple of weeks of life. Moreover, the quality of evidence to address these questions is variable and includes retrospective analyses, cohort studies, and clinical trials conducted at single and multiple sites. Another prohibitive element to comparing results between clinical investigations is the variable definition of cholestasis. While some trials utilize cutoff values of 1 mg/dL, 2 mg/dL, or 3 mg/dL, others use CB to total serum bilirubin ratios to define cholestasis.

Further complicating matters, one must also recognize that altering either the composition or the dose of an ILE will influence an infant's exposure to the various ILE constituents. A reduction in soybean oil will cause a coinciding reduction in phytosterol content as well as provisions of specific PUFAs and vitamin E isomers. If a particular ILE dose or product reduces the risk of cholestasis, it should be acknowledged that randomization will not elucidate whether any specific

ILE constituent is implicated in this risk reduction, but rather that the entirety of the ILE is implicated.

ILE DOSE REDUCTION AND CHOLESTASIS PREVENTION

Evaluations of ILE dose reduction rely upon case-control studies as well as randomized clinical trials. In studies comparing surgical infants who received 1 g/kg/d of SO ILE to historical controls treated with the standard dose of SO ILE (~2–3 g/kg/d), the group that received 1 g/kg/d had a lower incidence of cholestasis.[37] When considering safety, SO ILE dose reductions lower than 1 g/kg/d are associated with an EFAD and decreased energy provision.[28,37] Even when cholestasis is not avoided, lower doses appear to mitigate higher CB concentrations.[28,37,38]

ILE dose and cholestasis risk have been evaluated in nonsurgical and surgical infant populations through clinical trials. In infants born ≤29 weeks without a primary gastrointestinal surgical diagnosis, a maximum dose of 1 g/kg/d versus 3 g/kg/d of SO ILE led to no difference in cholestasis rates, CB changes over time, and growth between groups.[39] Two trials in neonates with intestinal surgical diseases randomized infants to a maximum dose of 1 g/kg/d or 3 g/kg/d of SO ILE. In both studies, dose did not influence cholestasis rates. However, in contrast to the study in preterm infants, infants with gastrointestinal disorders receiving the lower dose of SO ILE had a slower rise in CB over time.[18,19,39] It should be noted that only in the study by Calkins et al. was this change over time statistically significant (p = 0.02, Calkins et al. vs. p = 0.1, Rollins et al.).[18,19] In a separate trial of surgical infants randomized to 1 g/kg/d versus 2 g/kg/d of SO ILE, cholestasis rates were similar when the two groups were compared.[40] Consistent with previously mentioned studies, infants randomized to the lower SO ILE dose had a significantly slower CB change (0.16 mg/dL/week vs. 0.19 mg/dL/week, p = 0.0005).[18,19,40] While there is a paucity of data on SO ILE dose reduction and neurodevelopment, studies have not identified any adverse effects on neurodevelopment.[41–43]

Additional clinical trials have attempted to investigate whether a slight decrease in ILE dose may be of benefit. Incorporating comparisons of both ILE dose (2.5 g/kg/d vs. 3.5 g/kg/d) and composition (SO,MCT,OO,FO ILE vs. SO ILE), ILE dose was not associated with cholestasis in infants born <1250 g.[44]

It should be noted that doses <2.2–2.5 g/kg/d of SO,MCT,OO,FO ILE are associated with the development of an EFAD in very preterm infants.[45] When doses of 2.8 g/kg/d versus 3.8 g/kg/d of SO ILE were compared, cholestasis rates were also similar in infants born <29 weeks.[46] However, that clinical trial also randomized subjects to different doses of amino acids and carbohydrates.[47] Hence independent effects of the ILE cannot be discerned.

ILE COMPOSITION AND CHOLESTASIS PREVENTION

To evaluate the effect of ILE composition on cholestasis prevention, surgical neonates were randomized to either SO ILE (n = 10) or FO ILE (n = 9), both dosed at 1 g/kg/d.[43] CB concentrations, liver function tests, and cholestasis rates were similar between groups at an interim analysis, which coincided with the early termination of the study. The study was terminated early due to the unexpected low rate of cholestasis. Randomized trials have evaluated the effects of altering ILE composition in nonsurgical preterm infants where cholestasis is often a secondary outcome. These studies have compared SO,MCT,OO,FO ILE, 100% SO ILE, and other composite ILEs without fish oil.[44,48–51] In these trials, cholestasis rates are comparable between groups.[44,48–51]

Effects of SO,MCT,OO,FO ILE or other combinations of ILEs have been evaluated in clinical trials in nonsurgical, preterm infants. In a randomized controlled study of 223 extremely preterm infants by Repa et al., infants received SO,MCT,OO,FO ILE or SO ILE at equivalent doses. Rates of cholestasis (defined as a CB >1.5 mg/dL) were similar between groups (11% SO,MCT,OO,FO ILE vs. 18% SO ILE).[50] In another randomized controlled trial of very-low-birth-weight infants, there was no difference in cholestasis rates when infants who received SO,MCT,OO,FO ILE were compared to infants who received SO ILE (4% in both groups).[52] Considering the short duration of PN (PN duration 11–24 days), low rates of cholestasis would be expected. As a result, these studies were not adequately powered to detect a difference in that primary outcome, cholestasis. It is also unclear whether these results would be different if the studies included infants who later developed IF.

Meta-analyses have failed to demonstrate that SO,MCT,OO,FO ILE alters cholestasis risk.[53–55] A Cochrane Database systematic review showed no benefit of any specific ILE composition, either with or without fish oil, for cholestasis prevention in preterm infants, inclusive of infants with and without surgical diagnoses.[54,55] This review accounted for variable definitions of cholestasis. The review included trials with any definition of cholestasis and then separately analyzed trials that defined cholestasis as a CB ≥2 mg/dL. Findings of no difference based on ILE composition were consistent throughout the analyses. The database separately analyzed outcomes for infants born late preterm and term with similar negative findings. In contrast to the analyses of preterm infants, the studies available for analysis of infants born late preterm or term only included infants with gastrointestinal surgical diseases.[54,55]

IV LIPID EMULSIONS AND CHOLESTASIS TREATMENT

When implementing a change in ILE in response to cholestasis development, it is vital to recognize the expected time course of change in biochemical markers. In children with even modest elevations in CB, serial sampling shows that complete resolution (i.e., levels consistently <2 mg/dL) may take several weeks to months.[4,12,13,15] When an ILE is replaced by FO ILE, CB often increases or plateaus prior to decreasing.[4,13,15]

A series of five infants with SBS were treated with a composite ILE of olive and soybean oils in conjunction with FO ILE, each administered at 1 g/kg/d.[56] The combination ILE was initiated at various times in relation to cholestasis development. In some instances, the combination ILE was initiated prior to cholestasis while in other instances it was initiated after cholestasis. The heterogeneity of those patients and CB trajectories suggests the need for caution in firmly concluding benefit. A larger retrospective evaluation of this same combination therapy in comparison to historical treatment with SO ILE concluded that the combined therapy led to improved outcomes based on decreased overall mortality and mortality due to liver failure.[57] It is noteworthy that the comparison infants who received SO ILE were born during a 20-year span, starting in 1985. Clinical, nutritional, and surgical care of infants with IF and IFALD has changed considerably over that period.

In contrast, multiple studies have demonstrated that FO ILE biochemically reverses pediatric IFALD.[4,6,12–15]

In multicenter analyses, infants with IFALD were pair-matched (2:1) based on postmenstrual age (PMA) and baseline CB. Mortality was not different between infants with IFALD who were managed with FO ILE versus SO ILE.[13,14] However, liver failure was more likely in the SO ILE group. Moreover, the aspartate transaminase to platelet ratio index (APRI), a biomarker for liver fibrosis, decreased with FO ILE and increased with SO ILE. Consistent with these results, rates for cholestasis resolution were significantly higher in infants receiving FO ILE compared to those receiving SO ILE (65% vs. 16%).[14] Lastly, infants treated with FO ILE were less likely to receive a liver-inclusive transplant compared to those treated with SO ILE (4% vs. 12%).[14]

Few clinical trials have addressed randomization of infants with already established cholestasis to differing ILE regimens. In one study, preterm infants with cholestasis were randomized to SO ILE or FO ILE at equivalent doses (1.5 g/kg/d). The trial was discontinued at interim analysis (n = 32) because of a lack of equipoise and increased awareness of the theorized benefit of FO ILE. There was no difference in the primary outcome, resolution of IFALD.[11] However, the FO ILE group had a markedly slower rise in CB than the SO ILE group that was statistically significant (0.6 μmol/L/week vs. 13.5 μmol/L/week). A separate trial compared SO ILE to SO,MCT,OO,FO ILE in infants with established cholestasis.[58] With an intention to treat analysis, infants had similar CB levels at the study end. When the analysis excluded an infant in the SO ILE group who was deemed an outlier based on a high CB concentration, infants randomized to SO,MCT,OO,FO ILE had significantly lower CB concentrations. In this study, the ILE dose was reduced per protocol as enteral feedings advanced, and the mean dose administered during the trial was generally >2 g/kg/d for all infants.[58]

Safety concerns are paramount when intervening in a neonatal population with altered hepatic function and other comorbidities. During early utilization of FO ILE in infants, concerns of perioperative bleeding were reported. This was attributed to ARA-induced impaired platelet function (Fig. 6.3). In a piglet model, decreased ARA production of thromboxane A2 and increased platelet reaction time were noted with FO ILE.[59] In contrast, in a larger study of infants with advanced IFALD, FO ILE was associated with a decreased incidence of bleeding compared to SO ILE. In a regression analysis, a higher baseline CB and SO ILE treatment were associated with bleeding.[5] While FO ILE may theoretically increase an infant's risk for bleeding, FO ILE treats IFALD, which is a significant risk factor for bleeding. Clinicians should always be cautious when the cell membrane PUFA composition is altered in critically ill infants at risk of hematologic abnormalities and clinical bleeding.

Summary

ILEs are a critical part of nutrition in the NICU. Considering the variety of ILEs available, clinicians should have an understanding of the various oil sources and roles that fatty acids, phytosterols, and vitamin E play in neonatal liver health. Clinicians must balance each ILE's nutritional value with its potential contribution to IFALD. When deliberating an ILE's risks and benefits, both true and theoretical, clinicians should consider the infant's gestational age and inherent risk for IF and IFALD. Such considerations will vary based on the population (i.e., nonsurgical preterm infants vs. infants at risk for or with IF) and presence of established liver injury. Despite advancements in ILE development, what constitutes the optimal ILE has yet to be defined for infants in the NICU. Clinical and research collaboration is needed to advance the field of neonatal nutrition to ensure that preterm infants and infants with IF receive optimal PN while minimizing the adverse effects resulting from exposure to long-term PN and ILE use.

REFERENCES

1. Dick MC, Mowat AP. Hepatitis syndrome in infancy—an epidemiological survey with 10 year follow up. *Arch Dis Child.* 1985;60(6):512–516. doi:10.1136/adc.60.6.512.
2. Feldman AG, Sokol RJ. Neonatal cholestasis: emerging molecular diagnostics and potential novel therapeutics. *Nat Rev Gastroenterol Hepatol.* 2019;16(6):346–360. doi:10.1038/s41575-019-0132-z.
3. Fawaz R, Baumann U, Ekong U, et al. Guideline for the evaluation of cholestatic jaundice in infants: joint recommendations of the North American Society for Pediatric Gastroenterology, Hepatology, and Nutrition and the European Society for Pediatric Gastroenterology, Hepatology, and Nutrition. *J Pediatr Gastroenterol Nutr.* 2017;64(1):154–168. doi:10.1097/MPG.0000000000001334.
4. Gura KM, Lee S, Valim C, et al. Safety and efficacy of a fish-oil-based fat emulsion in the treatment of parenteral nutrition-associated liver disease. *Pediatrics.* 2008;121(3):e678–e686. doi:10.1542/peds.2007-2248.

5. Gura KM, Calkins KL, Premkumar MH, Puder M. Use of intravenous soybean and fish oil emulsions in pediatric intestinal failure-associated liver disease: a multicenter integrated analysis report on extrahepatic adverse events. *J Pediatr.* 2022;241: 173–180.e1. doi:10.1016/j.jpeds.2021.10.030.

6. Calkins KL, Dunn JC, Shew SB, et al. Pediatric intestinal failure-associated liver disease is reversed with 6 months of intravenous fish oil. *JPEN J Parenter Enteral Nutr.* 2014; 38(6):682–692. doi:10.1177/0148607113495416.

7. Calkins KL, DeBarber A, Steiner RD, et al. Intravenous fish oil and pediatric intestinal failure-associated liver disease: changes in plasma phytosterols, cytokines, and bile acids and erythrocyte fatty acids. *JPEN J Parenter Enteral Nutr.* 2018;42(3): 633–641. doi:10.1177/0148607117709196.

8. El Kasmi KC, Anderson AL, Devereaux MW, et al. Toll-like receptor 4-dependent Kupffer cell activation and liver injury in a novel mouse model of parenteral nutrition and intestinal injury. *Hepatology.* 2012;55(5):1518–1528. doi:10.1002/hep.25500.

9. El Kasmi KC, Anderson AL, Devereaux MW, et al. Phytosterols promote liver injury and Kupffer cell activation in parenteral nutrition-associated liver disease. *Sci Transl Med.* 2013; 5(206):206ra137. doi:10.1126/scitranslmed.3006898.

10. Ng K, Stoll B, Chacko S, et al. Vitamin E in new-generation lipid emulsions protects against parenteral nutrition-associated liver disease in parenteral nutrition-fed preterm pigs. *JPEN J Parenter Enteral Nutr.* 2016;40(5):656–671. doi:10.1177/0148607114567900.

11. Lam HS, Tam YH, Poon TC, et al. A double-blind randomised controlled trial of fish oil-based versus soy-based lipid preparations in the treatment of infants with parenteral nutrition-associated cholestasis. *Neonatology.* 2014;105(4):290–296. doi:10.1159/000358267.

12. Premkumar MH, Carter BA, Hawthorne KM, King K, Abrams SA. High rates of resolution of cholestasis in parenteral nutrition-associated liver disease with fish oil-based lipid emulsion monotherapy. *J Pediatr.* 2013;162(4):793–798.e1. doi:10.1016/j.jpeds.2012.10.019.

13. Gura K, Premkumar MH, Calkins KL, Puder M. Intravenous fish oil monotherapy as a source of calories and fatty acids promotes age-appropriate growth in pediatric patients with intestinal failure-associated liver disease. *J Pediatr.* 2020;219: 98–105.e4. doi:10.1016/j.jpeds.2019.12.065.

14. Gura KM, Premkumar MH, Calkins KL, Puder M. Fish oil emulsion reduces liver injury and liver transplantation in children with intestinal failure-associated liver disease: a multicenter integrated study. *J Pediatr.* 2021;230:46–54.e2. doi:10.1016/j.jpeds.2020.09.068.

15. Wang C, Venick RS, Shew SB, et al. Long-term outcomes in children with intestinal failure-associated liver disease treated with 6 months of intravenous fish oil followed by resumption of intravenous soybean oil. *JPEN J Parenter Enteral Nutr.* 2019;43(6):708–716. doi:10.1002/jpen.1463.

16. Lauriti G, Zani A, Aufieri R, et al. Incidence, prevention, and treatment of parenteral nutrition-associated cholestasis and intestinal failure-associated liver disease in infants and children: a systematic review. *JPEN J Parenter Enteral Nutr.* 2014;38(1): 70–85. doi:10.1177/0148607113496280.

17. Modi BP, Galloway DP, Gura K, et al. ASPEN definitions in pediatric intestinal failure. *JPEN J Parenter Enteral Nutr.* 2022;46(1):42–59. doi:10.1002/jpen.2232.

18. Calkins KL, Havranek T, Kelley-Quon LI, et al. Low-dose parenteral soybean oil for the prevention of parenteral nutrition-associated liver disease in neonates with gastrointestinal disorders. *JPEN J Parenter Enteral Nutr.* 2017;41(3): 404–411. doi:10.1177/0148607115588334.

19. Rollins MD, Ward RM, Jackson WD, et al. Effect of decreased parenteral soybean lipid emulsion on hepatic function in infants at risk for parenteral nutrition-associated liver disease: a pilot study. *J Pediatr Surg.* 2013;48(6):1348–1356. doi:10.1016/j.jpedsurg.2013.03.040.

20. Fell GL, Cho BS, Dao DT, et al. Fish oil protects the liver from parenteral nutrition-induced injury via GPR120-mediated PPARγ signaling. *Prostaglandins Leukot Essent Fatty Acids.* 2019;143:8–14. doi:10.1016/j.plefa.2019.02.003.

21. Spector AA, Kim HY. Discovery of essential fatty acids. *J Lipid Res.* 2015;56(1):11–21. doi:10.1194/jlr.R055095.

22. Kalish BT, Le HD, Gura KM, Bistrian BR, Puder M. A metabolomic analysis of two intravenous lipid emulsions in a murine model. *PLoS One.* 2013;8(4):e59653. doi:10.1371/journal.pone.0059653.

23. Kalish BT, Le HD, Fitzgerald JM, et al. Intravenous fish oil lipid emulsion promotes a shift toward anti-inflammatory proresolving lipid mediators. *Am J Physiol Gastrointest Liver Physiol.* 2013;305(11):G818–G828. doi:10.1152/ajpgi.00106.2013.

24. Clandinin MT, Chappell JE, Leong S, Heim T, Swyer PR, Chance GW. Extrauterine fatty acid accretion in infant brain: implications for fatty acid requirements. *Early Hum Dev.* 1980;4(2):131–138. doi:10.1016/0378-3782(80)90016-x.

25. Robinson DT, Carlson SE, Murthy K, Frost B, Li S, Caplan M. Docosahexaenoic and arachidonic acid levels in extremely low birth weight infants with prolonged exposure to intravenous lipids. *J Pediatr.* 2013;162(1):56–61. doi:10.1016/j.jpeds.2012.06.045.

26. Martin CR, Dasilva DA, Cluette-Brown JE, et al. Decreased postnatal docosahexaenoic and arachidonic acid blood levels in premature infants are associated with neonatal morbidities. *J Pediatr.* 2011;159(5):743–749.e1–2. doi:10.1016/j.jpeds.2011.04.039.

27. Lagerstedt SA, Hinrichs DR, Batt SM, Magera MJ, Rinaldo P, McConnell JP. Quantitative determination of plasma c8-c26 total fatty acids for the biochemical diagnosis of nutritional and metabolic disorders. *Mol Genet Metab.* 2001;73(1):38–45. doi:10.1006/mgme.2001.3170.

28. Cober MP, Killu G, Brattain A, Welch KB, Kunisaki SM, Teitelbaum DH. Intravenous fat emulsions reduction for patients with parenteral nutrition-associated liver disease. *J Pediatr.* 2012;160(3):421–427. doi:10.1016/j.jpeds.2011.08.047.

29. Gura KM, Parsons SK, Bechard LJ, Kneuertz PJ, Presley CJ, Bridges JFP. Use of a fish oil-based lipid emulsion to treat essential fatty acid deficiency in a soy allergic patient receiving parenteral nutrition. *Clin Nutr.* 2005;24(5):839–847. doi:10.1016/j.clnu.2005.05.020.

30. Ong ML, Venick RS, Shew SB, et al. Intravenous fish oil and serum fatty acid profiles in pediatric patients with intestinal failure-associated liver disease. *JPEN J Parenter Enteral Nutr.* 2019;43(6):717–725. doi:10.1002/jpen.1532.

31. Correani A, Pignotti A, Marinelli L, et al. Plasma phytosterol half-life and levels are increased in very low birth weight preterm infants with parenteral nutrition-associated cholestasis. *Lipids.* 2018;53(7):717–725. doi:10.1002/lipd.12072.

32. Nghiem-Rao TH, Tunc I, Mavis AM, et al. Kinetics of phytosterol metabolism in neonates receiving parenteral nutrition. *Pediatr Res.* 2015;78(2):181–189. doi:10.1038/pr.2015.78.

33. Kurvinen A, Nissinen MJ, Gylling H, et al. Effects of long-term parenteral nutrition on serum lipids, plant sterols, cholesterol

metabolism, and liver histology in pediatric intestinal failure. *J Pediatr Gastroenterol Nutr.* 2011;53(4):440–446. doi:10.1097/MPG.0b013e3182212130.

34. Mutanen A, Nissinen MJ, Lohi J, Heikkilä P, Gylling H, Pakarinen MP. Serum plant sterols, cholestanol, and cholesterol precursors associate with histological liver injury in pediatric onset intestinal failure. *Am J Clin Nutr.* 2014;100(4):1085–1094. doi:10.3945/ajcn.114.088781.

35. Jain AK, Stoll B, Burrin DG, Holst JJ, Moore DD. Enteral bile acid treatment improves parenteral nutrition-related liver disease and intestinal mucosal atrophy in neonatal pigs. *Am J Physiol Gastrointest Liver Physiol.* 2012;302(2):G218–G224. doi:10.1152/ajpgi.00280.2011.

36. Guthrie G, Tackett B, Stoll B, Martin C, Olutoye O, Burrin DG. Phytosterols synergize with endotoxin to augment inflammation in Kupffer cells but alone have limited direct effect on hepatocytes. *JPEN J Parenter Enteral Nutr.* 2018;42(1):37–48. doi:10.1177/0148607117722752.

37. Sanchez SE, Braun LP, Mercer LD, Sherrill M, Stevens J, Javid PJ. The effect of lipid restriction on the prevention of parenteral nutrition-associated cholestasis in surgical infants. *J Pediatr Surg.* 2013;48(3):573–578. doi:10.1016/j.jpedsurg.2012.08.016.

38. Nehra D, Fallon EM, Carlson SJ, et al. Provision of a soy-based intravenous lipid emulsion at 1 g/kg/d does not prevent cholestasis in neonates. *JPEN J Parenter Enteral Nutr.* 2013;37(4):498–505. doi:10.1177/0148607112453072.

39. Levit OL, Calkins KL, Gibson LC, et al. Low-dose intravenous soybean oil emulsion for prevention of cholestasis in preterm neonates. *JPEN J Parenter Enteral Nutr.* 2016;40(3):374–382. doi:10.1177/0148607114540005.

40. Gupta K, Wang H, Amin SB. Soybean-oil lipid minimization for prevention of intestinal failure-associated liver disease in late-preterm and term infants with gastrointestinal surgical disorders. *JPEN J Parenter Enteral Nutr.* 2021;45(6):1239–1248. doi:10.1002/jpen.2004.

41. Blackmer AB, Warschausky S, Siddiqui S, et al. Preliminary findings of long-term neurodevelopmental outcomes of infants treated with intravenous fat emulsion reduction for the management of parenteral nutrition-associated cholestasis. *JPEN J Parenter Enteral Nutr.* 2015;39(1):34–46. doi:10.1177/0148607114551965.

42. Ong ML, Purdy IB, Levit OL, et al. Two-year neurodevelopment and growth outcomes for preterm neonates who received low-dose intravenous soybean oil. *JPEN J Parenter Enteral Nutr.* 2018;42(2):352–360. doi:10.1177/0148607116674482.

43. Nehra D, Fallon EM, Potemkin AK, et al. A comparison of 2 intravenous lipid emulsions: interim analysis of a randomized controlled trial. *JPEN J Parenter Enteral Nutr.* 2014;38(6):693–701. doi:10.1177/0148607113492549.

44. D'Ascenzo R, Savini S, Biagetti C, et al. Higher docosahexaenoic acid, lower arachidonic acid and reduced lipid tolerance with high doses of a lipid emulsion containing 15% fish oil: a randomized clinical trial. *Clin Nutr.* 2014;33(6):1002–1009. doi:10.1016/j.clnu.2014.01.009.

45. Gramlich L, Ireton-Jones C, Miles JM, Morrison M, Pontes-Arruda A. Essential fatty acid requirements and intravenous lipid emulsions. *JPEN J Parenter Enteral Nutr.* 2019;43(6):697–707. doi:10.1002/jpen.1537.

46. Morgan C, McGowan P, Herwitker S, Hart AE, Turner MA. Postnatal head growth in preterm infants: a randomized controlled parenteral nutrition study. *Pediatrics.* 2014;133(1):e120–e128. doi:10.1542/peds.2013-2207.

47. Morgan C, Herwitker S, Badhawi I, et al. SCAMP: standardised, concentrated, additional macronutrients, parenteral nutrition in very preterm infants: a phase IV randomised, controlled exploratory study of macronutrient intake, growth and other aspects of neonatal care. *BMC Pediatr.* 2011;11:53. doi:10.1186/1471-2431-11-53.

48. Göbel Y, Koletzko B, Böhles HJ, et al. Parenteral fat emulsions based on olive and soybean oils: a randomized clinical trial in preterm infants. *J Pediatr Gastroenterol Nutr.* 2003;37(2):161–167. doi:10.1097/00005176-200308000-00015.

49. Savini S, D'Ascenzo R, Biagetti C, et al. The effect of 5 intravenous lipid emulsions on plasma phytosterols in preterm infants receiving parenteral nutrition: a randomized clinical trial. *Am J Clin Nutr.* 2013;98(2):312–318. doi:10.3945/ajcn.112.056556.

50. Repa A, Binder C, Thanhaeuser M, et al. A mixed lipid emulsion for prevention of parenteral nutrition associated cholestasis in extremely low birth weight infants: a randomized clinical trial. *J Pediatr.* 2018;194:87–93.e1. doi:10.1016/j.jpeds.2017.11.012.

51. Wang Y, Zhou KJ, Tang QY, et al. Effect of an olive oil-based lipid emulsion compared with a soybean oil-based lipid emulsion on liver chemistry and bile acid composition in preterm infants receiving parenteral nutrition: a double-blind, randomized trial. *JPEN J Parenter Enteral Nutr.* 2016;40(6):842–850. doi:10.1177/0148607114566853.

52. Vlaardingerbroek H, Vermeulen MJ, Carnielli VP, Vaz FM, van den Akker CH, van Goudoever JB. Growth and fatty acid profiles of VLBW infants receiving a multicomponent lipid emulsion from birth. *J Pediatr Gastroenterol Nutr.* 2014;58(4):417–427. doi:10.1097/MPG.0000000000000280.

53. Park HW, Lee NM, Kim JH, Kim KS, Kim SN. Parenteral fish oil-containing lipid emulsions may reverse parenteral nutrition-associated cholestasis in neonates: a systematic review and meta-analysis. *J Nutr.* 2015;145(2):277–283. doi:10.3945/jn.114.204974.

54. Kapoor V, Malviya MN, Soll R. Lipid emulsions for parenterally fed preterm infants. *Cochrane Database Syst Rev.* 2019;6:CD013163. doi:10.1002/14651858.CD013163.pub2.

55. Kapoor V, Malviya MN, Soll R. Lipid emulsions for parenterally fed term and late preterm infants. *Cochrane Database Syst Rev.* 2019;6:CD013171. doi:10.1002/14651858.CD013171.pub2.

56. Lilja HE, Finkel Y, Paulsson M, Lucas S. Prevention and reversal of intestinal failure-associated liver disease in premature infants with short bowel syndrome using intravenous fish oil in combination with omega-6/9 lipid emulsions. *J Pediatr Surg.* 2011;46(7):1361–1367. doi:10.1016/j.jpedsurg.2010.12.021.

57. Angsten G, Finkel Y, Lucas S, Kassa AM, Paulsson M, Lilja HE. Improved outcome in neonatal short bowel syndrome using parenteral fish oil in combination with ω-6/9 lipid emulsions. *JPEN J Parenter Enteral Nutr.* 2012;36(5):587–595. doi:10.1177/0148607111430507.

58. Diamond IR, Grant RC, Pencharz PB, et al. Preventing the progression of intestinal failure-associated liver disease in infants using a composite lipid emulsion: a pilot randomized controlled trial of SMOFlipid. *JPEN J Parenter Enteral Nutr.* 2017;41(5):866–877. doi:10.1177/0148607115626921.

59. Dicken BJ, Bruce A, Samuel TM, Wales PW, Nahirniak S, Turner JM. Bedside to bench: the risk of bleeding with parenteral omega-3 lipid emulsion therapy. *J Pediatr.* 2014;164(3):652–654. doi:10.1016/j.jpeds.2013.10.066.

Chapter 7

Monitoring of Feeding Tolerance in Preterm Infants

Eric B. Ortigoza

Chapter Outline

Key Points

1. The current definition of feeding intolerance is based on nonspecific clinical signs and symptoms.
2. Research on feeding intolerance is limited by the lack of a more objective definition.
3. Current methods to monitor for feeding tolerance in the NICU are nonspecific and poor predictors of gastrointestinal pathology.
4. Emerging technologies to monitor for feeding tolerance show promise but need further development.
5. The integration of emerging noninvasive technologies with laboratory analyses of bacterial colonization, microbiota-derived metabolites, and gut hormones may help us understand the mechanisms of gastrointestinal development and feeding tolerance.

Introduction

Preterm infants who tolerate enteral nutrition have more favorable outcomes.[1–4] Yet, feeding a very premature baby via the enteral route can be challenging, particularly if the baby is born weighing less than 1500 grams.[3] These premature babies require either a nasogastric or orogastric feeding tube because they are unable to coordinate sucking, swallowing, and breathing. Effective integration of these skills is necessary for safe oral feeding.[5]

Because of gastrointestinal immaturity and the risk of feeding intolerance, enteral feeds via a gavage feeding tube are advanced slowly. Soon after birth, intravenous nutrition is necessary until full enteral nutrition is achieved. The practice of initiating and advancing enteral feeds can vary significantly among clinicians. Furthermore, feeding guidelines differ among NICUs. Some clinicians employ a slow, cautious approach, while others employ a faster approach.

In addition to variable feeding guidelines and practices, current clinical measures for monitoring feeding tolerance (gastric residual volume, abdominal circumference, bowel sounds, emesis, stool patterns, apnea, bradycardia, and desaturation) are nonspecific and poor indicators of gut maturity, tolerance, and feeding readiness.[6] As a result, the interpretation of these findings can be subjective, leading to clinical interventions that vary among clinicians. There is great concern among some clinicians that a fast feeding advancement may lead to necrotizing enterocolitis (NEC),[7] the most common gastrointestinal cause of morbidity and mortality affecting predominantly very-low-birth-weight preterm infants.[8] The concern for NEC and the use of these nonspecific, unreliable measures contribute to delays, slow advancement, and frequent interruptions of enteral feeds in babies who otherwise may tolerate a faster advancement. This delay leads to prolonged intravenous nutrition that results in complications such as cholestasis, infection, and increased hospital stay and cost.[2–4] However, no specific, reliable measure to monitor for feeding tolerance currently exists. Therefore, we depend on these unreliable clinical techniques that are poor predictors of tolerance and feeding readiness. Objective measures of feeding tolerance are needed for better assessment of gastrointestinal maturity and prediction of feeding readiness so that feeds can be advanced quickly and safely to help decrease morbidity and mortality in premature infants.

Feeding Intolerance in Preterm Infants

Feeding intolerance is a combination of clinical signs suggestive of an inability by the patient to tolerate enteral nutrition.[6] The definition of feeding intolerance varies among different authors. The most comprehensive definition in the literature is "the inability to digest enteral feedings presented as gastric residual volume more than 50%, abdominal distension or emesis or

both, and the disruption of the patient's feeding plan."[9] However, this definition of feeding intolerance is based on nonspecific clinical signs such as gastric residual volume, abdominal distension, and emesis. It does not provide the clinician with an instrument to differentiate between developmental feeding intolerance (DFI) resulting from gastrointestinal immaturity and dysmotility and pathologic feeding intolerance (PFI), which is associated with the ileus due to several conditions including NEC, spontaneous intestinal perforation, and bowel obstruction. Additionally, the "inability to follow a feeding plan" or guideline may depend on clinician preference or hesitancy, which can be unrelated to the presence of feeding intolerance. For example, the feeding plan may be altered if the clinician routinely stops enteral feeding during administration of indomethacin or pressors and during a sepsis evaluation or a procedure. Thus a more objective, specific definition of feeding intolerance is needed to guide clinical care and further research.

Feeding intolerance remains a major cause of morbidity in preterm infants, resulting in prolonged need for parenteral (intravenous) nutrition and central line access, which can lead to sepsis, cholestasis, prolonged length of hospital stay, malnutrition, and poor neurodevelopmental outcomes.[2–4] In most cases, feeding intolerance represents a developmental condition that is related to anatomical and functional immaturity of the gastrointestinal tract; however, its clinical presentation can overlap with that of more serious gastrointestinal pathology.[6] As a result, the clinician must interpret the clinical and prognostic significance of nonspecific clinical signs and symptoms, which is one of the most uncertain and unidentified problems in the nutritional management of preterm infants. Often, these nonspecific signs are interpreted incorrectly as PFI, leading to the inappropriate and prolonged cessation of enteral feeding or the limitation of feeding advancement in preterm infants who do not have any gastrointestinal pathology. The evaluation for PFI also exposes infants to the risks of intravenous antibiotics and radiographs.[10] Thus morbidity that is associated with feeding intolerance is likely a result of our inability to differentiate DFI from PFI.

The lack of objective biomarkers makes it difficult to diagnose feeding intolerance and predict gastrointestinal pathology. There is a critical need to develop specific, reliable, and objective biomarkers that are validated to differentiate DFI from PFI in preterm infants. Development of these biomarkers will serve as a cornerstone for future research on early detection and treatment of PFI.

Current Clinical Assessment of Feeding Tolerance

The clinical assessment of feeding tolerance in preterm infants is limited by nonspecific measures. The following subsections describe the most common tools that are used daily in NICUs to monitor for feeding tolerance.

GASTRIC RESIDUAL VOLUME

The immature gastrointestinal tract of preterm infants is characterized by pregavage stomach residuals that may indicate poor gastric emptying, gastroduodenal hypomotility, and gastroduodenal reflux.[6] Because gastric residuals characterize the preterm immature gastrointestinal tract, gastric residual volume should not represent a diagnostic sign of a pathologic condition. It is influenced by feeding method (continuous, near-continuous, or intermittent bolus), infant position,[11] and tube-feeding position and gauge.[12] Therefore the routine measurement of gastric residual volume is mostly inaccurate and not a reliable predictor of feeding intolerance. The role of gastric residual color (clear, milky, bilious, blood-stained, or hemorrhagic) is just as inconsistent in its role for predicting serious gastrointestinal pathology such as NEC.[13–15] Furthermore, the practice of checking gastric residuals raises concern about safety and the potential for trauma to the gastric mucosa as well as loss of valuable gastric acid and enzymes.

ABDOMINAL CIRCUMFERENCE/GIRTH

Measuring the abdominal circumference is a routine practice in the NICU to monitor for feeding tolerance. A common sign seen in premature babies is *abdominal distension*, defined as an increase in abdominal girth or as dilated loops of the bowel. This may be assessed clinically or radiologically; however, abdominal distension has a poor predictive value for feeding outcomes, even when accounting for use of continuous positive airway pressure (CPAP), which can increase abdominal circumference.[16,17]

BOWEL SOUNDS

The auscultation of bowel sounds is an imprecise clinical sign.[18,19] Motility and bowel sounds vary substantially among patients depending on timing of auscultation and feeding state. In addition, there is variability among clinicians with detection of bowel sounds.[20]

EMESIS

The presence of emesis or vomiting is nonspecific to feeding intolerance and may be a result of many different etiologies. Because of immaturity of the gastrointestinal tract, we expect preterm infants to have poor gastric emptying, gastroduodenal hypomotility, and gastroduodenal reflux.[6] These findings can lead to residual volume present in the stomach that can reflux into the esophagus and be regurgitated orally. Also, because gastroesophageal reflux (GER) is physiologic and common in preterm infants, it can also result in regurgitation similar to emesis.[21] Regurgitation secondary to GER is not indicative of feeding intolerance. The color of the vomitus is also nonspecific to feeding intolerance. Although bile-stained vomitus in a full-term neonate can be a symptom of bowel obstruction,[22] in preterm infants bile-stained vomitus may also be related to immaturity due to gastroduodenal hypomotility and gastroduodenal reflux.

STOOL PATTERNS

Spontaneous meconium evacuation can be prolonged in premature infants. Meconium retention has been associated with a delay in establishing enteral feeds.[23–26] Some have suggested that this delay may be due to meconium obstructing the distal intestine.[27,28] However, this delay may be secondary to immature intestinal motility or limited (or lack of) enteral nutrition during the first days after birth. Therefore the time to spontaneous meconium evacuation may be confounded by different feeding guidelines.

Hypermagnesemia at birth, secondary to antenatal magnesium sulfate administration, has been associated with early feeding intolerance in preterm infants,[29] especially at doses >80 g.[30] Two proposed mechanisms include reduced gastrointestinal motility and limited magnesium sulfate clearance. Magnesium can replace calcium in smooth muscle cells, disrupting actin and myosin interactions, thus reducing contractility. Additionally, the effects of magnesium may be prolonged because of limited clearance secondary to immature renal function.[30,31] Antenatal magnesium does not significantly affect intestinal blood flow but seems to attenuate the increasing trend of intestinal blood flow in the early postnatal days. However, the impact of this finding on clinical outcomes has not been demonstrated.[32] Findings from a meta-analysis do not support clear associations between antenatal magnesium sulfate and adverse neonatal outcomes such as feeding intolerance.[33] Further research is required to firmly establish a relationship.[29,33]

Some clinicians have suggested the use of enemas and suppositories to expedite meconium evacuation with the intention of promoting feeding tolerance; however, randomized controlled trials did not produce conclusive results.[34–37] Therefore this practice is not supported by evidence and may cause unintentional adverse events including an increase in the incidence of NEC.[35,36]

The presence of blood in the stool may be concerning for NEC; however, it is nonspecific. It may also be a sign of food protein–induced enterocolitis, a non–IgE-mediated syndrome resulting in hypersensitivity to food allergens such as cow's milk and soy proteins.[38] Blood in the stool also may be secondary to anal fissures secondary to constipation or instrumental trauma due to rectal stimulation or enemas/suppositories. Thus routine fecal occult blood testing is nonspecific and does not predict pathology such as NEC.[39]

APNEA, BRADYCARDIA, AND DESATURATION

The monitoring of feeding tolerance often includes observing the heart rate, respiratory rate, and oxygen saturation. Cardiorespiratory events such as apnea, bradycardia, and desaturation sometimes lead to withholding of enteral feeds.[40] However, cardiorespiratory events are very common in preterm infants and are secondary to immaturity of respiratory control. In fact, apnea of prematurity is one of the most common diagnoses in the NICU.[41] These clinical signs and symptoms are not indicative of feeding intolerance and may be related to a variety of other conditions, including late-onset sepsis (LOS).

GER is frequently blamed for cardiorespiratory events that are related to enteral feeding. However, evidence suggests that GER is not associated with apnea of prematurity, and treatment of presumed or proven GER solely for the reduction in apnea events is not supported by currently available evidence.[41]

Gavage tube feeding itself can have some physiologic effects in babies, including a transient rise in postprandial oxygen consumption,[42] decreased oxygenation,[43–47] increased heart rate,[42] decreased functional residual capacity,[48] and decreased lung volumes.[49] Additionally, the speed of administration of enteral feeds can have an effect on heart rate, respiratory rate, and oxygen saturation. Faster administration of a bolus gavage feed (via push) has been shown to increase respiratory rate and decrease heart rate after feeding, compared to slower bolus gavage feed (via gravity).[50] It is postulated that these cardiorespiratory events are related to the volume displacement caused by feeds introduced into the stomach.[46] Fast gastric feeding may also lead to vagal stimulation resulting in bradycardia and apnea, especially in low-birth-weight infants.[51] Small, sick infants may be prone to respiratory instability during intermittent gavage feeding versus continuous tube feeds.[45] Generally, apnea, bradycardia, and desaturation are not specific and are poor predictors of feeding tolerance.

Emerging Technologies to Monitor Feeding Tolerance

Current technologies that are applied in the evaluation of the neonatal gastrointestinal tract include plain radiography, contrast studies, and scintigraphy. Plain radiography is used commonly in the NICU for assessment of NEC, bowel perforation, and bowel obstruction. However, radiography provides limited information about gastrointestinal motility and feeding readiness because it provides a snapshot of a single time point. Contrast studies provide functional information about gastric emptying or intestinal transit, but they require contrast to be administered in the gastrointestinal tract and require fluoroscopy that can increase radiation exposure. Scintigraphy is not used commonly in preterm infants but may provide information about gut motility. It uses a gamma camera to detect radionuclide tracers as they move through the gastrointestinal tract. Its limitations include poor image resolution, difficult interpretation, and the need to move the patient out of the NICU. Additionally, radiation exposure is a disadvantage to plain radiography, contrast studies, and scintigraphy. Thus these technologies limit the evaluation of feeding readiness and tolerance because of safety concerns, lack of validation, and practicality. Development of better modalities is needed.

For a preterm infant to achieve full enteral feedings quickly and safely, we need a bedside technology that can provide objective, quantitative information that will help the clinician in the evaluation for feeding tolerance and readiness. Currently, no noninvasive technology exists; therefore we depend on nonspecific clinical measures that slow down enteral feeding advancement. With additional development, the following technological methods may be able to monitor for feeding tolerance and provide the clinician with objective information to help differentiate DFI from PFI. Emerging technologies include ultrasonography, intraluminal manometry, high-frequency heart rate variability, electrogastrography, electronic bowel sound/acoustics monitoring, and abdominal near-infrared spectroscopy (see Table 7.1).

ULTRASONOGRAPHY

Abdominal ultrasonography may be an alternative to the technologies described previously because it lacks exposure to radiation. Ultrasonography can be used to estimate gastric emptying by calculating gastric volume. Changes in splanchnic blood flow can be evaluated by Doppler ultrasound (to measure blood flow velocities and pulsatility index in the superior mesenteric artery).[52–54] These changes can be observed in response to enteral feeding, acute bowel inflammation, and bowel ischemia. Ultrasonography may be useful to detect pneumatosis and portal venous air in preterm infants with NEC.[55] A limitation of this technology is that the presence of intraluminal air can cause significant artifacts. In addition, it requires sophisticated equipment, a skilled sonographer, and an individual trained to interpret the results.

INTRALUMINAL MANOMETRY

Intraluminal manometry measures intraluminal pressure via a catheter that is passed through the nose and into the stomach and small intestine. This catheter can measure the changes in intraluminal pressure that reflect contractions of the gastrointestinal tract. Manometry has been a useful tool in the study of gastrointestinal motility.[56–58] Manometry catheters can contain either a water-perfused or a solid-state pressure transducer. In a water-perfused catheter system, the catheter contains multiple individual channels and is perfused with distilled water driven by a pneumatic perfusion pump. In a solid-state catheter system, pressure transducers are mounted within the manometric catheter and are at the point of measurement.[59] The solid-state catheter system is easier to use but is more expensive and fragile. The water-perfusion system is less expensive, more flexible, and thinner than solid-state systems, allowing

TABLE 7.1	Pros and Cons of Emerging Technologies for Monitoring Feeding Tolerance	
Emerging Technology	**Pros**	**Cons**
Ultrasonography	Noninvasive	Abdominal air causes image artifacts Requires skilled sonographer
Intraluminal manometry	Detection of gastrointestinal contractions	Tube insertion through nose or mouth Catheters can be expensive
High-frequency heart rate variability	Noninvasive	Needs additional validation
Electrogastrography	Noninvasive	Noise and motion artifacts Normative values needed
Electronic bowel sound/acoustics monitoring	Noninvasive	Needs complex denoising algorithms
Abdominal near-infrared spectroscopy	Noninvasive	Trend monitor Needs validation for abdominal use

for use in children; however, it takes more time to set up and can be technically demanding. Both systems must be disinfected after each use.

Although manometry has been used to evaluate enteral feeding tolerance in preterm infants,[57] its invasive nature prevents its routine use in premature infants. Because the catheter must be inserted inside the gastrointestinal lumen, it raises concerns about its safety to vulnerable infants who already have a feeding tube in place. For this technology to work on our tiniest patients in the NICU, catheters must have a small diameter, be low in cost, and be disposable and integrated with feeding tubes.

HIGH-FREQUENCY HEART RATE VARIABILITY

This method uses electrocardiographic data from cardiorespiratory monitors to measure natural fluctuating interbeat intervals of the heart, which reflect modulation of the autonomic nervous system.[60] Higher heart rate variability (HRV) is associated with well-functioning neural regulation, stress adaptation, and better outcomes in several neonatal diseases,[61–63] whereas low HRV is associated with physiologic instability, inflammation, and sepsis.[64–67] High-frequency HRV (HF-HRV) is indicative of parasympathetic or cardiac vagal tone and low-frequency HRV (LF-HRV) is indicative of mixed parasympathetic and sympathetic influences.[64,66] Tonic vagal efferent activity regulates motility and secretion of the upper gastrointestinal tract and intestinal immune defenses.[68,69] A low vagal tone (decrease in HF-HRV) was demonstrated in preterm infants who developed feeding intolerance or NEC.[70] With further development, this may be a promising noninvasive modality for monitoring of feeding tolerance.

ELECTROGASTROGRAPHY

Cutaneous electrogastrography (EGG) is a noninvasive tool to measure gastric myoelectrical activity using electrodes that are placed on the abdominal skin. Gastric myoelectrical activity is driven by the interstitial cells of Cajal, which are the pacemaker cells of the stomach.[71] These cells generate normal slow-wave activities of the stomach with an electrical frequency of two to four waves or cycles per minute (cpm).[72–74] Noninvasive, cutaneous EGG slow-wave measurements correlate with invasive, serosal EGG slow-wave measurements.[75]

EGG has been utilized in newborns to measure postnatal developmental changes in gastric myoelectrical activity.[76–83] The gastric rhythm of the EGG myoelectrical activity is similar between preterm and term infants, but the amplitude is reduced in preterm infants.[84] Term babies who are breastfed have more adult-like fasting slow-wave activities than formula-fed term babies at 6 months of age.[85] Other studies have used EGG to show that standard formulas supplemented with prebiotics or probiotics may mimic breast milk from a functional standpoint, improving gastric motility in preterm babies.[86–88] EGG can also measure gastric dysrhythmias, such as bradygastria (frequencies <2 cpm) and tachygastria (frequencies 4–9 cpm). Tachygastria has been reported in many preterm infants,[89,90] suggesting that it may be more common in the setting of gastric immaturity. Also, tachygastria has been associated with gastric hypomotility and functional gastrointestinal disorders in older children and adults.[91] Thus the relationship between tachygastria and feeding intolerance secondary to immaturity in preterm infants remains a gap in knowledge. Although few studies have used EGG to assess for feeding tolerance, its noninvasive nature makes it an attractive bedside modality for monitoring gastrointestinal motility in preterm babies.

ELECTRONIC BOWEL SOUND/ACOUSTICS MONITORING

Bowel sounds are the result of vibrations and contractions of the walls of the gastrointestinal tract while propelling liquid and gas within the lumen. Qualitative features of bowel sounds include bursts and rushes. Bursts include pops and clicks that are associated with intestinal mixing, whereas rushes are associated with peristalsis. Although clinical auscultation of bowel sounds is nonspecific, subjective, and unreliable,[92–94] quantitative analysis of bowel sounds may provide a more objective interpretation of the acoustics of the gastrointestinal tract that are associated with motility.

In adults, computerized bowel sound analysis has been used to investigate intestinal obstruction,[95,96] acute abdomen,[97] irritable bowel syndrome,[98–100] small-volume ascites,[101] delayed gastric emptying,[102,103] and postoperative ileus.[104,105] In children, a relative scarcity of research exists in computerized bowel sound analysis even though it is noninvasive and a natural advancement of traditional bowel auscultation.

Tomomasa and colleagues demonstrated that infants with pyloric stenosis had a gastrointestinal sound index that was significantly lower than in healthy control infants.[106] Most recently, continuous bowel sound monitoring has been utilized to study postnatal gastrointestinal development in preterm infants.[80] Further research should focus on developing normative data on preterm infants at different gestational ages and the changes that occur with maturation. Progress in this area will allow for the study of bowel sounds in preterm infants with feeding intolerance.

The utility of electronic bowel sound monitoring in ICUs has high potential but the progress of clinical research on electronic bowel sound/acoustics analysis has been slow.[107–109] Additional research is needed on denoising algorithms to help eliminate artifacts from noisy settings.[110–112] Nonetheless, computerized analysis of bowel sounds shows promise as a potential tool for monitoring feeding tolerance and for diagnosis of gastrointestinal disorders.[113]

ABDOMINAL NEAR-INFRARED SPECTROSCOPY

Near-infrared spectroscopy (NIRS) is available in many ICUs to evaluate cerebral circulation and the changes in cerebral oxyhemoglobin during treatment for respiratory failure and cardiac disease. NIRS equipment can be applied to other body parts such as the flank and abdomen. Abdominal NIRS measures regional tissue oxygenation continuously at the bedside. Routine measurement of mesenteric oxygenation may identify infants at risk for disease and contribute to prevention.

Studies using abdominal NIRS in preterm infants demonstrated maturational changes in mesenteric oxygenation. In one study, for the first 3 postnatal weeks there was an increase in the abdominal baseline of the regional oxygen saturation (rSO_2) from 32% to 66% in stable preterm infants of 29 to 34 weeks gestation.[114] Another study demonstrated that rSO_2 increases with postmenstrual age (PMA).[80] These findings may be related to significant basal changes in intestinal vascular resistance that occur during the first month after birth.[115] Because a strong association has been described between hemodynamic changes in preterm infants and feeding intolerance,[2,116] it makes sense to monitor the gastrointestinal system for feeding tolerance. A study investigated the postprandial changes of mesenteric oxygenation due to feeding.[117] For the preterm infants between 32 and 35 6/7 weeks who were stable and tolerating orogastric feeds, rSO_2 increased significantly one hour after feeding.

The relationship between mesenteric oxygenation and gastrointestinal motility needs to be delineated further. A higher rSO_2 was demonstrated in infants with increased peristaltic activity visualized by ultrasound imaging compared to infants with decreased intestinal motility.[118] Further research to assess this potential relationship will allow for the integration of abdominal NIRS with other noninvasive technologies to monitor gastrointestinal motility, such as EGG and electronic bowel sound/acoustics monitoring.[80]

Because NIRS is noninvasive and now readily available in NICUs, abdominal NIRS has been proposed as a monitoring tool to diagnose NEC; however, results have been inconsistent in small studies.[119–121] In a small observational cohort study of 40 neonates, the authors concluded that NIRS has potential value in the prediction of splanchnic ischemia.[122] Similarly, another study demonstrated that low splanchnic oxygenation in the first week of life during continuous feeding may predict NEC.[123] There have also been individual case reports using NIRS noting that significant mesenteric oxygen desaturation was associated with NEC.[124]

Current NIRS devices are useful as trend monitors. High interpatient variability causes difficulties in the definition of critical values of oxygen parameters. The main reason for this is the introduction of movement artifacts and uncertain optical path length factors, especially in the abdominal measurements. Measurement accuracy should be improved for NIRS to become a more useful method. Further research is required to develop this tool to monitor for feeding tolerance.

Potential Role for the Analysis of Bacterial Colonization, Microbiota-Derived Metabolites, and Gut Hormones

The integration of emerging noninvasive technologies with laboratory analyses of bacterial colonization, microbiota-derived metabolites, and gut hormones would be a significant step forward in understanding the mechanisms of gastrointestinal development and feeding tolerance. In addition, it may also lead to specific, objective biomarkers that may help in the differentiation between DFI and PFI.

GUT MICROBIOME PROFILING

Prior studies have described the relationship between the microbiome and the development of NEC, notably by an expansion of *Proteobacteria* and decreased *Firmicutes*.[125] In a recent study, *Klebsiella* from the phylum *Proteobacteria* was described as a potential diagnostic biomarker for DFI in preterm infants.[126] Using 16S rRNA sequencing techniques, results from that study demonstrated that the relative abundance of *Klebsiella* was significantly higher in preterm infants with feeding intolerance than in preterm infants without feeding intolerance. Further, once the feeding intolerance resolved, the relative abundance of *Klebsiella* significantly decreased in those infants who were previously diagnosed with intolerance. However, nonspecific clinical signs (gastric residual volume and abdominal distension) were used in that study to define feeding intolerance, which, as described earlier, is a significant limitation. A definition of feeding intolerance that is based on objective parameters is essential.

Microbiome profiling techniques include 16S rRNA sequencing and metagenomic shotgun sequencing. The *16S rRNA gene sequencing* technique is a common amplicon sequencing method used to identify phylogenies of bacteria in a complex community.[127,128] A limitation of 16S rRNA sequencing is that data are provided as a relative abundance and not as absolute quantities. Polymerase chain reaction (PCR) bias is seen with 16S rRNA sequencing, where specific gut microbiota taxa can be either over- or underrepresented depending on the choice of primers and the 16S rRNA variable region used for amplification. Therefore, based on 16S rRNA sequencing data analysis, select bacterial species/group quantitative PCR (qPCR) assays should be performed to confirm 16S rRNA sequencing results. *Metagenomic shotgun sequencing* has several advantages over 16S rRNA sequencing: (1) it eliminates PCR bias; (2) it has a higher degree of gut microbiome taxonomic resolution, particularly at the species level, which is important because bacteria belonging to the same genus can exhibit significantly different phenotypes or effects on the host; and (3) it provides insight into functional pathways, such as the metabolic potential of the microbiome.[129] Although metagenomic shotgun sequencing has several advantages over 16S rRNA sequencing, it is significantly more costly.

METABOLOMICS

The mechanism underlying the relationship between *Proteobacteria* such as *Klebsiella* and feeding intolerance remains unclear. A concomitant decrease in short-chain fatty acid–producing commensal bacteria (*Firmicutes* and *Bacteroidetes*) may help explain this finding. Specific intestinal microbiota–derived metabolites such as short-chain fatty acids (SCFAs) are important for gastrointestinal motility[130] and may help us understand the relationship between the microbiome and feeding intolerance. SCFAs stimulate enteroendocrine cells to produce the hormone peptide YY (PYY),[131] which then acts as a modulator for upper gastrointestinal motility.[132,133] To identify specific gut microbiota–derived metabolites that may play a critical role in modulating gut motility, unbiased shotgun metabolomics profiling can be performed. With this method, metabolites are first extracted from fecal samples and then analyzed with an ultra-high-performance liquid chromatography-tandem mass spectroscopy (UPLC-MS/MS). Compounds are identified by automated comparison to reference chemical library entries with subsequent visual inspection for quality control.[129] Instead of unbiased shotgun metabolomics profiling, more targeted analyses are also available.

GUT HORMONE CONCENTRATIONS

Gut hormones influence gut maturation, gastrointestinal motility, nutrient absorption, appetite, and energy homeostasis.[10,134] Serum gastric inhibitory polypeptide (GIP) and PYY concentrations are associated with fewer days to achieve full enteral feedings in preterm infants.[10] GIP is the main humoral effector of the enteroinsular axis, inducing insulin release in response to luminal carbohydrate, and is also active in fatty acid metabolism.[135] Higher serum GIP concentrations may be a physiologic marker of an intact gut hormone axis and maturity in nutrient processing.[10] PYY acts in gastric motility inhibition and peptide suppression.[136] Higher serum concentrations of PYY are associated with fewer days to achieve full enteral feedings, suggesting a potential role as a regulator of gastrointestinal transit.[10] A limitation is that blood collection from these preterm infants is required for serum analyses of gut hormone concentrations. However, analyses are done by enzyme-linked immunosorbent assay (ELISA), which requires approximately 25 microliters of serum.

Summary

Enteral feeding of the premature infant can be challenging because of feeding intolerance secondary to gastrointestinal immaturity. Current methods to monitor for tolerance are nonspecific and poor predictors of pathology. Research on feeding intolerance is limited by the lack of a more objective definition. Emerging technologies to monitor for feeding tolerance show promise but need further development. The integration of emerging noninvasive technologies with laboratory analyses of bacterial colonization, microbiota-derived metabolites, and gut hormones would help us understand the mechanisms of gastrointestinal development and feeding tolerance. In addition, it may also lead to the development of specific, objective biomarkers to help differentiate DFI from PFI with the goal of safely advancing enteral feeds more quickly, thereby decreasing morbidity in preterm infants.

REFERENCES

1. Ehrenkranz RA, Das A, Wrage LA, et al. Early nutrition mediates the influence of severity of illness on extremely LBW infants. *Pediatr Res.* 2011;69(6):522-529. doi:10.1203/PDR.0b013e318217f4f1.
2. Raiten DJ, Steiber AL, Carlson SE, et al. Working group reports: evaluation of the evidence to support practice guidelines for nutritional care of preterm infants—the Pre-B Project. *Am J Clin Nutr.* 2016;103(2):648S-678S. doi:10.3945/ajcn.115.117309.
3. Neu J, Zhang L. Feeding intolerance in very-low-birthweight infants: what is it and what can we do about it? *Acta Paediatr Suppl.* 2005;94(449):93-99. doi:10.1080/08035320510043628.
4. Moore TA, Pickler RH. Feeding intolerance, inflammation, and neurobehaviors in preterm infants. *J Neonatal Nurs.* 2017; 23(3):134-141. doi:10.1016/j.jnn.2016.09.009.
5. Jadcherla SR. Advances with neonatal eerodigestive science in the pursuit of safe swallowing in infants: invited review. *Dysphagia.* 2017;32(1):15-26. doi:10.1007/s00455-016-9773-z.
6. Fanaro S. Feeding intolerance in the preterm infant. *Early Hum Dev.* 2013;89(suppl 2):S13-S20. doi:10.1016/j.earlhumdev.2013.07.013.
7. Masoli D, Dominguez A, Tapia JL, Uauy R, Fabres J. Enteral feeding and necrotizing enterocolitis: does time of first feeds and rate of advancement matter? *J Pediatr Gastroenterol Nutr.* 2021; 72(5):763-768. doi:10.1097/mpg.0000000000003069.
8. Bazacliu C, Neu J. Necrotizing enterocolitis: long term complications. *Curr Pediatr Rev.* 2019;15(2):115-124. doi:10.2174/15 73396315666190312093119.
9. Moore TA, Wilson ME. Feeding intolerance: a concept analysis. *Adv Neonatal Care.* 2011;11(3):149-154. doi:10.1097/ANC.0b013e31821ba28e.
10. Shanahan KH, Yu X, Miller LG, Freedman SD, Martin CR. Early serum gut hormone concentrations associated with time to full enteral feedings in preterm infants. *J Pediatr Gastroenterol Nutr.* 2018;67(1):97-102. doi:10.1097/MPG.0000000000001987.
11. Bankhead R, Boullata J, Brantley S, et al. Enteral nutrition practice recommendations. *JPEN J Parenter Enteral Nutr.* 2009;33(2):122-167. doi:10.1177/0148607108330314.
12. Metheny NA, Stewart J, Nuetzel G, Oliver D, Clouse RE. Effect of feeding-tube properties on residual volume measurements in tube-fed patients. *JPEN J Parenter Enteral Nutr.* 2005;29(3): 192-197. doi:10.1177/0148607105029003192.
13. McClave SA, Snider HL. Clinical use of gastric residual volumes as a monitor for patients on enteral tube feeding. *JPEN J Parenter Enteral Nutr.* 2002;26(suppl 6):S43-S48; discussion S49-S50. doi:10.1177/014860710202600607.
14. Parker L, Torrazza RM, Li Y, Talaga E, Shuster J, Neu J. Aspiration and evaluation of gastric residuals in the neonatal intensive care unit: state of the science. *J Perinat Neonatal Nurs.* 2015;29(1): 51-59; quiz E2. doi:10.1097/JPN.0000000000000080.
15. Mihatsch WA, von Schoenaich P, Fahnenstich H, et al. The significance of gastric residuals in the early enteral feeding advancement of extremely low birth weight infants. *Pediatrics.* 2002;109(3):457-459. doi:10.1542/peds.109.3.457.
16. Schanler RJ, Shulman RJ, Lau C, Smith EO, Heitkemper MM. Feeding strategies for premature infants: randomized trial of gastrointestinal priming and tube-feeding method. *Pediatrics.* 1999;103(2):434-439. doi:10.1542/peds.103.2.434.
17. Shulman RJ, Ou CN, Smith EO. Evaluation of potential factors predicting attainment of full gavage feedings in preterm infants. *Neonatology.* 2011;99(1):38-44. doi:10.1159/000302020.
18. Baid H. A critical review of auscultating bowel sounds. *Br J Nurs.* 2009;18(18):1125-1129. doi:10.12968/bjon.2009.18.18.44555.
19. Reintam Blaser A, Starkopf L, Deane AM, Poeze M, Starkopf J. Comparison of different definitions of feeding intolerance: a retrospective observational study. *Clin Nutr.* 2015;34(5): 956-961. doi:10.1016/j.clnu.2014.10.006.
20. Yen K, Karpas A, Pinkerton HJ, Gorelick MH. Interexaminer reliability in physical examination of pediatric patients with abdominal pain. *Arch Pediatr Adolesc Med.* 2005;159(4): 373-376. doi:10.1001/archpedi.159.4.373.
21. Lopez-Alonso M, Moya MJ, Cabo JA, et al. Twenty-four-hour esophageal impedance-pH monitoring in healthy preterm neonates: rate and characteristics of acid, weakly acidic, and weakly alkaline gastroesophageal reflux. *Pediatrics.* 2006;118(2):e299-e308. doi:10.1542/peds.2005-3140.
22. Mohinuddin S, Sakhuja P, Bermundo B, et al. Outcomes of full-term infants with bilious vomiting: observational study of a retrieved cohort. *Arch Dis Child.* 2015;100(1):14-17. doi:10.1136/archdischild-2013-305724.
23. Verma A, Dhanireddy R. Time of first stool in extremely low birth weight (< or = 1000 grams) infants. *J Pediatr.* 1993;122(4): 626-629. doi:10.1016/S0022-3476(05)83550-4.
24. Meetze WH, Palazzolo VL, Bowling D, Behnke M, Burchfield DJ, Neu J. Meconium passage in very-low-birth-weight infants. *JPEN J Parenter Enteral Nutr.* 1993;17(6):537-540. doi:10.117 7/0148607193017006537.

25. Siddiqui MM, Drewett M, Burge DM. Meconium obstruction of prematurity. *Arch Dis Child Fetal Neonatal Ed*. 2012;97(2): F147-F150. doi:10.1136/adc.2010.190157.

26. Bekkali N, Hamers SL, Schipperus MR, et al. Duration of meconium passage in preterm and term infants. *Arch Dis Child Fetal Neonatal Ed*. 2008;93(5):F376-F379. doi:10.1136/adc.2008.138024.

27. Shim SY, Kim HS, Kim DH, et al. Induction of early meconium evacuation promotes feeding tolerance in very low birth weight infants. *Neonatology*. 2007;92(1):67-72. doi:10.1159/000100804.

28. Shinohara T, Tsuda M, Koyama N. Management of meconium-related ileus in very low-birthweight infants. *Pediatr Int*. 2007;49(5):641-644. doi:10.1111/j.1442-200X.2007.02457.x.

29. Junqueira EO, Marba STM, Caldas JPS. Hypermagnesemia and feeding intolerance in preterm infants: a cohort study. *JPEN J Parenter Enteral Nutr*. 2022;46(5):1054-1060. doi:10.1002/jpen.2336.

30. Belden MK, Gnadt S, Ebert A. Effects of maternal magnesium sulfate treatment on neonatal feeding tolerance. *J Pediatr Pharmacol Ther*. 2017;22(2):112-117. doi:10.5863/1551-6776-22.2.112.

31. Havranek T, Ashmeade TL, Afanador M, Carver JD. Effects of maternal magnesium sulfate administration on intestinal blood flow velocity in preterm neonates. *Neonatology*. 2011;100(1): 44-49. doi:10.1159/000319049.

32. Gursoy T, Imamoglu EY, Ovali F, Karatekin G. Effects of antenatal magnesium exposure on intestinal blood flow and outcome in preterm neonates. *Am J Perinatol*. 2015;32(11): 1064-1069. doi:10.1055/s-0035-1548541.

33. Shepherd E, Salam RA, Manhas D, et al. Antenatal magnesium sulphate and adverse neonatal outcomes: a systematic review and meta-analysis. *PLoS Med*. 2019;16(12):e1002988. doi:10.1371/journal.pmed.1002988.

34. Sáenz de Pipaón Marcos M, Teresa Montes Bueno M, Sanjosé B, Gil M, Parada I, Amo P. Randomized controlled trial of prophylactic rectal stimulation and enemas on stooling patterns in extremely low birth weight infants. *J Perinatol*. 2013;33(11): 858-860. doi:10.1038/jp.2013.86.

35. Haiden N, Norooz F, Klebermass-Schrehof K, et al. The effect of an osmotic contrast agent on complete meconium evacuation in preterm infants. *Pediatrics*. 2012;130(6):e1600-e1606. doi:10.1542/peds.2011-3634.

36. Livingston MH, Shawyer AC, Rosenbaum PL, Williams C, Jones SA, Walton JM. Glycerin enemas and suppositories in premature infants: a meta-analysis. *Pediatrics*. 2015;135(6): 1093-1106. doi:10.1542/peds.2015-0143.

37. Ibrahim T, Li Wei C, Bautista D, Sriram B, Xiangzhen Fay L, Rajadurai VS. Saline enemas versus glycerin suppositories to promote enteral feeding in premature infants: a pilot randomized controlled trial. *Neonatology*. 2017;112(4):347-353. doi:10.1159/000477999.

38. Lenfestey MW, de la Cruz D, Neu J. Food protein-induced enterocolitis instead of necrotizing enterocolitis? A neonatal intensive care unit case series. *J Pediatr*. 2018;200:270-273. doi:10.1016/j.jpeds.2018.04.048.

39. Pickering A, White R, Davis NL. Routine fecal occult blood testing does not predict necrotizing enterocolitis in very low birth weight neonates. *J Neonatal Perinatal Med*. 2016;9(2): 171-178. doi:10.3233/npm-16915120.

40. Kuzma-O'Reilly B, Duenas ML, Greecher C, et al. Evaluation, development, and implementation of potentially better practices in neonatal intensive care nutrition. *Pediatrics*. 2003;111 (4 Pt 2):e461-e470.

41. Eichenwald EC, Committee on Fetus and Newborn, American Academy of Pediatrics. Apnea of prematurity. *Pediatrics*. 2016; 137(1). doi:10.1542/peds.2015-3757.

42. Mukhtar AI, Stothers JK. Cardiovascular effects of nasogastric tube feeding in the healthy preterm infant. *Early Hum Dev*. 1982;6(1):25-30. doi:10.1016/0378-3782(82)90054-8.

43. Krauss AN, Brown J, Waldman S, Gottlieb G, Auld PA. Pulmonary function following feeding in low-birth-weight infants. *Am J Dis Child*. 1978;132(2):139-142. doi:10.1001/archpedi.1978. 02120270037008.

44. Hammerman C, Kaplan M. Oxygen saturation during and after feeding in healthy term infants. *Biol Neonate*. 1995;67(2): 94-99. doi:10.1159/000244149.

45. Blondheim O, Abbasi S, Fox WW, Bhutani VK. Effect of enteral gavage feeding rate on pulmonary functions of very low birth weight infants. *J Pediatr*. 1993;122(5 Pt 1):751-755. doi:10.1016/s0022-3476(06)80021-1.

46. Yu VY. Cardiorespiratory response to feeding in newborn infants. *Arch Dis Child*. 1976;51(4):305-309. doi:10.1136/adc.51.4.305.

47. Wilkinson A, Yu VY. Immediate effects of feeding on blood-gases and some cardiorespiratory functions of ill newborn infants. *Lancet*. 1974;1(7866):1083-1085. doi:10.1016/s0140-6736(74)90558-3.

48. Heldt GP. The effect of gavage feeding on the mechanics of the lung, chest wall, and diaphragm of preterm infants. *Pediatr Res*. 1988;24(1):55-58. doi:10.1203/00006450-198807000-00014.

49. Pitcher-Wilmott R, Shutack JG, Fox WW. Decreased lung volume after nasgogastric feeding of neonates recovering from respiratory disease. *J Pediatr*. 1979;95(1):119-121. doi:10.1016/s0022-3476(79)80103-1.

50. Dawson JA, Summan R, Badawi N, Foster JP. Push versus gravity for intermittent bolus gavage tube feeding of preterm and low birth weight infants. *Cochrane Database Syst Rev*. 2021;8:CD005249. doi:10.1002/14651858.CD005249.pub3.

51. Kindley AD, Harris F. Heart rate changes during gauge feeding of neonates. *Early Hum Dev*. 1980;4(4):387-392. doi:10.1016/0378-3782(80)90043-2.

52. Sancak S, Arman D, Gursoy T, Topcuoglu S, Karatekin G, Ovalı F. Intestinal blood flow by Doppler ultrasound: the impact of clarithromycin treatment for feeding intolerance in preterm neonates. *J Matern Fetal Neonatal Med*. 2016;29(11): 1853-1856. doi:10.3109/14767058.2015.1066327.

53. Deeg KH. Sonographic and doppler sonographic diagnosis of necrotizing enterocolitis in preterm infants and newborns [Sonografische und dopplersonografische Diagnose der nekrotisierenden Enterokolitis bei Fruh- und Neugeborenen]. *Ultraschall Med*. 2019;40(3):292-318. doi:10.1055/a-0879-8110.

54. Robel-Tillig E, Knüpfer M, Pulzer F, Vogtmann C. Blood flow parameters of the superior mesenteric artery as an early predictor of intestinal dysmotility in preterm infants. *Pediatr Radiol*. 2004;34(12):958-962. doi:10.1007/s00247-004-1285-6.

55. van Druten J, Khashu M, Chan SS, Sharif S, Abdalla H. Abdominal ultrasound should become part of standard care for early diagnosis and management of necrotizing enterocolitis: a narrative review. *Arch Dis Child Fetal Neonatal Ed*. 2019;104(5): F551-F559. doi:10.1136/archdischild-2018-316263.

56. Soffer EE. Small bowel motility: ready for prime time? *Curr Gastroenterol Rep*. 2000;2(5):364-369. doi:10.1007/s11894-000-0035-7.

57. Berseth CL, Nordyke CK. Manometry can predict feeding readiness in preterm infants. *Gastroenterology*. 1992;103(5): 1523-1528. doi:10.1016/0016-5085(92)91173-2.

58. Arbizu R, Freiberg B, Rodriguez L. Lower gastrointestinal functional and motility disorders in children. *Pediatr Clin North Am.* 2021;68(6):1255-1271. doi:10.1016/j.pcl.2021.07.010.

59. Bredenoord AJ, Hebbard GS. Technical aspects of clinical high-resolution manometry studies. *Neurogastroenterol Motil.* 2012;24(suppl 1):5-10. doi:10.1111/j.1365-2982.2011.01830.x.

60. Liu HL, Garzoni L, Herry C, et al. Can monitoring fetal intestinal inflammation using heart rate variability analysis signal incipient necrotizing enterocolitis of the neonate? *Pediatr Crit Care Med.* 2016;17(4):e165-e176. doi:10.1097/pcc.0000000000000643.

61. Metzler M, Govindan R, Al-Shargabi T, et al. Pattern of brain injury and depressed heart rate variability in newborns with hypoxic ischemic encephalopathy. *Pediatr Res.* 2017;82(3):438-443. doi:10.1038/pr.2017.94.

62. Bohanon FJ, Mrazek AA, Shabana MT, et al. Heart rate variability analysis is more sensitive at identifying neonatal sepsis than conventional vital signs. *Am J Surg.* 2015;210(4):661-667. doi:10.1016/j.amjsurg.2015.06.002.

63. Sullivan BA, McClure C, Hicks J, Lake DE, Moorman JR, Fairchild KD. Early heart rate characteristics predict death and morbidities in preterm infants. *J Pediatr.* 2016;174:57-62. doi:10.1016/j.jpeds.2016.03.042.

64. Gardner FC, Adkins CS, Hart SE, Travagli RA, Doheny KK. Preterm stress behaviors, autonomic indices, and maternal perceptions of infant colic. *Adv Neonatal Care.* 2018;18(1):49-57. doi:10.1097/anc.0000000000000451.

65. Heart rate variability. Standards of measurement, physiological interpretation, and clinical use. Task Force of the European Society of Cardiology and the North American Society of Pacing and Electrophysiology. *Eur Heart J.* 1996;17(3):354-381.

66. Laborde S, Mosley E, Thayer JF. Heart rate variability and cardiac vagal tone in psychophysiological research—recommendations for experiment planning, data analysis, and data reporting. *Front Psychol.* 2017;8:213. doi:10.3389/fpsyg.2017.00213.

67. Al-Shargabi T, Reich D, Govindan RB, et al. Changes in autonomic tone in premature infants developing necrotizing enterocolitis. *Am J Perinatol.* 2018;35(11):1079-1086. doi:10.1055/s-0038-1639339.

68. Meister AL, Doheny KK, Travagli RA. Necrotizing enterocolitis: it's not all in the gut. *Exp Biol Med (Maywood).* 2020;245(2):85-95. doi:10.1177/1535370219891971.

69. Tracey KJ. The inflammatory reflex. *Nature.* 2002;420(6917):853-859. doi:10.1038/nature01321.

70. Meister AL, Gardner FC, Browning KN, Travagli RA, Palmer C, Doheny KK. Vagal tone and proinflammatory cytokines predict feeding intolerance and necrotizing enterocolitis risk. *Adv Neonatal Care.* 2021;21(6):452-461. doi:10.1097/ANC.0000000000000959.

71. Owyang C, Hasler WL. Physiology and pathophysiology of the interstitial cells of Cajal: from bench to bedside. VI. Pathogenesis and therapeutic approaches to human gastric dysrhythmias. *Am J Physiol Gastrointest Liver Physiol.* 2002;283(1):G8-G15. doi:10.1152/ajpgi.00095.2002.

72. Coleski R, Hasler WL. Directed endoscopic mucosal mapping of normal and dysrhythmic gastric slow waves in healthy humans. *Neurogastroenterol Motil.* 2004;16(5):557-565. doi:10.1111/j.1365-2982.2004.00542.x.

73. Lin Z, Sarosiek I, Forster J, Damjanov I, Hou Q, McCallum RW. Association of the status of interstitial cells of Cajal and electrogastrogram parameters, gastric emptying and symptoms in patients with gastroparesis. *Neurogastroenterol Motil.* 2010;22(1):56-61.e10. doi:10.1111/j.1365-2982.2009.01365.x.

74. Chen J. A computerized data analysis system for electrogastrogram. *Comput Biol Med.* 1992;22(1-2):45-57. doi:10.1016/0010-4825(92)90051-n.

75. Chen JD, Schirmer BD, McCallum RW. Serosal and cutaneous recordings of gastric myoelectrical activity in patients with gastroparesis. *Am J Physiol.* 1994;266(1 Pt 1):G90-G98. doi:10.1152/ajpgi.1994.266.1.G90.

76. Devanarayana NM, de Silva DG, de Silva HJ. Gastric myoelectrical and motor abnormalities in children and adolescents with functional recurrent abdominal pain. *J Gastroenterol Hepatol.* 2008;23(11):1672-1677. doi:10.1111/j.1440-1746.2008.05529.x.

77. Chang FY. Electrogastrography: basic knowledge, recording, processing and its clinical applications. *J Gastroenterol Hepatol.* 2005;20(4):502-516. doi:10.1111/j.1440-1746.2004.03751.x.

78. Lin Z, Chen JD, Schirmer BD, McCallum RW. Postprandial response of gastric slow waves: correlation of serosal recordings with the electrogastrogram. *Dig Dis Sci.* 2000;45(4):645-651. doi:10.1023/a:1005434020310.

79. Parkman HP, Hasler WL, Barnett JL, Eaker EY, American Motility Society Clinical GI Motility Testing Task Force. Electrogastrography: a document prepared by the gastric section of the American Motility Society Clinical GI Motility Testing Task Force. *Neurogastroenterol Motil.* 2003;15(2):89-102. doi:10.1046/j.1365-2982.2003.00396.x.

80. Ortigoza EB, Cagle J, Chien JH, Oh S, Brown LS, Neu J. Electrogastrography, near-infrared spectroscopy, and acoustics to measure gastrointestinal development in preterm babies. *J Pediatr Gastroenterol Nutr.* 2018;66(6):e146-e152. doi:10.1097/MPG.0000000000001867.

81. Chen JD, Co E, Liang J, et al. Patterns of gastric myoelectrical activity in human subjects of different ages. *Am J Physiol.* 1997;272(5 Pt 1):G1022-G1027. doi:10.1152/ajpgi.1997.272.5.G1022.

82. Liang J, Co E, Zhang M, Pineda J, Chen JD. Development of gastric slow waves in preterm infants measured by electrogastrography. *Am J Physiol.* 1998;274(3 Pt 1):G503-G508. doi:10.1152/ajpgi.1998.274.3.G503.

83. Patterson M, Rintala R, Lloyd DA. A longitudinal study of electrogastrography in normal neonates. *J Pediatr Surg.* 2000;35(1):59-61. doi:10.1016/s0022-3468(00)80014-7.

84. Zhang J, Ouyang H, Zhu HB, et al. Development of gastric slow waves and effects of feeding in pre-term and full-term infants. *Neurogastroenterol Motil.* 2006;18(4):284-291. doi:10.1111/j.1365-2982.2006.00756.x.

85. Riezzo G, Castellana RM, De Bellis T, Laforgia F, Indrio F, Chiloiro M. Gastric electrical activity in normal neonates during the first year of life: effect of feeding with breast milk and formula. *J Gastroenterol.* 2003;38(9):836-843. doi:10.1007/s00535-003-1158-z.

86. Indrio F, Riezzo G, Raimondi F, Bisceglia M, Cavallo L, Francavilla R. The effects of probiotics on feeding tolerance, bowel habits, and gastrointestinal motility in preterm newborns. *J Pediatr.* 2008;152(6):801-806. doi:10.1016/j.jpeds.2007.11.005.

87. Indrio F, Riezzo G, Raimondi F, Bisceglia M, Cavallo L, Francavilla R. Effects of probiotic and prebiotic on gastrointestinal motility in newborns. *J Physiol Pharmacol.* 2009;60(suppl 6):27-31.

88. Indrio F, Riezzo G, Raimondi F, et al. Prebiotics improve gastric motility and gastric electrical activity in preterm newborns. *J Pediatr Gastroenterol Nutr.* 2009;49(2):258-261. doi:10.1097/MPG.0b013e3181926aec.

89. Cucchiara S, Salvia G, Scarcella A, et al. Gestational maturation of electrical activity of the stomach. *Dig Dis Sci.* 1999;44(10):2008-2013. doi:10.1023/a:1026666100878.

90. Riezzo G, Indrio F, Montagna O, et al. Gastric electrical activity and gastric emptying in term and preterm newborns. *Neurogastroenterol Motil.* 2000;12(3):223-229. doi:10.1046/j.1365-2982.2000.00203.x.

91. Ouyang H, Xing J, Chen JD. Tachygastria induced by gastric electrical stimulation is mediated via alpha- and beta-adrenergic pathway and inhibits antral motility in dogs. *Neurogastroenterol Motil.* 2005;17(6):846-853. doi:10.1111/j.1365-2982.2005.00696.x.

92. Breum BM, Rud B, Kirkegaard T, Nordentoft T. Accuracy of abdominal auscultation for bowel obstruction. *World J Gastroenterol.* 2015;21(34):10018-10024. doi:10.3748/wjg.v21.i34.10018.

93. Felder S, Margel D, Murrell Z, Fleshner P. Usefulness of bowel sound auscultation: a prospective evaluation. *J Surg Educ.* 2014;71(5):768-773. doi:10.1016/j.jsurg.2014.02.003.

94. Dumas J, Hill KM, Adrezin RS, et al. Feasibility of an electronic stethoscope system for monitoring neonatal bowel sounds. *Conn Med.* 2013;77(8):467-471.

95. Ching SS, Tan YK. Spectral analysis of bowel sounds in intestinal obstruction using an electronic stethoscope. *World J Gastroenterol.* 2012;18(33):4585-4592. doi:10.3748/wjg.v18.i33.4585.

96. Yoshino H, Abe Y, Yoshino T, Ohsato K. Clinical application of spectral analysis of bowel sounds in intestinal obstruction. *Dis Colon Rectum.* 1990;33(9):753-757. doi:10.1007/BF02052320.

97. Sugrue M, Redfern M. Computerized phonoenterography: the clinical investigation of a new system. *J Clin Gastroenterol.* 1994;18(2):139-144.

98. Craine BL, Silpa ML, O'Toole CJ. Two-dimensional positional mapping of gastrointestinal sounds in control and functional bowel syndrome patients. *Dig Dis Sci.* 2002;47(6):1290-1296. doi:10.1023/a:1015318413638.

99. Craine BL, Silpa ML, O'Toole CJ. Enterotachogram analysis to distinguish irritable bowel syndrome from Crohn's disease. *Dig Dis Sci.* 2001;46(9):1974-1979. doi:10.1023/a:1010651602095.

100. Craine BL, Silpa M, O'Toole CJ. Computerized auscultation applied to irritable bowel syndrome. *Dig Dis Sci.* 1999;44(9):1887-1892. doi:10.1023/a:1018859110022.

101. Liatsos C, Hadjileontiadis LJ, Mavrogiannis C, Patch D, Panas SM, Burroughs AK. Bowel sounds analysis: a novel noninvasive method for diagnosis of small-volume ascites. *Dig Dis Sci.* 2003;48(8):1630-1636. doi:10.1023/a:1024788428692.

102. Kim KS, Seo JH, Song CG. Non-invasive algorithm for bowel motility estimation using a back-propagation neural network model of bowel sounds. *Biomed Eng Online.* 2011;10:69. doi:10.1186/1475-925x-10-69.

103. Kim KS, Seo JH, Ryu SH, Kim MH, Song CG. Estimation algorithm of the bowel motility based on regression analysis of the jitter and shimmer of bowel sounds. *Comput Methods Programs Biomed.* 2011;104(3):426-434. doi:10.1016/j.cmpb.2011.02.014.

104. Kaneshiro M, Kaiser W, Pourmorady J, et al. Postoperative gastrointestinal telemetry with an acoustic biosensor predicts ileus vs. uneventful GI recovery. *J Gastrointest Surg.* 2016;20(1):132-139; discussion 139. doi:10.1007/s11605-015-2956-3.

105. Spiegel BM, Kaneshiro M, Russell MM, et al. Validation of an acoustic gastrointestinal surveillance biosensor for postoperative ileus. *J Gastrointest Surg.* 2014;18(10):1795-1803. doi:10.1007/s11605-014-2597-y.

106. Tomomasa T, Morikawa A, Sandler RH, et al. Gastrointestinal sounds and migrating motor complex in fasted humans. *Am J Gastroenterol.* 1999;94(2):374-381. doi:10.1111/j.1572-0241.1999.00862.x.

107. Nowak JK, Nowak R, Radzikowski K, Grulkowski I, Walkowiak J. Automated bowel sound analysis: an overview. *Sensors (Basel).* 2021;21(16):5294. doi:10.3390/s21165294.

108. Li B, Wang JR, Ma YL. Bowel sounds and monitoring gastrointestinal motility in critically ill patients. *Clin Nurse Spec.* 2012;26(1):29-34. doi:10.1097/NUR.0b013e31823bfab8.

109. Li B, Tang S, Ma YL, Tang J, Wang B, Wang JR. Analysis of bowel sounds application status for gastrointestinal function monitoring in the intensive care unit. *Crit Care Nurs Q.* 2014;37(2):199-206. doi:10.1097/cnq.0000000000000019.

110. Allwood G, Du X, Webberley KM, Osseiran A, Marshall BJ. Advances in acoustic signal processing techniques for enhanced bowel sound analysis. *IEEE Rev Biomed Eng.* 2019;12:240-253. doi:10.1109/RBME.2018.2874037.

111. Kolle K, Aftab MF, Andersson LE, Fougner AL, Stavdahl O. Data driven filtering of bowel sounds using multivariate empirical mode decomposition. *Biomed Eng Online.* 2019;18(1):28. doi:10.1186/s12938-019-0646-1.

112. Bilionis I, Apostolidis G, Charisis V, Liatsos C, Hadjileontiadis L. Non-invasive detection of bowel sounds in real-life settings using spectrogram zeros and autoencoding. *Annu Int Conf IEEE Eng Med Biol Soc.* 2021;2021:915-919. doi:10.1109/embc46164.2021.9630783.

113. Inderjeeth AJ, Webberley KM, Muir J, Marshall BJ. The potential of computerised analysis of bowel sounds for diagnosis of gastrointestinal conditions: a systematic review. *Syst Rev.* 2018;7(1):124. doi:10.1186/s13643-018-0789-3.

114. McNeill S, Gatenby JC, McElroy S, Engelhardt B. Normal cerebral, renal and abdominal regional oxygen saturations using near-infrared spectroscopy in preterm infants. *J Perinatol.* 2011;31(1):51-57. doi:10.1038/jp.2010.71.

115. Reber KM, Nankervis CA, Nowicki PT. Newborn intestinal circulation. Physiology and pathophysiology. *Clin Perinatol.* 2002;29(1):23-39. doi:10.1016/s0095-5108(03)00063-0.

116. Clyman R, Wickremasinghe A, Jhaveri N, et al. Enteral feeding during indomethacin and ibuprofen treatment of a patent ductus arteriosus. *J Pediatr.* 2013;163(2):406-411. doi:10.1016/j.jpeds.2013.01.057.

117. Dave V, Brion LP, Campbell DE, Scheiner M, Raab C, Nafday SM. Splanchnic tissue oxygenation, but not brain tissue oxygenation, increases after feeds in stable preterm neonates tolerating full bolus orogastric feeding. *J Perinatol.* 2009;29(3):213-218. doi:10.1038/jp.2008.189.

118. Akotia DH, Durham JT, Arnell KM, Petruzzelli DL, Katheria AC. Relationship between near-infrared spectroscopy and transabdominal ultrasonography: noninvasive monitoring of intestinal function in neonates. *Med Sci Monit.* 2016;22:61-68. doi:10.12659/msm.895730.

119. Corvaglia L, Martini S, Battistini B, Rucci P, Faldella G, Aceti A. Splanchnic oxygenation at first enteral feeding in preterm infants: correlation with feeding intolerance. *J Pediatr Gastroenterol Nutr.* 2017;64(4):550-554. doi:10.1097/MPG.0000000000001308.

120. Dani C, Corsini I, Generoso M, Gozzini E, Bianconi T, Pratesi S. Splanchnic tissue oxygenation for predicting feeding tolerance in preterm infants. *JPEN J Parenter Enteral Nutr.* 2015;39(8):935-940. doi:10.1177/0148607114538671.

121. Le Bouhellec J, Prodhomme O, Mura T, et al. Near-infrared spectroscopy: a tool for diagnosing necrotizing enterocolitis at onset of symptoms in preterm neonates with acute gastrointestinal symptoms? *Am J Perinatol.* 2020;38(S 01):e299-e308. doi:10.1055/s-0040-1710033.

122. Fortune PM, Wagstaff M, Petros AJ. Cerebro-splanchnic oxygenation ratio (CSOR) using near infrared spectroscopy may be able to predict splanchnic ischaemia in neonates. *Intensive Care Med.* 2001;27(8):1401-1407. doi:10.1007/s001340100994.

123. Palleri E, Wackernagel D, Wester T, Bartocci M. Low splanchnic oxygenation and risk for necrotizing enterocolitis in extremely preterm newborns. *J Pediatr Gastroenterol Nutr.* 2020;71(3):401-406. doi:10.1097/mpg.0000000000002761.

124. Stapleton GE, Eble BK, Dickerson HA, Andropoulos DB, Chang AC. Mesenteric oxygen desaturation in an infant with congenital heart disease and necrotizing enterocolitis. *Tex Heart Inst J.* 2007;34(4):442-444.

125. Pammi M, Cope J, Tarr PI, et al. Intestinal dysbiosis in preterm infants preceding necrotizing enterocolitis: a systematic review and meta-analysis. *Microbiome.* 2017;5(1):31. doi:10.1186/s40168-017-0248-8.

126. Yuan Z, Yan J, Wen H, Deng X, Li X, Su S. Feeding intolerance alters the gut microbiota of preterm infants. *PLoS One.* 2019;14(1):e0210609. doi:10.1371/journal.pone.0210609.

127. Fan D, Coughlin LA, Neubauer MM, et al. Activation of HIF-1alpha and LL-37 by commensal bacteria inhibits Candida albicans colonization. *Nat Med.* 2015;21(7):808-814. doi:10.1038/nm.3871.

128. Simms-Waldrip TR, Sunkersett G, Coughlin LA, et al. Antibiotic-induced depletion of anti-inflammatory clostridia is associated with the development of graft-versus-host disease in pediatric stem cell transplantation patients. *Biol Blood Marrow Transplant.* 2017;23(5):820-829. doi:10.1016/j.bbmt.2017.02.004.

129. Frankel AE, Coughlin LA, Kim J, et al. Metagenomic shotgun sequencing and unbiased metabolomic profiling identify specific human gut microbiota and metabolites associated with immune checkpoint therapy efficacy in melanoma patients. *Neoplasia.* 2017;19(10):848-855. doi:10.1016/j.neo.2017.08.004.

130. Cherbut C, Aube AC, Blottiere HM, Galmiche JP. Effects of short-chain fatty acids on gastrointestinal motility. *Scand J Gastroenterol Suppl.* 1997;222:58-61. doi:10.1080/00365521.1997.11720720.

131. Larraufie P, Martin-Gallausiaux C, Lapaque N, et al. SCFAs strongly stimulate PYY production in human enteroendocrine cells. *Sci Rep.* 2018;8(1):74. doi:10.1038/s41598-017-18259-0.

132. Khandekar N, Berning BA, Sainsbury A, Lin S. The role of pancreatic polypeptide in the regulation of energy homeostasis. *Mol Cell Endocrinol.* 2015;418(Pt 1):33-41. doi:10.1016/j.mce.2015.06.028.

133. Cherbut C. Motor effects of short-chain fatty acids and lactate in the gastrointestinal tract. *Proc Nutr Soc.* 2003;62(1):95-99. doi:10.1079/PNS2002213.

134. Lucas A, Bloom SR, Green AA. Gastrointestinal peptides and the adaptation to extrauterine nutrition. *Can J Physiol Pharmacol.* 1985;63(5):527-537. doi:10.1139/y85-092.

135. McIntosh CHS, Widenmaier S, Kim SJ. Glucose-dependent insulinotropic polypeptide (gastric inhibitory polypeptide; GIP). In: *Vitamins & Hormones.* Cambridge, MA: Academic Press; 2009:409-471.

136. Cooper JA. Factors affecting circulating levels of peptide YY in humans: a comprehensive review. *Nutr Res Rev.* 2014;27(1):186-197. doi:10.1017/s0954422414000109.

Chapter 8

Human Milk Bioactives and Roles in the GI Tract

Lisa Stinson, Josef Neu and Donna Tracy Geddes

Chapter Outline

Key Points

- In addition to nutrients, human milk contains myriad bioactive components that promote development of neonatal intestinal immunity.
- A range of bioactive proteins in human milk function in protection against infection, immuno-modulation, and nutrient utilization.
- Human milk growth factors and hormones modulate growth and development of the intestines and have immunomodulatory effects.
- Human milk oligosaccharides promote a healthy intestinal microbiome and protect infants from infection.
- Human milk exposes infants to maternal bacteria and their metabolites, which have immune-modulating effects.
- Research on human milk extracellular vesicles and miRNA is relatively new; however, emerging data suggest these components play important roles in programming intestinal immune ontogeny.
- Bioactive factors in human milk are particularly important for preterm infants, for whom prenatal intestinal development is interrupted.
- Human milk bioactive factors are unique and many are lacking and/or inactive in bovine milk and infant formula.
- Milk processing techniques, such as pasteurization, impact the activity of various milk bioactive substances.

Introduction

In addition to providing the gold standard of nutrition for infants,[1] human milk also contains numerous components that are considered bioactive.

These are not utilized directly for nutritional purposes and instead provide for specialized needs of the infant, such as immunoprotection and immunomodulation, metabolic homeostasis, digestion, regulatory activities, and microbial colonization. These factors are usually not found in commercial formulas unless specifically added. Additionally, many are not found in banked donor milk due to inactivation during pasteurization or storage.[2–4] Given the personalized nature of human milk and the communicative role of milk in the co-adapting mother-infant-milk triad,[5] bioactive factors in donor milk may not be dynamically interactive with the infant. Thus mother's own milk (MoM) plays an important role in guiding early intestinal development.

This chapter summarizes some of the important and well-known bioactive components found in human milk, how they synergize with the intrinsically programmed development of the intestine during neonatal life, and how they are affected by maternal and environmental factors. We apply a special focus on preterm infants, born before 37 weeks of gestational age, and how they differ from those born at term.

Ontogeny of Intestinal Immunity

The development of the intestinal immune system begins *in utero* (Fig. 8.1). This prior immune development is critical given that, at birth, the neonate is challenged with extraordinary bacterial and antigenic exposures.[6] Several maturational events occur during fetal development, providing the neonate with an armamentarium of immunologic weapons that protect the intestinal mucosal surface from invasion by pathogens and allow immunomodulation for tolerance to potentially beneficial microorganisms and antigenic nutrients. While the hallmarks of a well-functioning intestinal immune system, including mononuclear leukocytes in the lamina propria and organized gut-associated lymphoid tissue, are identifiable by 200 days gestation, these do not reach functional maturity until 4 to 6 months after birth.[7–10] Many of the mechanisms through which this maturation occurs are intrinsic to the intestine; however, extrinsic stimuli, such as those provided by human milk, augment the intrinsic mechanisms. This is particularly

important for infants born preterm, who have not had the full complement of *in utero* development.

Human milk promotes the development of the intestinal immune system and protects preterm infants against adverse consequences. These include intestinal injuries and dysfunction (often placed under the umbrella term *necrotizing enterocolitis* or *NEC*), chronic lung disease, infection, sepsis, and retinopathy of prematurity. Interactions between human milk bioactive components and the developing neonate also play a major role in later neurodevelopment, food allergy, inflammatory bowel disease, metabolic syndrome, and even transgenerational outcomes.

WHAT'S SPECIAL ABOUT THE PRETERM INFANT

Many aspects of the innate immune system are present at the time of term birth, but many are lacking when the infant is born preterm.[11] At birth, even in infants born at term, the adaptive immune system is not yet trained and hence relies on transplacental passage of maternal IgG during the last three months of gestation in addition to maternal antibodies provided via breastfeeding.[12] The immune response to gut pathogens in term newborns requires protein components from mother's milk to efficiently fulfill toll-like receptor (TLR) binding and signal transduction.[13] Innate immune functions in the fetus are developmentally regulated during pregnancy; hence, the preterm infant has a high propensity to be at risk of developing severe infections.[12]

The significantly higher risk of infection for preterm infants is influenced by several factors (Fig. 8.2).[14] Infants born preterm have reduced proportions of peripheral blood lymphocytes, fewer Paneth cells, reduced production of antimicrobial peptides, a patchy intestinal mucus layer, higher permeability of the epithelial tight junctions, and lower counts of phagocytic peripheral monocytes.[15] Additionally, passive immunity transferred to the fetus via the placenta increases with gestational age.

Breastfeeding

Breastfeeding has been shown to reduce infant mortality by 12% compared to formula feeding and to be greatly beneficial in both short- and long-term disease prevention.[16] Numerous mechanisms related to

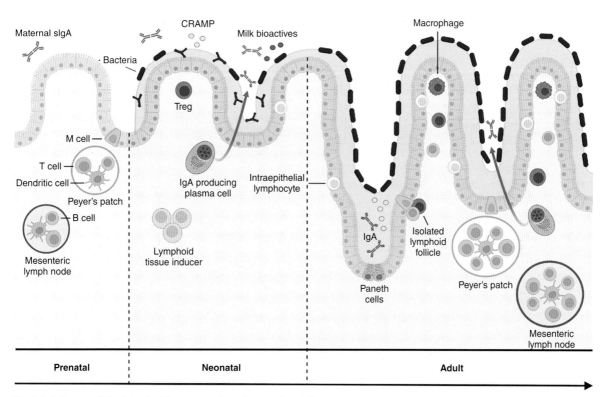

Fig. 8.1 Ontogeny of the intestinal immune system. Compared to full-term neonates, preterm neonates have few Paneth cells, reduced antimicrobial peptides, less mucosal covering, and higher permeability of the epithelial tight junctions. *CRAMP*, Cathelicidin-related antimicrobial peptide; *Treg*, regulatory T cell. Adapted from Brandtzaeg P. Role of the intestinal immune system in health. In: Baumgart DC, ed. *Crohn's Disease and Ulcerative Colitis: From Epidemiology and Immunobiology to a Rational Diagnostic and Therapeutic Approach.* Cham: Springer International Publishing; 2017: 23-56.

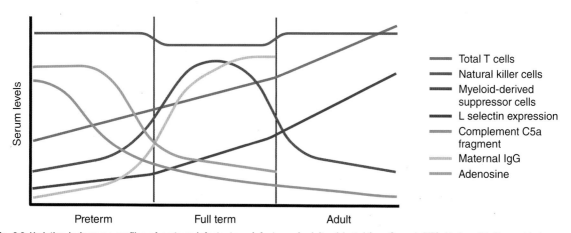

Fig. 8.2 Variation in immune profiles of preterm infants, term infants, and adults. Adapted from Sampah MES, Hackam DJ. Dysregulated mucosal immunity and associated pathogeneses in preterm neonates. *Front Immunol.* 2020;11:899. doi:10.3389/fimmu.2020.00899.

immune, nutritional, and bioactive components of human milk have been reported to account for this beneficial effect.

Human milk is a dynamic biofluid that is responsive to infant and mammary health status. Temporal changes to human milk composition occur over the course of lactation (from colostrum to mature milk), over a day (circadian rhythms), and even over the course of a feed. Some bioactive factors of human milk are at a higher concentration in colostrum (the "first milk") due to open tight junctions between mammary epithelial cells during this period (Table 8.1).[17] Among these, immunoglobulins and immune cells provide passive immunity transfer from the mother. The high concentration of these protective factors in colostrum provides early protection during the vulnerable neonatal period. Transfer of maternal cells is also thought to help with immune responses and tissue repair.

Human Milk Bioactive Components

Human milk contains a variety of bioactive factors such as hormones, cytokines, leukocytes, immunoglobulins, lactoferrin, lysozyme, stem cells, oligosaccharides (HMOs), microbiota, metabolites, and microRNAs (Table 8.1). Understanding the roles of human milk bioactive factors on immune function provides a scientific basis upon which to build breastfeeding recommendations. It may also enhance subsequent health in those infants who can only formula feed by providing modifications to formulas that provide some of the benefits incurred by human milk. However, there is still much to learn about interactions between the various human milk components and the mechanisms underlying their health benefits. Here we will discuss the major bioactive components of human milk and their role in intestinal ontogeny and immune development.

TABLE 8.1   Bioactive Components of Human Milk and Their Function[a]

Human Milk Component	Function	Concentration in Colostrum	Concentration in Mature Milk
Lactoferrin	Immunomodulation, antiviral, antibacterial, iron metabolism	5.8 g/L	2 g/L
Lysozyme	Antibacterial and antiviral	0.36 g/L	0.4 g/L
Microbes	Infant microbiome colonization, infant immune training	10^6 cells/mL	10^6 cells/mL
Exosomes	Cell-to-cell communication, carriers of "cargo" such as nucleic acids and proteins	1.62 particles/mL	0.4 particles/mL
Immunoglobulins	Transfer of immunity from mother to infants, aggregation of bacteria for immune exclusion, entrapment of bacteria via hydrophily, reduction of bacterial motility via binding to flagella	IgA: 7.8 g/L IgG: 0.5 g/L	IgA: 1 g/L IgG: 0.05 g/L
Enzymes	Digestion, absorption, mitigation of inflammation	Amylase: 4.1 U/L Lipoprotein lipase: 624 mU/L	Amylase: 2.9 U/L Lipoprotein lipase: 534 mU/L
Growth factors	Maturation of intestinal mucosa, neuronal growth, stimulation of cell proliferation and maturation, angiogenesis	EGF: 366 ng/mL TGF-α: 84 ng/mL VEGF: 23 mg/L	EGF: 191 ng/mL TGF-α: 140 ng/mL VEGF: 14 mg/L
Oligosaccharides	Prebiotic stimulation of bacterial growth, decoy pathogen receptors, immune modulation	20–30 g/L	5–15 g/L
miRNAs	Modulation of immune pathways, microbial colonization, oxidative stress, inflammation, development	782 known 67 unique	805 known 89 unique

[a]Many of these compounds are targets of active research for addition to commercial formulas due to their potentially beneficial activities.
EGF, Epidermal growth factor; *VEGF*, vascular endothelial growth factor.

Proteins and Peptides

It is well recognized that breastfed infants have fewer infections than formula-fed infants. Several human milk proteins have been shown to be involved in protecting against infection (Fig. 8.3).[20,21] These are discussed in the subsections that follow.

LACTOFERRIN

After whey and casein, lactoferrin is the most abundant protein in breast milk. Its role is multifaceted (Fig. 8.4): it plays a major role in immunity of the infant, prevents infection, is involved in iron metabolism, has antiinflammatory properties, and is an antioxidant.

In the early 1970s, human milk was found to have bacteriostatic activity against *Escherichia coli*.[20] The active agent, lactoferrin, was found to be a protein with high affinity for iron. Lactoferrin can sequester environmental iron required for pathogen survival. This action confers a bacteriostatic effect that inhibits the growth or reproduction of bacteria. As a corollary, the growth of those bacteria that do not require much iron is enhanced. Many of these taxa that do not require iron are beneficial to humans, such as *Lactobacillus* and *Bifidobacterium*. Lactoferrin also has a direct bactericidal function.[21] With its high positive ionic charge, lactoferrin can form a complex with lipopolysaccharide (LPS), a highly negatively charged bacterial cell wall component, creating holes in the outer membrane of Gram-negative bacteria. These membrane breaches can be fatal for bacteria and can allow penetration of another human milk protein, lysozyme, which degrades the proteoglycan matrix and kills the bacterium.[22]

In addition to its antibacterial activities, lactoferrin also has important antiviral properties. The antiviral action of lactoferrin is mediated through its ability to block viral entry into host cells. It does this by binding to heparan sulfate glycosaminoglycan cell receptors or by binding directly to viral particles.[23] As such, lactoferrin's antiviral action is important during the initial

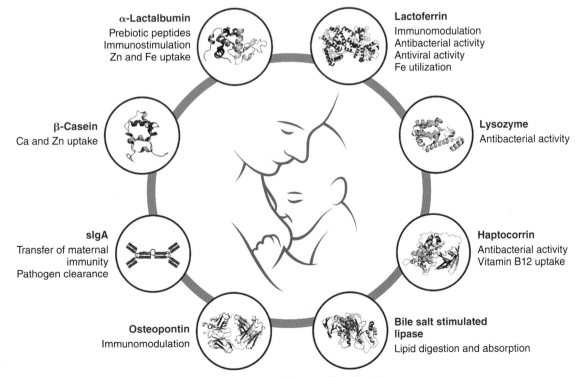

Fig. 8.3 Bioactive proteins in human milk and their functions.

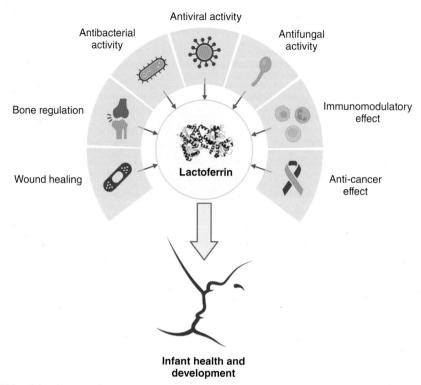

Fig. 8.4 The manifold functions of human milk lactoferrin in infant health and development. Adapted from Elzoghby AO, Abdelmoneem MA, Hassanin IA, et al. Lactoferrin, a multi-functional glycoprotein: active therapeutic, drug nanocarrier & targeting ligand. *Biomaterials*. 2020;263:120355. doi:10.1016/j.biomaterials.2020.120355.

phase of infection. Highly relevant to the recent CO-VID-19 pandemic is evidence that lactoferrin can bind to at least some of the receptors used by coronaviruses and thereby block their entry.[24] Thus lactoferrin may contribute to protection from COVID-19 infection in breastfed infants.

The iron-binding capacity of lactoferrin increases intestinal iron absorption. Each lactoferrin molecule can bind two iron ions. Lactoferrin molecules enter intestinal epithelial cells via their own receptor, then release their bound iron into the cell for transportation to the circulation via transferrin.[25] Lactoferrin thereby aids in iron uptake from human milk, which is notably low in iron.

Lactoferrin levels change as milk matures. Colostrum has higher concentrations in both term and preterm milk.[26,27] Preterm milk tends to maintain higher levels of lactoferrin over time, providing prolonged protection from infection for these vulnerable infants.[27] Concentrations of lactoferrin similar to those

found in human milk increase intestinal cell proliferation, whereas lower concentrations increase intestinal cell differentiation.[18,28] The implications for this finding are that the intestinal mucosa of breastfed infants is more developed than that of formula-fed infants. Increased mucosal development caused by lactoferrin may therefore increase the mucosal surface and enhance the uptake of iron as well as other nutrients.

Lactoferrin is also present in cow's milk; however, studies *in vitro* have shown that human milk is more effective in preventing bacterial growth than cow's milk.[29] Studies investigating the addition of cow's milk lactoferrin to breast milk, donor human milk, and infant formula have shown no differences in late outcomes of preterm infants between treated and control infants.[30–32]

LYSOZYME

Widely distributed in tears, saliva, and milk,[33,34] lysozyme plays important roles as a nonspecific immune factor.[35] *Lysozyme*, first described by Alexander Fleming in 1922,[36] is an enzyme that catalyzes the hydrolysis of 1,4 beta linkages between sugar molecules found in peptidoglycan, which is the major component of the Gram-positive bacterial cell wall. This hydrolysis of peptidoglycan compromises the integrity of bacterial cell walls causing lysis (or disintegration) of the bacteria, hence its name. In addition to its bactericidal effects on Gram-positive bacteria, it acts synergistically with lactoferrin to destroy Gram-negative bacteria. Following penetration of the cell wall by lactoferrin, lysozyme can enter the cell and disrupt cellular respiration.[37]

The lysozyme content of human milk ranges from 3 to 3000 μg/mL, and the typical concentration is about 200–400 μg/mL.[38,39] Cow's milk comparatively contains only minute quantities of lysozyme and has a lower activity compared to human milk.[40,41] Reduced lysozyme sulfate levels have been associated with bronchopulmonary dysplasia in preterm newborns.[42] The relevance of this association between lysozyme, which is found in high concentrations in human milk, and a lower incidence of bronchopulmonary dysplasia seen in preterm infants is of interest, but causality has not yet been proven.

BILE SALT–STIMULATED LIPASE

Lipid digestion is critical for infant development. Milk fat is partially hydrolyzed in the stomach and further hydrolyzed in the upper small intestine. The major lipases aiding fat digestion in the newborn small intestine are pancreatic lipase and bile salt-stimulated lipase (BSSL) derived from the exocrine pancreas and milk, respectively.[43] The relative role of the milk-derived lipase is not clear; however, it is known that pancreatic lipase production and secretion in the first several weeks after birth is limited.[44,45] Thus human milk BSSL may compensate for the low endogenous capacity to digest lipids in early life. BSSL hydrolyzes triglycerides, diglycerides, and monoglycerides found in human milk, which are extremely important for preterm infant health.[46] However, heat pasteurization of donor human milk, which is routinely fed to preterm infants, destroys BSSL, leading to reduced lipid absorption.[47] Therefore alternative pasteurization methods, such as high-pressure processing and UV-C irradiation, are currently being explored.

OSTEOPONTIN

Osteopontin (OPN), also called *bone sialoprotein*, is found primarily in bone matrix but also various other organs. OPN is involved in normal physiologic processes and plays a critical role in normal bone mineralization and in response to external stress.[48] It anchors osteoclasts to the surface of bones and is involved in the process of bone resorption.[49]

In addition to its function in bone, OPN possesses immunomodulatory, cell attachment, migration, proliferation, and differentiation functions.[50] OPN is synthesized by a variety of tissues and appears in almost all body fluids, including human milk,[51] where it is one of the five most abundant milk proteins.[18] OPN concentrations are higher in colostrum (~178 mg/L) than in mature milk (~54 mg/L).[52] Compared to human milk, bovine milk and infant formula contain significantly less OPN: ~18 and ~9 mg/L in bovine milk and infant formula, respectively.[53] Studies with a commercial formula supplemented with bovine OPN found that infants fed formula with supplemental bovine osteopontin (bOPN) exhibited lower serum levels of inflammatory cytokines[54] and an immune cell profile more similar to that of breastfed infants than to that of infants fed regular formula.[55] The consequences of these findings for infant health and/or protection against disease are yet to be elucidated.

IMMUNOGLOBULINS

Immunoglobulins are glycoprotein molecules produced by activated B cells and plasma cells in response to antigens. Maternal immunoglobulins provide passive immunity to infants via transfer across the placenta and transfer via breastfeeding. There are five different types of immunoglobulins: IgA, IgG, IgM, IgE, and IgD. IgG is the only Ig that crosses the placenta with the majority being transferred in the last 20 weeks of pregnancy.[56] In human milk all types of immunoglobulins are present, but the most abundant are secretory IgA (sIgA) followed by IgG.[57] sIgA serves as the first line of defense in the infant intestine.[58] sIgA in milk is partially digested in the stomach of both preterm and term infants and continues to the lower intestine where it provides immunity.[59] While sIgA levels in human milk decrease over the first 12 weeks after birth,[60] the cells that produce sIgA in the infant's intestine increase 10 to 20 times over the first 6 months after birth,[61] thus markedly diminishing the reliance on human milk sIgA.

IgG, the main immunoglobulin found in serum, is found in low concentrations in human milk but increases over time[62] and is higher in the milk of exclusively breastfeeding mothers compared to those who are nonexclusively breastfeeding. It is thought that human milk IgG plays a role in decreasing infections in infants.

IgM is also transferred to infants via human milk and in contrast to sIgA is partially digested by term infants while not digested by preterm infants. IgM is thought to provide protection against infections via opsonization of antigens for complement fixation and subsequent destruction.[63]

Banked donor milk contains significantly lower concentrations of IgA, sIgA, IgM, and IgG. This is thought to be important to infants receiving donor milk while in the NICU due to its frequent use. Immunoglobulins in donor milk are impacted by the lactation stage of mothers who donate (often >6 months postnatal), resulting in lower levels of some of these immunoglobulins. In addition, donor milk is also subjected to Holder pasteurization, which denatures immunoglobulins—in particular IgM and IgG, which are more sensitive to Holder pasteurization than IgA.[64] It is critical to note that donor milk as well as frozen MoM may not provide optimal immune protection for the infant. Through the enteromammary system, maternal immunity can be transferred to the breastfed infant, but if the exposure happened at a time remote from the time the milk was collected, this response would not be optimal since the infant only receives antibodies against the antigens to which the mother has already been exposed.[65]

BIOACTIVE PROTEINS INVOLVED IN NUTRIENT UTILIZATION

Nutrient utilization from human milk is known to be high. Therefore concentrations of nutrients in human milk are used for setting minimum concentrations of nutrients in infant formula. Several proteins in human milk have been shown to facilitate the uptake of nutrients (Fig. 8.3). The nutrient utilization properties of lactoferrin (iron absorption) and BSSL (lipid metabolism) have been discussed previously in this chapter.

Here we will focus on other proteins involved in nutrient utilization.

ALPHA-LACTALBUMIN

Alpha-lactalbumin (α-lactalbumin) comprises 10% to 20% of the protein in human milk. It has a specific binding site for calcium and another binding site for essential trace elements such as iron and zinc.[18] The uptake of iron is enhanced in infant rhesus monkeys fed infant formula with added bovine α-lactalbumin compared with regular formula. Although the mechanisms remain poorly understood, peptides from α-lactalbumin formed during digestion retain their binding capacity and facilitate the uptake of micronutrients by the mucosal cell.

HAPTOCORRIN

All vitamin B_{12} in human milk is bound to haptocorrin. Using cultured intestinal epithelial cells, it was found that uptake of radiolabeled vitamin B_{12} was increased by human haptocorrin, suggesting that haptocorrin may facilitate the absorption of vitamin B_{12} in young infants, a period when the production of intrinsic B_{12} is immature.[18]

BETA-CASEIN

Beta-casein forms several phosphopeptides during digestion. Several of these bind divalent cations such as calcium and zinc, and it has been suggested that they facilitate the absorption of these nutrients.[18]

Growth Factors and Hormones in Human Milk

Several hormones and growth factors are found in human milk that serve as bioactive agents, with functions in intestinal growth and development (Table 8.2).

GROWTH FACTORS

Growth and development of the intestines is strongly influenced by human milk. Both breastfeeding and weaning drive epithelial growth and differentiation, with breastfeeding promoting intestinal crypt fission and weaning promoting crypt hyperplasia.[9] These two events, influenced by growth factors provided in human milk,[8] significantly increase the surface area of the intestines.

TABLE 8.2   Growth Factors and Hormones of Human Milk and Their Function in the Intestine

Component	Functions
Epidermal growth factor	Stimulation of cell proliferation, maturation, and healing of the intestinal mucosa
Neuronal growth factors	Development of the enteric nervous system in newborns
Insulin-like growth factor	Stimulation of erythropoiesis, prevention of oxidative stress damage
Vascular endothelial growth factor	Regulation of angiogenesis
Erythropoietin	Responsible for increasing red blood cells
Adiponectin	Regulation of metabolism and suppression of inflammation
Leptin	Regulation of intestinal motility, absorption of macronutrients, stimulation of gut mucosal cell proliferation, inhibition of apoptosis

Several growth factors in human milk are important for infant intestinal development. Epidermal growth factor (EGF) plays a critical role in cell proliferation, prevention of apoptosis, intestinal maturation, and repair.[66,67] EGF survives infant gastric digestion and has bioactivity within the intestine. EGF levels are 2000 times higher in colostrum than in mature milk and decrease with lactation.[67,68] EGF levels are also higher in preterm milk,[67,68] again highlighting the dynamic and responsive nature of mother's milk.

Human milk also contains neural growth factors, including brain-derived neurotrophic factor (BDNF) and glial cell line–derived neurotrophic factor (GDNF), which function in the development and maturation of the infant enteric nervous system (ENS). BDNF has been shown to influence peristalsis while GDNF stimulates neural outgrowth and survival.

Angiogenesis is regulated by vascular endothelial growth factor (VEGF) and its antagonists. Human milk VEGF therefore likely contributes to the development of infant intestinal vasculature.[69]

Insulin-like growth factor (IGF)-1 and IGF-2 are abundant in colostrum and decrease with lactation. IGF is taken up in its bioactive form by the intestine and transported to the blood.[70] IGF-1 protects the intestinal epithelium against damage caused by oxidative stress. Furthermore, it stimulates erythropoiesis and helps increase the red cell mass.[71]

A number of human milk growth factors are thought to be particularly beneficial for preterm infants. For instance, VGEF, which is notably lower in preterm compared to term milk, may play a role in prevention of retinopathy of prematurity,[72] and erythropoietin stimulates red blood cell production and is

thought to help prevent anemia of prematurity.[73] Additionally, EGF has been shown to be a key factor in the development of NEC. Evidence from animal studies demonstrates that EGF receptor knockout mice develop intestinal necrosis similar to neonatal NEC, and that supplementation with EGF can prevent NEC in a rat model of the condition.[74–77] In preterm neonates, serum, urine, and salivary EGF levels correlate positively with gestational age at delivery and negatively with NEC incidence.[78–80] Thus exposure to human milk growth factors may be a mechanism by which protection is conferred to the premature infant.

HORMONES

Human milk also contains hormones, such as leptin, adiponectin, ghrelin, and insulin, which play important roles in metabolism, energy homeostasis, and appetite control.

While leptin receives much attention for its impacts on the central nervous system (CNS), particularly the hypothalamus where it regulates appetite, growing evidence demonstrates a diverse range of functions for leptin in the gastrointestinal tract.[81] These include impacts on gastric emptying and small intestine motility, macronutrient absorption, and intestinal mucosal cell proliferation.[81] In neonatal piglets, leptin stimulates the development of intestinal mucosal morphometry and promotes proliferation of mucosal epithelial cells.[82] Further, leptin has immunomodulatory, inflammatory, and antiinflammatory effects and may play a role in healing ischemic injury in the gastrointestinal tract.[81] It is therefore of great interest in the context of preterm neonates.

Another important appetite-regulating hormone in human milk is adiponectin. Adiponectin regulates insulin sensitivity and has been shown to influence gastric emptying times in breastfed infants.[83] Additionally, adiponectin is able to attenuate inflammatory responses by modulating signaling pathways across a range of cell types.[84,85]

Carbohydrates

LACTOSE

Lactose, the primary sugar in human milk, provides osmotic pressure to increase volume. As with many components in human milk that have multiple roles, lactose may be considered a bioactive component, especially in preterm infants who have low lactase activity in the intestinal tract. Unhydrolyzed lactose is fermented by microbes in the distal intestine, resulting in the production of short-chain fatty acids (SCFAs),[86] which play important roles in mucosal immunity and interepithelial junction integrity.[87]

HUMAN MILK OLIGOSACCHARIDES

After lactose, human milk oligosaccharides (HMOs) represent the highest concentration of carbohydrate in human milk.[88,89] HMOs are the third most abundant solid component of human milk, with more than 200 structures identified. These complex sugars are indigestible to the infant and are not considered a macronutrient. Instead, they arrive in the intestine intact, where they act as prebiotics for the local microbiota, particularly bifidobacteria ("bifidogenic" role). As such, they promote a favorable intestinal microbiome for infants that is low in complexity and dominated by *Bifidobacterium* species. Development of the immune system is contingent on the microbial composition of the gastrointestinal tract,[90] highlighting the important role of HMOs. Like nondigestible fiber for adults, HMOs have raised considerable interest in terms of their function and potential for supplementation.

Since the discovery of HMOs in human milk[91] there has been a growing interest in their physiologic, immunologic, and epigenetic roles and how they relate to the microbial ecosystem in human milk and in the infant gastrointestinal tract.[92] In addition to serving as substrate for microbial metabolism, they function as antiadhesive and antimicrobial factors.[92] HMOs act as decoy receptors, binding potential pathogens such as *Pseudomonas aeruginosa*, *Salmonella enterica*,

and enteropathogenic *Escherichia coli*.[93] They have also been shown to prevent the growth and biofilm formation of *Streptococcus agalactiae* (Group B Streptococcus), the leading cause of pneumonia, meningitis, and sepsis in infants.[94,95] Further, by promoting a *Bifidobacterium*-dominated gut microbiome, HMOs support colonization resistance against pathogens. As such, HMOs are associated with a lower risk of various types of infections.[96]

HMOs are not only found in relatively high concentrations, but they also exhibit relatively high diversity compared to bovine milk oligosaccharides.[97] Bovine milk contains relatively few oligosaccharides and at far lower levels. Therefore there has been increasing interest in supplementing infant formula with selected HMOs, particularly 2'-FL.

HMOs are derived from simpler mono and disaccharides such as lactose. Elongation monosaccharides consist of galactose, N-acetyl-galactosamine, fucose, and sialic acid. Elongation with these mono and disaccharides is brought about by a series of enzymes found in the lactating mammary gland. Biological functions of oligosaccharides are closely related to their conformation, which is constructed via an elongation that is achieved by an enzymatic attachment of GlcNAc residues linked in ß1-3 or in ß1-6 linkage to a Gal residue followed by further addition of Gal in a ß-1-3 or ß-1-4 bond.[97,98]

HMO profiles vary in milk from mothers who give birth to preterm versus term infants,[97] with stage of lactation (colostrum, transitional, mature) being a key parameter affecting HMO composition. Maternal genetic polymorphisms in the Lewis blood groups are associated with structural differences in HMOs and their level of secretion.[99] HMO profiles differ dramatically based on Lewis blood group (FUT2 and FUT3 maternal polymorphisms). The prevalence of FUT2 negative genotypes varies across different geographies. Environmental and maternal factors may also contribute to HMO variability, but these are not currently well understood.[99]

Breastfed infants have a significantly higher abundance of *Bifidobacterium* species in their gut compared to formula-fed infants.[100] The dominance of bifidobacteria in the breastfed infant gut is highly relevant for intestinal development. HMO-promoted bifidobacteria, along with other HMO-fermenting species, such as *Bacteroides* species, metabolize HMOs to create SCFAs and other immune-modulating metabolites such as indoles. *Bifidobacteria longum* subspecies *infantis* (*B. infantis*), the most abundant species in the breastfed infant gut microbiome, has been shown to produce indole-3-lactic acid (ILA) when grown on HMOs.[101] ILA significantly attenuates inflammation in intestinal epithelial cells.[101] It is highly suspected that these activities are very relevant for the development of immune competence. Therefore HMOs are integral to the beneficial effect of a healthy infant gut microbiome.

In addition to their effect on the infant gut microbiota, HMOs may guide tolerogenic programming of the infant immune system to prevent the development of allergies and other immune-mediated illnesses.[102] HMOs may also provide protection against intestinal injury, with studies in preterm infants and animal models supporting this theory.[103] However, studies of oligosaccharide administration in preterm infants have been underpowered, and thus further research is required to support the contention that these agents may protect against intestinal injuries seen in preterm infants. Nevertheless, HMOs, which are not affected by heat pasteurization, may help explain the protective effect of human milk against NEC in preterm infants.

HMOs have also been investigated in relation to infant growth.[104,105] Studies linking HMOs and growth suggest that specific oligosaccharides may act via the microbiota in affecting infant body composition and growth. At this juncture, various proposed hypotheses and possible mechanistic pathways for HMOs have not been adequately tested.

Many functional processes in the brain depend on sialic acid bound to proteins and glycolipids. Human milk contains high levels of sialic acid primarily in the form of sialyllactose HMOs (predominantly 3'-SL and 6'-SL). Emerging evidence suggests that HMO-derived sialic acid may impact neurodevelopment in breastfed infants; however, these findings require further investigation.[106,107]

Microbiome

Numerous studies dating back more than a century demonstrated that bacteria are common in milk of healthy ruminants. However, milk microbes were traditionally viewed from a pathogenic perspective. More recently, human milk microbiota have been considered as normal commensal microbes that may play an important role in development of the infant gastrointestinal tract and immune development. Human milk harbors a low-diversity, low-biomass microbiome, which is commonly dominated by *Staphylococcus* and *Streptococcus* species, followed by other genera, such as *Veillonella*, *Corynebacterium*, *Propionibacterium*, and *Bifidobacterium*.[108] A small percent of human milk microbes colonize the infant gut, particularly *Bifidobacteria*.[109] Transfer of commensal bacteria from mother to infant via milk contributes to optimal early gut microbiome establishment, which underpins lifelong health. The early life gut microbiome plays important roles in programming immune tolerance and maturation, metabolic functions, and intestinal epithelial barrier function.[110,111] As such, aberrations to early microbiome colonization have been associated with the development of a wide range of noncommunicable diseases.[112] Interestingly, recent studies have suggested that a significant portion of the bacteria in human milk are nonviable and are coated in sIgA.[113,114] These bacteria would be unable to colonize the infant gut; however, they may still have a biological function in infant immune maturation. Exposure to nonliving or IgA-bound bacteria may present the developing mucosal immune system with an opportunity to encounter a range of microbes in a nonthreatening form, guiding immune education and tolerance.

Maternal and infant factors, including lactational stage, maternal pregestational body mass index (BMI), maternal gestational weight, mode of delivery, geographical location, antibiotics, parity, infant sex, and method of breastfeeding, influence the composition of the milk microbiome.[115] Donor milk is largely devoid of these microbes, and studies have suggested the possibility of "refaunation" of donor milk using small aliquots of fresh MoM samples incubated with donor milk for varying time periods.[116] Another consideration for preterm infants is the use of stored MoM, which is common in NICU settings. Cold storage (both refrigeration and freezing) has been shown to alter the viable microbiome profile of fresh milk.[4]

Human Milk Microbial Metabolites

Human milk contains a vast number of metabolites produced by either the mammary or maternal gut microbiota that are relevant for mammary and infant health.[117] While numerous studies have characterized the composition of the milk and infant microbiota, relatively little study has been performed on microbial metabolites in human milk. This is an important research gap, as metabolites are the effectors through which microbes impact host health.[118] Here we briefly discuss key metabolites of interest in infant intestinal ontogeny (Fig. 8.5). From the information provided, it is clear that characterizing the bacterial taxa present in human milk does not provide the same level of functional information that integration of metabolomic and metagenomic information does. Additional integration with epigenetic data will further expand our understanding of the role of the microbiome and its metabolic products in infant development. This will provide important new information related to developmental potential, aid in the development of predictive biomarkers, and provide preventive strategies against future disease.

SHORT-CHAIN FATTY ACIDS

SCFAs, including butyrate, acetate, and propionate, result from bacterial fermentation of fiber in the maternal gut and may reach the mammary gland through the bloodstream. SCFAs are also produced by the infant gut microbiota upon their metabolism of HMOs. These metabolites play multifaceted roles in human homeostasis via their interactions with the immune and neuroendocrine systems, contributing to the immunologic, metabolic, and neurologic programming of the host.[119] In particular, they promote expansion and differentiation of regulatory T cells, inhibit inflammation, promote intestinal barrier integrity, regulate lipid metabolism and glucose homeostasis, and influence epigenetic imprinting.[120,121] Emerging evidence from animal models suggests that supplementation of pregnant and lactating mothers with fiber, prebiotics, or SCFAs protects offspring from developing allergic disease.[122–124] Human milk SCFAs have also been linked to infant body composition in the first year of life.[125]

INDOLES

As products of tryptophan metabolism by intestinal bacteria, indoles interact with the aryl hydrocarbon

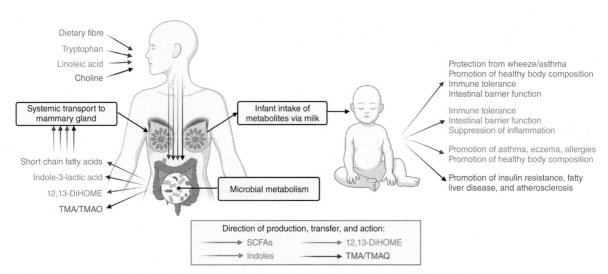

Fig. 8.5 Potential impacts of maternally derived microbial metabolites on developmental programming in the breastfed infant. *12,13-DiHOME*, 12,13-Dihydroxy-9Z-octadecenoic acid; *SCFAs*, short-chain fatty acids; *TMA*, trimethylamine; *TMAO*, trimethylamine N-oxide. Sourced from Stinson LF, Geddes DT. Microbial metabolites: the next frontier in human milk. *Trends Microbiol.* 2022;30(5):408-410. doi:10.1016/j.tim.2022.02.007.

receptor (AhR) and farnesoid X receptors (FXRs)[119] and thereby play integral roles in innate immunity, intestinal epithelial barrier integrity, and suppression of inflammation. AhR is a ligand-activated transcription factor that integrates environmental, dietary, microbial, and metabolic cues to control complex transcription. FXRs play a critical role in regulating bile acid, carbohydrate, and lipid metabolism. FXRs also possess potent antiinflammatory and antifibrotic properties. Of particular interest is ILA, which is being explored as a defense against NEC for preterm infants due to its powerful antiinflammatory properties.[126]

Human milk is the only source of tryptophan for the exclusively breastfed infant; however, to date no study has reported the presence of indoles in human milk. Typical human milk and infant gut bifidobacterial species have been shown to produce ILA from tryptophan, and ILA production is increased when these species are grown on HMOs.[101,127] Further, breastfed infants have higher levels of ILA in their stool compared to formula-fed infants.[128] ILA therefore is likely to be produced by infant gut or milk bifidobacteria.

Human Milk Extracellular Vesicles

Extracellular vesicles (EVs) are lipid bilayer bound particles that are released from cells. EVs consist of a variety of subtypes, including exosomes, microvesicles (MVs), ectosomes, and apoptotic bodies, and can be differentiated using methods such as ultracentrifugation.[129] EVs play important roles in cell-to-cell communication by delivering proteins, nucleic acids, and metabolites to recipient cells (Fig. 8.6).[130] EVs are increasingly recognized for their functions within both the innate and adaptive immune systems, including mediation of inflammation, promotion of intestinal barrier integrity, antigen presentation, and activation of B and T cells.[131] Human milk contains EVs with a range of functional properties that play roles in gut maturation, immunomodulation, mitigation of intestinal damage, and defense against viral infection.[132] In vitro studies have demonstrated that milk-derived EVs survive simulated gastric and intestinal digestion and may thereby directly impact infant intestinal physiology.[133] Infant formula completely lacks EVs, while bovine milk contains EVs that differ in profile and function to those found in human milk.[133]

miRNA

miRNAs are small noncoding RNAs (~22 nucleotides) that regulate posttranscriptional expression of genes primarily by destabilizing mRNA thus inhibiting

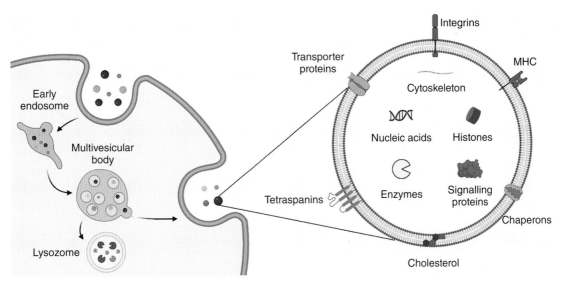

Fig. 8.6 Extracellular vesicle biogenesis and cargo. *MHC*, Major histocompatibility complex.

protein translation.[134,135] Compared to other body fluids, human milk is exceptionally rich in miRNA.[136]

Human milk miRNAs are packaged in exosomes that can survive the chemical conditions of the intestine and be absorbed by the intestinal epithelium.[137,138] It is thought that these miRNAs are derived from mammary gland immune cells.[139] These miRNAs are also thought to regulate the innate immune response via TLR4 signaling and macrophage activation.[140,141]

Another role for exosome mediated miRNA is a novel mechanism of genetic exchange via cargo delivery between maternal mammary epithelium and infant intestinal cells. From the intestinal cells, miRNA may be transferred into the infant bloodstream to cells in other tissues. The transfer of this genetic material to the infant can affect gene transcription and regulation of cellular events in several tissues, contributing to the immune programming.[142]

We are just beginning to understand the specific roles of human milk miRNAs. There is currently a need to develop a better understanding of how these affect the intestinal microbiota and infant intestinal immune system.

Summary

Human milk bioactive factors program the infant mucosal immune system and guide intestinal development. The bioactive substances within human milk are of great benefit to the preterm infant intestine, protecting against infection, inflammation, and injury. Many of the bioactive components in human milk are missing or are at far lower levels in bovine milk and infant formula, highlighting the importance of species-specific nutrition. Further, milk processing methods, such as pasteurization or cold storage, alter the composition and functionality of human milk bioactive factors. This is a significant consideration for preterm infants, who are commonly fed stored MoM or pasteurized donor human milk. Synergies between human milk bioactive components likely contribute to the myriad health benefits of this dynamic biofluid. Therefore integrated analyses are required to better understand interactions between various human milk bioactive factors within the infant.

REFERENCES

1. Walker A. Breast milk as the gold standard for protective nutrients. *J Pediatr.* 2010;156(suppl 2):S3-S7. doi:10.1016/j.jpeds.2009.11.021.
2. Paulaviciene IJ, Liubsys A, Eidukaite A, Molyte A, Tamuliene L, Usonis V. The effect of prolonged freezing and Holder pasteurization on the macronutrient and bioactive protein compositions of human milk. *Breastfeed Med.* 2020;15(9):583-588. doi:10.1089/bfm.2020.0219.
3. Guerra AF, Mellinger-Silva C, Rosenthal A, Luchese RH. Hot topic: holder pasteurization of human milk affects some bioactive proteins. *J Dairy Sci.* 2018;101(4):2814-2818. doi:10.3168/jds.2017-13789.
4. Stinson LF, Trevenen ML, Geddes DT. Effect of cold storage on the viable and total bacterial populations in human milk. *Nutrients.* 2022;14(9):1875. doi:10.3390/nu14091875.
5. Bode L, Raman AS, Murch SH, Rollins NC, Gordon JI. Understanding the mother-breastmilk-infant "triad." *Science.* 2020;367(6482):1070-1072. doi:10.1126/science.aaw6147.
6. Conroy ME, Walker WA. Intestinal immune health. *Nestle Nutr Workshop Ser Pediatr Program.* 2008;62:111-121; discussion 21-25. doi:10.1159/000146255.
7. Montgomery RK, Mulberg AE, Grand RJ. Development of the human gastrointestinal tract: twenty years of progress. *Gastroenterology.* 1999;116(3):702-731. doi:10.1016/s0016-5085(99)70193-9.
8. Hirai C, Ichiba H, Saito M, Shintaku H, Yamano T, Kusuda S. Trophic effect of multiple growth factors in amniotic fluid or human milk on cultured human fetal small intestinal cells. *J Pediatr Gastroenterol Nutr.* 2002;34(5):524-528. doi:10.1097/00005176-200205000-00010.
9. Cummins AG, Thompson FM. Effect of breast milk and weaning on epithelial growth of the small intestine in humans. *Gut.* 2002;51(5):748-754. doi:10.1136/gut.51.5.748.
10. Rognum TO, Thrane S, Stoltenberg L, Vege A, Brandtzaeg P. Development of intestinal mucosal immunity in fetal life and the first postnatal months. *Pediatr Res.* 1992;32(2):145-149. doi:10.1203/00006450-199208000-00003.
11. Van Belkum M, Mendoza Alvarez L, Neu J. Preterm neonatal immunology at the intestinal interface. *Cell Mol Life Sci.* 2020;77(7):1209-1227. doi:10.1007/s00018-019-03316-w.
12. Nussbaum C, Sperandio M. Innate immune cell recruitment in the fetus and neonate. *J Reprod Immunol.* 2011;90(1):74-81. doi:10.1016/j.jri.2011.01.022.
13. Goldman AS. The immune system in human milk and the developing infant. *Breastfeed Med.* 2007;2(4):195-204. doi:10.1089/bfm.2007.0024.
14. Goldman AS, Chheda S. The immune system in human milk: a historic perspective. *Ann Nutr Metab.* 2021;77(4):189-196. doi:10.1159/000516995.
15. Milcic TL. The complete blood count. *Neonatal Netw.* 2010;29(2):109-115. doi:10.1891/0730-0832.29.2.109.
16. Oddy WH. Breastfeeding protects against illness and infection in infants and children: a review of the evidence. *Breastfeed Rev.* 2001;9(2):11-18.
17. Stelwagen K, Singh K. The role of tight junctions in mammary gland function. *J Mammary Gland Biol Neoplasia.* 2014;19(1):131-138. doi:10.1007/s10911-013-9309-1.
18. Lönnerdal B. Bioactive proteins in human milk: health, nutrition, and implications for infant formulas. *J Pediatr.* 2016;173(suppl):S4-S9. doi:10.1016/j.jpeds.2016.02.070.
19. Lönnerdal B. Bioactive proteins in human milk: mechanisms of action. *J Pediatr.* 2010;156(suppl 2):S26-S30. doi:10.1016/j.jpeds.2009.11.017.

20. Bullen JJ. Iron-binding proteins and other factors in milk responsible for resistance to *Escherichia coli*. In: Elliott K, Knight J, eds. *Ciba Foundation Symposium 42 - Acute Diarrhoea in Childhood*. 1976. https://doi.org/10.1002/9780470720240.ch9.

21. Arnold RR, Cole MF, McGhee JR. A bactericidal effect for human lactoferrin. *Science*. 1977;197(4300):263-265. doi:10.1126/science.327545.

22. Ellison RT 3rd, Giehl TJ. Killing of gram-negative bacteria by lactoferrin and lysozyme. *J Clin Invest*. 1991;88(4):1080-1091. doi:10.1172/JCI115407.

23. Berlutti F, Pantanella F, Natalizi T, et al. Antiviral properties of lactoferrin—a natural immunity molecule. *Molecules*. 2011;16(8):6992-7018. doi:10.3390/molecules16086992.

24. Bolat E, Eker F, Kaplan M, et al. Lactoferrin for COVID-19 prevention, treatment, and recovery. *Front Nutr*. 2022;9:992733. doi:10.3389/fnut.2022.992733.

25. Suzuki YA, Lonnerdal B. Characterization of mammalian receptors for lactoferrin. *Biochem Cell Biol*. 2002;80(1):75-80. doi:10.1139/o01-228.

26. Albenzio M, Santillo A, Stolfi I, et al. Lactoferrin levels in human milk after preterm and term delivery. *Am J Perinatol*. 2016;33(11):1085-1089. doi:10.1055/s-0036-1586105.

27. Hirai Y, Kawakata N, Satoh K, et al. Concentrations of lactoferrin and iron in human milk at different stages of lactation. *J Nutr Sci Vitaminol (Tokyo)*. 1990;36(6):531-544. doi:10.3177/jnsv.36.531.

28. Buccigrossi V, de Marco G, Bruzzese E, et al. Lactoferrin induces concentration-dependent functional modulation of intestinal proliferation and differentiation. *Pediatr Res*. 2007;61(4):410-414. doi:10.1203/pdr.0b013e3180332c8d.

29. Yang Z, Jiang R, Chen Q, et al. Concentration of lactoferrin in human milk and its variation during lactation in different Chinese populations. *Nutrients*. 2018;10(9):1235. doi:10.3390/nu10091235.

30. Griffiths J, Jenkins P, Vargova M, et al. Enteral lactoferrin to prevent infection for very preterm infants: the ELFIN RCT. *Health Technol Assess*. 2018;22(74):1-60. doi:10.3310/hta22740.

31. Griffiths J, Jenkins P, Vargova M, et al. Enteral lactoferrin supplementation for very preterm infants: a randomised placebo-controlled trial. *Lancet*. 2019;393(10170):423-433. doi:10.1016/S0140-6736(18)32221-9.

32. Asztalos EV, Barrington K, Lodha A, Tarnow-Mordi W, Martin A. Lactoferrin infant feeding trial_Canada (LIFT_Canada): protocol for a randomized trial of adding lactoferrin to feeds of very-low-birth-weight preterm infants. *BMC Pediatr*. 2020;20(1):40. doi:10.1186/s12887-020-1938-0.

33. Mason DY, Taylor CR. The distribution of muramidase (lysozyme) in human tissues. *J Clin Pathol*. 1975;28(2):124-132. doi:10.1136/jcp.28.2.124.

34. Hankiewicz J, Swierczek E. Lysozyme in human body fluids. *Clin Chim Acta*. 1974;57(3):205-209. doi:10.1016/0009-8981(74)90398-2.

35. Ogundele MO. A novel anti-inflammatory activity of lysozyme: modulation of serum complement activation. *Mediators Inflamm*. 1998;7(5):363-365. doi:10.1080/09629359890893.

36. Fleming A. On a remarkable bacteriolytic element found in tissues and secretions. Proceedings of the Royal Society of London Series B, Containing Papers of a Biological Character. 1922;93(653):306-317.

37. Ibrahim HR, Imazato K, Ono H. Human lysozyme possesses novel antimicrobial peptides within its N-terminal domain that target bacterial respiration. *J Agric Food Chem*. 2011;59(18):10336-10345. doi:10.1021/jf2020396.

38. Chandan RC, Shahani KM, Holly RG. Lysozyme content of human milk. *Nature*. 1964;204:76-77. doi:10.1038/204076a0.

39. Montagne P, Cuillière ML, Molé C, Béné MC, Faure G. Changes in lactoferrin and lysozyme levels in human milk during the first twelve weeks of lactation. *Adv Exp Med Biol*. 2001;501:241-247. doi:10.1007/978-1-4615-1371-1_30.

40. Piccinini R, Binda E, Belotti M, Casirani G, Zecconi A. Comparison of blood and milk non-specific immune parameters in heifers after calving in relation to udder health. *Vet Res*. 2005;36(5-6):747-757. doi:10.1051/vetres:2005030.

41. Ito Y, Yamada H, Nakamura M, Yoshikawa A, Ueda T, Imoto T. The primary structures and properties of non-stomach lysozymes of sheep and cow, and implication for functional divergence of lysozyme. *Eur J Biochem*. 1993;213(2):649-658. doi:10.1111/j.1432-1033.1993.tb17805.x.

42. Revenis ME, Kaliner MA. Lactoferrin and lysozyme deficiency in airway secretions: association with the development of bronchopulmonary dysplasia. *J Pediatr*. 1992;121(2):262-270. doi:10.1016/s0022-3476(05)81201-6.

43. He X, McClorry S, Hernell O, Lönnerdal B, Slupsky CM. Digestion of human milk fat in healthy infants. *Nutr Res*. 2020;83:15-29. doi:10.1016/j.nutres.2020.08.002.

44. Cleghorn G, Durie P, Benjamin L, Dati F. The ontogeny of serum immunoreactive pancreatic lipase and cationic trypsinogen in the premature human infant. *Biol Neonate*. 1988;53(1):10-16. doi:10.1159/000242756.

45. Manson WG, Weaver LT. Fat digestion in the neonate. *Arch Dis Child Fetal Neonatal Ed*. 1997;76(3):F206-F211. doi:10.1136/fn.76.3.f206.

46. Lönnerdal B. Bioactive proteins in breast milk. *J Paediatr Child Health*. 2013;49(suppl 1):1-7. doi:10.1111/jpc.12104.

47. Andersson Y, Sävman K, Blackberg L, Hernell O. Pasteurization of mother's own milk reduces fat absorption and growth in preterm infants. *Acta Paediatr*. 2007;96(10):1445-1449. doi:10.1111/j.1651-2227.2007.00450.x.

48. McKee MD, Addison WN, Kaartinen MT. Hierarchies of extracellular matrix and mineral organization in bone of the craniofacial complex and skeleton. *Cells Tissues Organs*. 2005;181(3-4):176-188. doi:10.1159/000091379.

49. Choi ST, Kim JH, Kang EJ, et al. Osteopontin might be involved in bone remodelling rather than in inflammation in ankylosing spondylitis. *Rheumatology (Oxford)*. 2008;47(12):1775-1779. doi:10.1093/rheumatology/ken385.

50. Denhardt DT, Guo X. Osteopontin: a protein with diverse functions. *FASEB J*. 1993;7(15):1475-1482.

51. Rangaswami H, Bulbule A, Kundu GC. Osteopontin: role in cell signaling and cancer progression. *Trends Cell Biol*. 2006;16(2):79-87. doi:10.1016/j.tcb.2005.12.005.

52. Jiang R, Lönnerdal B. Osteopontin in human milk and infant formula affects infant plasma osteopontin concentrations. *Pediatr Res*. 2019;85(4):502-505. doi:10.1038/s41390-018-0271-x.

53. Schack L, Lange A, Kelsen J, et al. Considerable variation in the concentration of osteopontin in human milk, bovine milk, and infant formulas. *J Dairy Sci*. 2009;92(11):5378-5385. doi:10.3168/jds.2009-2360.

54. West CE, Kvistgaard AS, Peerson JM, Donovan SM, Peng YM, Lönnerdal B. Effects of osteopontin-enriched formula on lymphocyte subsets in the first 6 months of life: a randomized controlled trial. *Pediatr Res*. 2017;82(1):63-71. doi:10.1038/pr.2017.77.

55. Lönnerdal B, Kvistgaard AS, Peerson JM, Donovan SM, Peng YM. Growth, nutrition, and cytokine response of breast-fed infants and infants fed formula with added bovine osteopontin. *J Pediatr Gastroenterol Nutr.* 2016;62(4):650-657. doi:10.1097/MPG.0000000000001005.

56. Malek A, Sager R, Kuhn P, Nicolaides KH, Schneider H. Evolution of maternofetal transport of immunoglobulins during human pregnancy. *Am J Reprod Immunol.* 1996;36(5):248-255. doi:10.1111/j.1600-0897.1996.tb00172.x.

57. Peitersen B, Bohn L, Andersen H. Quantitative determination of immunoglobulins, lysozyme, and certain electrolytes in breast milk during the entire period of lactation, during a 24-hour period, and in milk from the individual mammary gland. *Acta Pædiatr Scand.* 1975;64(5):709-717. doi:10.1111/j.1651-2227.1975.tb03909.x.

58. Silvey KJ, Hutchings AB, Vajdy M, Petzke MM, Neutra MR. Role of immunoglobulin A in protection against reovirus entry into Murine Peyer's patches. *J Virol.* 2001;75(22):10870-10879. doi:10.1128/JVI.75.22.10870-10879.2001.

59. Demers-Mathieu V, Underwood MA, Beverly RL, Nielsen SD, Dallas DC. Comparison of human milk immunoglobulin survival during gastric digestion between preterm and term infants. *Nutrients.* 2018;10(5):631. doi:10.3390/nu10050631.

60. Ballabio C, Bertino E, Coscia A, et al. Immunoglobulin-A profile in breast milk from mothers delivering full term and preterm infants. *Int J Immunopathol Pharmacol.* 2007;20(1):119-128. doi:10.1177/039463200702000114.

61. Perkkiö M, Savilahti E. Time of appearance of immunoglobulin-containing cells in the mucosa of the neonatal intestine. *Pediatr Res.* 1980;14(8):953-955. doi:10.1203/00006450-198008000-00012.

62. Abuidhail J, Al-Shudiefat AAR, Darwish M. Alterations of immunoglobulin G and immunoglobulin M levels in the breast milk of mothers with exclusive breastfeeding compared to mothers with non-exclusive breastfeeding during 6 months postpartum: the Jordanian cohort study. *Am J Hum Biol.* 2019;31(1):e23197. doi:10.1002/ajhb.23197.

63. Demers-Mathieu V, Huston RK, Markell AM, et al. Differences in maternal immunoglobulins within mother's own breast milk and donor breast milk and across digestion in preterm infants. *Nutrients.* 2019;11(4):920. doi:10.3390/nu11040920.

64. Ford J, Law B, Marshall VM, Reiter B. Influence of the heat treatment of human milk on some of its protective constituents. *J Pediatr.* 1977;90(1):29-35. doi:10.1016/s0022-3476(77)80759-2.

65. Rodríguez JM, Fernández L, Verhasselt V. The gut-breast axis: programming health for life. *Nutrients.* 2021;13(2):606. doi:10.3390/nu13020606.

66. Ballard O, Morrow AL. Human milk composition: nutrients and bioactive factors. *Pediatr Clin North Am.* 2013;60(1):49-74. doi:10.1016/j.pcl.2012.10.002.

67. Dvorak B, Fituch CC, Williams CS, Hurst NM, Schanler RJ. Increased epidermal growth factor levels in human milk of mothers with extremely premature infants. *Pediatr Res.* 2003;54(1):15-19. doi:10.1203/01.PDR.0000065729.74325.71.

68. Dvorak B, Fituch CC, Williams CS, Hurst NM, Schanler RJ. Concentrations of epidermal growth factor and transforming growth factor-alpha in preterm milk. *Adv Exp Med Biol.* 2004;554:407-409. doi:10.1007/978-1-4757-4242-8_52.

69. DiBiasie A. Evidence-based review of retinopathy of prematurity prevention in VLBW and ELBW infants. *Neonatal Netw.* 2006;25(6):393-403. doi:10.1891/0730-0832.25.6.393.

70. Philipps AF, Dvorák B, Kling PJ, Grille JG, Koldovský O. Absorption of milk-borne insulin-like growth factor-I into portal blood of suckling rats. *J Pediatr Gastroenterol Nutr.* 2000;31(2):128-135. doi:10.1097/00005176-200008000-00008.

71. Kling PJ, Taing KM, Dvorak B, Woodward SS, Philipps AF. Insulin-like growth factor-I stimulates erythropoiesis when administered enterally. *Growth Factors.* 2006;24(3):218-223. doi:10.1080/08977190600783162.

72. Loui A, Eilers E, Strauss E, Pohl-Schickinger A, Obladen M, Koehne P. Vascular endothelial growth factor (VEGF) and soluble VEGF receptor 1 (sFlt-1) levels in early and mature human milk from mothers of preterm versus term infants. *J Hum Lact.* 2012;28(4):522-528. doi:10.1177/0890334412447686.

73. Soubasi V, Kremenopoulos G, Diamanti E, Tsantali C, Sarafidis K, Tsakiris D. Follow-up of very low birth weight infants after erythropoietin treatment to prevent anemia of prematurity. *J Pediatr.* 1995;127(2):291-297. doi:10.1016/s0022-3476(95)70313-6.

74. Miettinen PJ, Berger JE, Meneses J, et al. Epithelial immaturity and multiorgan failure in mice lacking epidermal growth factor receptor. *Nature.* 1995;376(6538):337-341. doi:10.1038/376337a0.

75. Clark JA, Doelle SM, Halpern MD, et al. Intestinal barrier failure during experimental necrotizing enterocolitis: protective effect of EGF treatment. *Am J Physiol Gastrointest Liver Physiol.* 2006;291(5):G938-G949. doi:10.1152/ajpgi.00090.2006.

76. Clark JA, Lane RH, Maclennan NK, et al. Epidermal growth factor reduces intestinal apoptosis in an experimental model of necrotizing enterocolitis. *Am J Physiol Gastrointest Liver Physiol.* 2005;288(4):G755-G762. doi:10.1152/ajpgi.00172.2004.

77. Dvorak B, Halpern MD, Holubec H, et al. Epidermal growth factor reduces the development of necrotizing enterocolitis in a neonatal rat model. *Am J Physiol Gastrointest Liver Physiol.* 2002;282(1):G156-G164. doi:10.1152/ajpgi.00196.2001.

78. Warner BB, Ryan AL, Seeger K, Leonard AC, Erwin CR, Warner BW. Ontogeny of salivary epidermal growth factor and necrotizing enterocolitis. *J Pediatr.* 2007;150(4):358-363. doi:10.1016/j.jpeds.2006.11.059.

79. Shin CE, Falcone RA Jr, Stuart L, Erwin CR, Warner BW. Diminished epidermal growth factor levels in infants with necrotizing enterocolitis. *J Pediatr Surg.* 2000;35(2):173-176; discussion 177. doi:10.1016/s0022-3468(00)90005-8.

80. Helmrath MA, Shin CE, Fox JW, Erwin CR, Warner BW. Epidermal growth factor in saliva and serum of infants with necrotising enterocolitis. *Lancet.* 1998;351(9098):266-267. doi:10.1016/S0140-6736(05)78271-4.

81. Yarandi SS, Hebbar G, Sauer CG, Cole CR, Ziegler TR. Diverse roles of leptin in the gastrointestinal tract: modulation of motility, absorption, growth, and inflammation. *Nutrition.* 2011;27(3):269-275. doi:10.1016/j.nut.2010.07.004.

82. Woliński J, Biernat M, Guilloteau P, Westrom BR, Zabielski R. Exogenous leptin controls the development of the small intestine in neonatal piglets. *J Endocrinol.* 2003;177(2):215-222. doi:10.1677/joe.0.1770215.

83. Gridneva Z, Kugananthan S, Hepworth AR, et al. Effect of human milk appetite hormones, macronutrients, and infant characteristics on gastric emptying and breastfeeding patterns of term fully breast-fed infants. *Nutrients.* 2016;9(1):15. doi:10.3390/nu9010015.

84. Choi HM, Doss HM, Kim KS. Multifaceted physiological roles of adiponectin in inflammation and diseases. *Int J Mol Sci.* 2020;21(4):1219. doi:10.3390/ijms21041219.

85. Ouchi N, Walsh K. Adiponectin as an anti-inflammatory factor. *Clin Chim Acta.* 2007;380(1-2):24-30. doi:10.1016/j.cca.2007.01.026.

86. Roy CC, Kien CL, Bouthillier L, Levy E. Short-chain fatty acids: ready for prime time? *Nutr Clin Pract.* 2006;21(4): 351-366. doi:10.1177/0115426506021004351.

87. Ney LM, Wipplinger M, Grossmann M, Engert N, Wegner VD, Mosig AS. Short chain fatty acids: key regulators of the local and systemic immune response in inflammatory diseases and infections. *Open Biol.* 2023;13(3):230014. doi:10.1098/rsob.230014.

88. Corona L, Lussu A, Bosco A, et al. Human milk oligosaccharides: a comprehensive review towards metabolomics. *Children (Basel).* 2021;8(9):804. doi:10.3390/children8090804.

89. Bode L. Human milk oligosaccharides: every baby needs a sugar mama. *Glycobiology.* 2012;22(9):1147-1162. doi:10.1093/glycob/cws074.

90. Plaza-Díaz J, Fontana L, Gil A. Human milk oligosaccharides and immune system development. *Nutrients.* 2018;10(8): 1038. doi:10.3390/nu10081038.

91. Polonovski M, Montreuil J. Chromatographic study of the polyosides of human milk. *C R Hebd Seances Acad Sci.* 1954;238(23):2263-2264.

92. Craft KM, Townsend SD. Mother knows best: deciphering the antibacterial properties of human milk oligosaccharides. *Acc Chem Res.* 2019;52(3):760-768. doi:10.1021/acs.accounts.8b00630.

93. Weichert S, Jennewein S, Hüfner E, et al. Bioengineered 2'-fucosyllactose and 3-fucosyllactose inhibit the adhesion of *Pseudomonas aeruginosa* and enteric pathogens to human intestinal and respiratory cell lines. *Nutr Res.* 2013;33(10): 831-838. doi:10.1016/j.nutres.2013.07.009.

94. Chambers SA, Moore RE, Craft KM, et al. A solution to antifolate resistance in group B Streptococcus: untargeted metabolomics identifies human milk oligosaccharide-induced perturbations that result in potentiation of trimethoprim. *mBio.* 2020;11(2):e00076-20. doi:10.1128/mBio.00076-20.

95. Ackerman DL, Craft KM, Doster RS, et al. Antimicrobial and antibiofilm activity of human milk oligosaccharides against *Streptococcus agalactiae, Staphylococcus aureus,* and *Acinetobacter baumannii. ACS Infect Dis.* 2018;4(3):315-324. doi:10.1021/acsinfecdis.7b00183.

96. Duijts L, Jaddoe VW, Hofman A, Moll HA. Prolonged and exclusive breastfeeding reduces the risk of infectious diseases in infancy. *Pediatrics.* 2010;126(1):e18-e25. doi:10.1542/peds.2008-3256.

97. Kunz C, Rudloff S, Baier W, Klein N, Strobel S. Oligosaccharides in human milk: structural, functional, and metabolic aspects. *Annu Rev Nutr.* 2000;20:699-722. doi:10.1146/annurev.nutr.20.1.699.

98. Smilowitz JT, Lebrilla CB, Mills DA, German JB, Freeman SL. Breast milk oligosaccharides: structure-function relationships in the neonate. *Ann Rev Nutr.* 2014;34:143-169. doi:10.1146/annurev-nutr-071813-105721.

99. Lefebvre G, Shevlyakova M, Charpagne A, et al. Time of lactation and maternal fucosyltransferase genetic polymorphisms determine the variability in human milk oligosaccharides. *Front Nutr.* 2020;7:574459. doi:10.3389/fnut.2020.574459.

100. Walker WA. Initial intestinal colonization in the human infant and immune homeostasis. *Ann Nutr Metab.* 2013;63(suppl 2):8-15. doi:10.1159/000354907.

101. Ehrlich AM, Pacheco AR, Henrick BM, et al. Indole-3-lactic acid associated with Bifidobacterium-dominated microbiota significantly decreases inflammation in intestinal epithelial cells. *BMC Microbiol.* 2020;20(1):357. doi:10.1186/s12866-020-02023-y.

102. Doherty AM, Lodge CJ, Dharmage SC, Dai X, Bode L, Lowe AJ. Human milk oligosaccharides and associations with immune-mediated disease and infection in childhood: a systematic review. *Front Pediatr.* 2018;6:91. doi:10.3389/fped.2018.00091.

103. Bode L. Human milk oligosaccharides in the prevention of necrotizing enterocolitis: a journey from in vitro and in vivo models to mother-infant cohort studies. *Front Pediatr.* 2018;6:385. doi:10.3389/fped.2018.00385.

104. Eriksen KG, Christensen SH, Lind MV, Michaelsen KF. Human milk composition and infant growth. *Curr Opin Clin Nutr Metab Care.* 2018;21(3):200-206. doi:10.1097/MCO.0000000000000466.

105. Cheema AS, Gridneva Z, Furst AJ, et al. Human milk oligosaccharides and bacterial profile modulate infant body composition during exclusive breastfeeding. *Int J Mol Sci.* 2022; 23(5):2865. doi:10.3390/ijms23052865.

106. Mudd AT, Fleming SA, Labhart B, et al. Dietary sialyllactose influences sialic acid concentrations in the prefrontal cortex and magnetic resonance imaging measures in corpus callosum of young pigs. *Nutrients.* 2017;9(12):1297. doi:10.3390/nu9121297.

107. Oliveros E, Martín M, Torres-Espínola F, et al. Human milk levels of 2-fucosyllactose and 6-sialyllactose are positively associated with infant neurodevelopment and are not impacted by maternal BMI or diabetic status. *J Nutr Food Sci.* 2021; 4(1):100024.

108. Stinson LF, Sindi ASM, Cheema AS, et al. The human milk microbiome: who, what, when, where, why, and how? *Nutr Rev.* 2021;79(5):529-543. doi:10.1093/nutrit/nuaa029.

109. Sindi AS, Geddes DT, Wlodek ME, Muhlhausler BS, Payne MS, Stinson LF. Can we modulate the breastfed infant gut microbiota through maternal diet? *FEMS Microbiol Rev.* 2021;45(5):fuab011. doi:10.1093/femsre/fuab011.

110. Toscano M, De Grandi R, Grossi E, Drago L. Role of the human breast milk-associated microbiota on the newborns' immune system: a mini review. *Front Microbiol.* 2017;8:2100. doi:10.3389/fmicb.2017.02100.

111. Latuga MS, Stuebe A, Seed PC. A review of the source and function of microbiota in breast milk. *Semin Reprod Med.* 2014;32(1):68-73. doi:10.1055/s-0033-1361824.

112. Stinson LF. Establishment of the early-life microbiome: a DOHaD perspective. *J Dev Orig Health Dis.* 2020;11(3): 201-210. doi:10.1017/S2040174419000588.

113. Stinson LF, Trevenen ML, Geddes DT. The viable microbiome of human milk differs from the metataxonomic profile. *Nutrients.* 2021;13(12):4445. doi:10.3390/nu13124445.

114. Dzidic M, Mira A, Artacho A, Abrahamsson TR, Jenmalm MC, Collado MC. Allergy development is associated with consumption of breastmilk with a reduced microbial richness in the first month of life. *Pediatr Allergy Immunol.* 2020; 31(3):250-257. doi:10.1111/pai.13176.

115. Moossavi S, Sepehri S, Robertson B, et al. Composition and variation of the human milk microbiota are influenced by maternal and early-life factors. *Cell Host Microbe.* 2019; 25(2):324-335.e4. doi:10.1016/j.chom.2019.01.011.

116. DeBose-Scarlett E, Bendixen MM, Lorca GL, Parker LA. Human milk microbes: strategies to improve delivery to the infant. *Semin Perinatol.* 2021;45(6):151451. doi:10.1016/j.semperi.2021.151451.

117. Gay MC, Koleva PT, Slupsky CM, et al. Worldwide variation in human milk metabolome: indicators of breast physiology and maternal lifestyle? *Nutrients.* 2018;10(9):1151. doi:10.3390/nu10091151.

118. Descamps HC, Herrmann B, Wiredu D, Thaiss CA. The path toward using microbial metabolites as therapies. *EBioMedicine*. 2019;44:747-754. doi:10.1016/j.ebiom.2019.05.063.

119. Stinson LF, Geddes DT. Microbial metabolites: the next frontier in human milk. *Trends Microbiol*. 2022;30(5):408-410. doi:10.1016/j.tim.2022.02.007.

120. Tan J, McKenzie C, Potamitis M, Thorburn AN, Mackay CR, Macia L. The role of short-chain fatty acids in health and disease. *Adv Immunol*. 2014;121:91-119. doi:10.1016/B978-0-12-800100-4.00003-9.

121. Thorburn AN, Macia L, Mackay CR. Diet, metabolites, and "western-lifestyle" inflammatory diseases. *Immunity*. 2014;40(6):833-842. doi:10.1016/j.immuni.2014.05.014.

122. Thorburn AN, McKenzie CI, Shen S, et al. Evidence that asthma is a developmental origin disease influenced by maternal diet and bacterial metabolites. *Nat Commun*. 2015;6:7320. doi:10.1038/ncomms8320.

123. Hogenkamp A, Knippels LM, Garssen J, van Esch BC. Supplementation of mice with specific nondigestible oligosaccharides during pregnancy or lactation leads to diminished sensitization and allergy in the female offspring. *J Nutr*. 2015;145(5):996-1002. doi:10.3945/jn.115.210401.

124. Hogenkamp A, Thijssen S, van Vlies N, Garssen J. Supplementing pregnant mice with a specific mixture of nondigestible oligosaccharides reduces symptoms of allergic asthma in male offspring. *J Nutr*. 2015;145(3):640-646. doi:10.3945/jn.114.197707.

125. Prentice PM, Schoemaker MH, Vervoort J, et al. Human milk short-chain fatty acid composition is associated with adiposity outcomes in infants. *J Nutr*. 2019;149(5):716-722. doi:10.1093/jn/nxy320.

126. Meng D, Sommella E, Salviati E, et al. Indole-3-lactic acid, a metabolite of tryptophan, secreted by *Bifidobacterium longum* subspecies infantis is anti-inflammatory in the immature intestine. *Pediatr Res*. 2020;88(2):209-217. doi:10.1038/s41390-019-0740-x.

127. Meng D, Sommella E, Salviati E, et al. Indole-3-lactic acid, a metabolite of tryptophan, secreted by Bifidobacterium longum subspecies infantis is anti-inflammatory in the immature intestine. *Pediatr Res*. 2020;88(2):209-217. doi:10.1038/s41390-019-0740-x.

128. Laursen MF, Sakanaka M, von Burg N, et al. Breastmilk-promoted bifidobacteria produce aromatic lactic acids in the infant gut. *Nat Microbiol*. 2021;6(11):1367-1382. doi:10.1038/s41564-021-00970-4.

129. O'Reilly D, Dorodnykh D, Avdeenko NV, et al. Perspective: the role of human breast-milk extracellular vesicles in child

130. Yokoi A, Ochiya T. Exosomes and extracellular vesicles: rethinking the essential values in cancer biology. *Semin Cancer Biol*. 2021;74:79-91. doi:10.1016/j.semcancer.2021.03.032.

131. Buzas EI. The roles of extracellular vesicles in the immune system. *Nat Rev Immunol*. 2023;23(4):236-250. doi:10.1038/s41577-022-00763-8.

132. Chutipongtanate S, Morrow AL, Newburg DS. Human milk extracellular vesicles: a biological system with clinical implications. *Cells*. 2022;11(15):2345. doi:10.3390/cells11152345.

133. Hu Y, Thaler J, Nieuwland R. Extracellular vesicles in human milk. *Pharmaceuticals (Basel)*. 2021;14(10):1050. doi:10.3390/ph14101050.

134. Cui J, Zhou B, Ross SA, Zempleni J. Nutrition, microRNAs, and human health. *Adv Nutr*. 2017;8(1):105-112. doi:10.3945/an.116.013839.

135. Zempleni J, Aguilar-Lozano A, Sadri M, et al. Biological activities of extracellular vesicles and their cargos from bovine and human milk in humans and implications for infants. *J Nutr*. 2017;147(1):3-10. doi:10.3945/jn.116.238949.

136. Weber JA, Baxter DH, Zhang S, et al. The microRNA spectrum in 12 body fluids. *Clin Chem*. 2010;56(11):1733-1741. doi:10.1373/clinchem.2010.147405.

137. Liao Y, Du X, Li J, Lönnerdal B. Human milk exosomes and their microRNAs survive digestion in vitro and are taken up by human intestinal cells. *Mol Nutr Food Res*. 2017;61(11). doi:10.1002/mnfr.201700082.

138. Kosaka N, Izumi H, Sekine K, Ochiya T. microRNA as a new immune-regulatory agent in breast milk. *Silence*. 2010;1(1):7. doi:10.1186/1758-907X-1-7.

139. Benmoussa A, Ly S, Shan ST, et al. A subset of extracellular vesicles carries the bulk of microRNAs in commercial dairy cow's milk. *J Extracell Vesicles*. 2017;6(1):1401897. doi:10.1080/20013078.2017.1401897.

140. Liu X, Zhan Z, Xu L, et al. MicroRNA-148/152 impair innate response and antigen presentation of TLR-triggered dendritic cells by targeting CaMKIIα. *J Immunol*. 2010;185(12):7244-7251. doi:10.4049/jimmunol.1001573.

141. Banerjee S, Xie N, Cui H, et al. MicroRNA let-7c regulates macrophage polarization. *J Immunol*. 2013;190(12):6542-6549. doi:10.4049/jimmunol.1202496.

142. Lönnerdal B. Human milk microRNAs/exosomes: composition and biological effects. *Nestle Nutr Inst Workshop Ser*. 2019;90:83-92. doi:10.1159/000490297.

Chapter 9

Donor Milk Nutrition for the Preterm Infant: Current Standards, Uses, and Transitions

Camilia R. Martin, Sarah N. Taylor, Kristin L. Santoro and Sarah E. Mahoney

Chapter Outline

Key Points

1. Pasteurized donor human milk is the preferred alternative feeding source when maternal milk is not available for preterm and low-birth-weight infants.
2. Holder pasteurization, freezing, and handling of donor human milk leads to decreased macronutrient content by reducing fat and protein levels. It also decreases many biologically active components that serve immunologic benefits. Some human milk immunoregulatory bioactives, such as human milk oligosaccharides, are preserved throughout these processes.
3. While studies are limited and results are variable, many researchers have reliably found lower in-hospital growth rates for infants fed predominately donor breast milk, both nonfortified and fortified, compared to infants fed preterm or term formula. These studies have not supported an effect of donor milk versus formula on long-term growth, neurodevelopment, or all-cause mortality.
4. Current randomized trials of donor human milk versus formula were not designed with necrotizing enterocolitis as the primary outcome; however, meta-analysis of the most current randomized clinical trials supports the use of donor human milk as a supplement to maternal milk for preterm infants, instead of formula, to decrease the risk of necrotizing enterocolitis.
5. Although research supports a potential cost benefit in the use of donor human milk in hospitals for preterm infants, the burden of cost is often cited as a barrier to access. Variable insurance reimbursement policies and limited human milk

banks nationwide contribute to shortages in donor human milk. Racial and economic inequities persist regarding access to donor human milk. Healthcare prescribers should work together to improve access for all patients who would benefit, especially those from diverse backgrounds.

6. While many Level III and IV newborn care facilities nationwide have established donor human milk programs, heterogeneity exists among eligibility and weaning criteria. Scientific evidence regarding best practices and timing for transition from donor human milk to formula is lacking. Further studies are warranted to aid in the development and adaptation of standardized donor human milk practice guidelines.

Introduction and Historical Background

Human milk provides nutritional and immunologic factors for optimal infant growth and development, yet not every mother is able to provide this resource to their infant.[1] When the gold standard of maternal milk (MM) is not available, infant formulas manufactured to approximate the macro- and micronutrients of human milk are available in most countries. Another option is donor human milk (DHM). The World Health Organization (WHO) and the American Academy of Pediatrics (AAP) guidelines recommend DHM rather than formula as the alternative feeding source when MM is not available.[1,2] Understanding the production of, options for, and evidence regarding DHM is key to providing this resource in the NICU.

Donation of human milk historically encompasses wet nursing, informal milk sharing, and milk banking.[3] In most contemporary NICUs, DHM is obtained formally from a bank with safety protocols to ensure the milk has no detectable microbes. Milk pasteurization and microbial testing are the primary methods by which a DHM bank achieves this goal.[4] Other methods to improve preservation of the immune activity of milk, such as ultraviolet irradiation or high-pressure processing without high heat, show promising results but are not yet clinically available.[5–7]

DIFFERENCES IN PASTEURIZATION TECHNIQUES

The mainstay of DHM banking is *Holder pasteurization (HoP)*, a method in which milk is heated to 62.5°C for 30 minutes.[4] Another common form of pasteurization is *vat pasteurization*, which is like HoP but differs in that the milk is heated in a large "vat" rather than in individual milk bottles and is heated to 63°C and for longer than 30 minutes. A third form is *retort processing*, which is a process that includes not only heat but also pressure, resulting in a commercially sterile milk product.[8–10] Although these processes remove or inactivate pathogens, they also decrease the biologically active components of human milk.[10] Investigation is ongoing to identify the best methods by which to remove infection risk while protecting immune components with processes that can be available in low- and middle-resource countries.[11]

DONOR HUMAN MILK STANDARDS

Formal milk banking has developed through regional standards set by organizations such as the Human Milk Banking Association of North America (HMBANA), the European Milk Bank Association, and the Brazilian Network of Human Milk Banks that has now been expanded as the Ibero-American Network of Human Milk Banks. These organizations set standards for safety including inclusion and exclusion of milk donors, milk handling, milk pooling, pasteurization, postpasteurization handling, and evaluation for microbial contamination. From a 2019 international symposium on human milk banking came a call for international guidance to ensure quality, safety, and equity in DHM as donor milk availability expands worldwide.[12]

CURRENT USE

Pasteurized DHM is recommended by the WHO and the AAP as the enteral nutrition to give to preterm or low-birth-weight infants when the mother's own milk is not available.[1,2,13] A growing number of hospitals also are providing donor milk to all newborns as a method to ensure an exclusive human milk diet during birth hospitalization.[14,15] Determining how these clinical guidelines and decisions are supported by evidence is critical to ensuring that this limited resource is available to those infants with the greatest need. Additionally, as the use of donor milk grows, the benefits and potential risks in all populations require investigation.

Evidence-Based Outcomes Related to Donor Human Milk

REDUCED RISK OF NECROTIZING ENTEROCOLITIS

Necrotizing enterocolitis (NEC) is a severe gastrointestinal inflammatory disease associated with death, short bowel syndrome (SBS), and later neurodevelopmental delay. For neonates, the risk of developing NEC inversely relates to the degree of prematurity. Cohort studies show an intake of MM is associated with a decreased risk of NEC.[16–19] Randomized trials have investigated whether DHM as a supplement to MM decreases the risk of NEC. The most recent *Cochrane Database of Systematic Reviews* meta-analysis of preterm or low-birth-weight infants fed either formula or DHM includes nine studies with a total of 1675 infants.[20] Four of the studies were performed in the 1980s and compared formula with unfortified DHM.[21–23] Four studies compared formula with fortified DHM, three with a cow's milk–based human milk fortifier (HMF)[24–26] and one with a DHM-based HMF.[27] The ninth study included in the meta-analysis compared formula and DHM with a primary outcome of days to reach full feed volume (150 mL/kg/d). The average time to full feeds was 12 days for both groups, and in the 70 infants studied, no NEC was diagnosed.[28] In the meta-analysis of the nine studies, the rate of NEC in infants receiving formula was 6.8% and in infants receiving DHM was 3.6%. The formula-fed group had higher risk of NEC: risk ratio (RR) of 1.87 with a 95% confidence interval (95% CI) of 1.23 to 2.85 and a number needed to treat for an additional harmful outcome of 33, classified as moderate certainty evidence.

When individually evaluating the four contemporary studies of preterm formula compared to fortified DHM, none of the studies were specifically powered to identify a difference in NEC outcomes.[24–27] Two included NEC in a cumulative outcome measure including infection and mortality,[24,26] one was powered for neurodevelopmental outcomes,[25] and the fourth was powered for a difference in parenteral nutrition days.[27] Individually, three of the four study results demonstrated no difference in NEC between formula- and DHM-fed preterm infants.[24,26,27] Furthermore, in three out of four of these studies, DHM was given as a supplement to MM; therefore these findings are not generalizable to populations of infants receiving

DHM as the sole source of breast milk. In a meta-analysis including 955 infants from all four studies, a difference in NEC of 9% in formula-fed infants compared to 5.5% in DHM-fed infants and a RR of 1.64 (95% CI 1.03, 2.61) with formula feeding was observed.[20] In all four of these studies, the definition of NEC is poorly defined. A meta-analysis was published in 2019 that reviewed all randomized trials published from January 1960 to January 2018 that specifically investigated the effect of DHM versus preterm formula on the most severe case of NEC, defined as *surgical NEC*, and found DHM was not protective against surgical NEC over preterm formula.[29] To summarize, due to several limitations in study design and a paucity of data, the evidence for a protective effect of DHM when supplemented with MM over preterm formula against NEC in preterm infants should be interpreted with caution, particularly in prevention of surgical NEC.

NO DIFFERENCE IN NEURODEVELOPMENT WITH DONOR HUMAN MILK COMPARED TO PRETERM FORMULA

MM composition includes specific micronutrients, fatty acids, and oligosaccharides that impact brain development, and many of these nutrients are preserved in DHM. On the other hand, preterm infants receiving formula instead of DHM exhibit a greater growth trajectory that predicts higher neurodevelopmental scores. Therefore an important question is whether DHM intake relates to better or worse cognitive outcomes for preterm infants. The GTA DoMINO (Greater Toronto Area Donor Milk for Improved Neurodevelopmental Outcomes) Feeding Group performed a randomized clinical trial with cognitive composite scores at 18 months obtained from Bayley Scales of Infant and Toddler Development, 3rd Edition (Bayley-III), as the primary outcome. In this study, the very-low-birth-weight infants receiving DHM exhibited no difference in neurodevelopment compared to infants receiving formula.[25] This study, along with a few older studies, is included in the meta-analysis, which also shows no difference in neurodevelopmental outcomes between DHM- and formula-feeding types.[20] A post hoc exploratory analysis of this study alone found an increased incidence of neuroimpairment scores in infants who received DHM over formula. There was no statistical difference in scores that was suggestive of cognitive disability between the two groups.[25]

HUMAN MILK DIET AND OTHER PRETERM INFANT OUTCOMES

As previously described, investigation of the impact of MM is limited due to the inability to randomize infants to receive or not to receive MM.[30] However, meta-analyses have been performed to investigate the effect of human milk (MM and DHM). In one meta-analysis, NEC was lower with intake of human milk (about a 4% reduction). Additionally, human milk intake was associated with a potential reduction in late-onset sepsis (LOS) and severe retinopathy of prematurity.[31] The role that DHM instead of formula plays in these outcomes is unclear since the risk difference for LOS and/or severe retinopathy of prematurity has not differed in randomized trials.[24–27]

OTHER POPULATIONS WITH POTENTIAL BENEFIT

With the known benefits of MM in gut physiology, DHM may confer benefit in other neonatal populations with diseases affecting the gastrointestinal tract. A single-institution retrospective cohort study of DHM as a supplement to MM for infants with gastroschisis or intestinal atresia demonstrated shorter length of hospital stay and fewer central line days.[32] Further study is needed to assess potential benefit in these high-risk neonatal populations.

Challenges and Limitations in Donor Milk Use

Despite the potential benefits of DHM for very-low-birth-weight infants when MM is not available, there are several challenges that are important for providers to consider regarding its use. Most concerning are the earlier studies that reported slower growth in infants receiving DHM over formula, including its association with decreased head circumference, which could have implications for future neurodevelopmental outcomes.[20] While later studies have shown improved growth rates after optimization of fortification and establishment of feeding protocols in neonatal settings,[33–35] other recent studies continue to show lagging growth in infants receiving feedings composed of a majority of DHM over MM.[36] These findings are largely attributable to (1) the changes in macronutrient content of DHM after standard handling and pasteurization practices and

(2) donor variability, including limited availability of donors with infants born preterm. This section reviews these challenges associated with DHM as well as limitations in supply, including cost-effectiveness analyses and inequities in access.

EFFECTS OF FREEZING AND PASTEURIZATION ON MACRONUTRIENTS

The procedures involved in DHM storage, pasteurization, and distribution likely lead to losses in human milk macronutrients and total energy content. Coliazy provided a recent comprehensive review of the literature that summarized the estimated losses in macronutrient content through each stepwise process of DHM production: multiple freezing cycles, HoP, and distribution/handling in multiple containers.[37] Two studies on the effects of freezing milk were highlighted that showed conflicting results. Ahrabi et al. found no effect of freezing DHM at −20°C for 9 months duration on energy and nutrient content.[38] In contrast, Garcia-Lara et al. compared dethawed milk after an initial freezing period of 90 days at −20°C, and again after pasteurization for 180 days at −20°C, to mimic current handling practices. This study showed a time-dependent reduction in fat and energy content, initially with a 9% decrease in fat after the first freezing cycle and an additional 2.7% decrease after the subsequent postpasteurization cycle. This led to an initial decrease in energy by 6 kcal/dL, followed by a 2.2% loss after the second freezing cycle.[39] During freezing and thawing cycles, free fatty acids are more susceptible to oxidation, after which they are not detected by the Miris Human Milk Analyzer (Miris AB), which was the methodology utilized by Garcia-Lara and colleagues.[39] This discrepancy in methodology may explain conflicting results from the study by Ahrabi. Variability also exists among the studies that investigated the effect of HoP on macronutrient content. The results of several recent studies are shown in Table 9.1.[39–43] Despite their heterogeneity, these studies collectively provide ample evidence that there are losses in fat and energy content after HoP, with variable reports of protein and lactose loss. Because the bactericidal effect of HoP is a necessary step in ensuring the safety of DHM samples, these nutritional losses must be considered when administering DHM to preterm infants. Providers routinely

TABLE 9.1 Reported Change in Fat, Protein, Lactose, and Total Energy Content in Donor Breast Milk After Holder Pasteurization				
First Author, Year	Fat	Protein	Lactose	Total Energy
Ley, 2011[40]	−2.8%	0%	0%	−6.2%
Adhisivam, 2019[41]	−25.0%	−12.5%	0%	−16%
Garcia-Lara, 2013[39]	−3.5%	0%	0%	−2.8%
Vieira, 2011[42]	−5.5%	−3.9%	0%	Not reported
Piemontese, 2019[43]	−4.8%	−2.5%	−0.9%	−2.5%

fortify donor milk to 24 kcal/oz and/or increase the volume of feeds to optimize growth patterns; however, these interventions have not been adequately studied.

EFFECTS OF FREEZING AND PASTEURIZATION ON BIOLOGICAL COMPONENTS

Beyond its nutritional value, human milk contains hundreds of biologically active components that provide immunologic and developmental benefits to infants. In addition to denaturing pathologic components in human milk, HoP causes disruptions in the protein structure of these beneficial components, leading to their partial or total inactivation. Maternal antibodies, particularly immunoglobulin A (IgA) and secretory immunoglobulin A (sIgA), are transmitted readily through human milk. HoP reduces quantities of sIgA, IgA, and some degree of other immunoglobulins.[44] Many studies have attempted to quantify this reduction. One recent study showed a reduction in IgA, immunoglobulin M (IgM), and lactoferrin by 30%, 36%, and 70%, respectively, and another approximated about a 50% loss in sIgA and IgA with processing and handling.[45,46] Lactoferrin is an iron-binding protein with antiviral and antibacterial properties.[47] It works synergistically with lysozyme, an enzyme that breaks down bacterial cell walls, that is also reduced through the process of HoP.[48] Digestive enzymes in human milk are also degenerated through HoP, including bile salt–stimulated lipase,[49] lipoprotein lipase, and amylase.[50] These enzymes likely serve particular benefit in both full-term and preterm infants in the first month of life with lower levels of pancreatic lipase and thus lower capacity for fat digestion.[51] This theoretical effect has been variably observed in clinical studies. In a small pilot study of patients who received raw human milk and pasteurized DHM, there was no effect of human milk type on gastric emptying or gastric lipolysis.[52] However, a larger observational cohort study found that very-low-birth-weight infants fed a majority of DHM versus those fed mostly MM were more likely to have feeding intolerance and poor growth.[36] Human milk contains an abundance of cytokines with predominately antiinflammatory effects. These cytokines possess wide variability in their degrees of resistance to the thermal effects of pasteurization, but many experience some degree of reduction in mature human milk after pasteurization, including interleukin (IL)-10, IL-1β, interferon (INF)-γ, IL-6, tumor necrosis factor alpha (TNF-α), and IL-8.[53] While theoretically shifting the balance between pro- and antiinflammatory cytokines could impact an infant's ability to combat infection, the clinical impact of these alterations in cytokine activity after HoP is unknown.

Despite the reductions in several components that offer immunologic and developmental benefits in DHM after HoP, several vital biological components with a role in immunologic defense and gastrointestinal development are preserved after HoP. Human milk oligosaccharides (HMOs) play an important role in intestinal health by competitively binding pathogens at the intestinal mucosa to prevent their invasion of the gut, and as prebiotics by stimulating the colonization of beneficial bacteria in the intestine.[54] Many studies have reliably demonstrated preservation of HMOs in DHM after HoP.[8,11,53,55] *Glycosaminoglycans* are polysaccharides that are found in human milk, with high concentrations in preterm human milk, and serve important antiinfectious functions by inhibiting pathogenic binding to the intestinal cell wall and promoting and regulating intestinal development. These compounds are preserved after HoP.[56] Gangliosides are glycosphingolipids that act as target receptors for bacterial adhesion, allowing for immune protection against bowel necrosis, inflammatory reactions, and NEC.[57] These compounds are also preserved after HoP and are present in DHM.[53] The preservation of these important compounds likely plays a role in the protective effect of DHM over formula in preventing NEC,[20] despite losses of other immunologic compounds in DHM after HoP.

EFFECTS OF INDIVIDUAL VARIATION IN DONOR HUMAN MILK

An additional challenge in the use of DHM is the degree of variability that naturally occurs in expressed human milk. Human milk composition can vary based on individual factors such as diet, health, and environmental exposures; based on the stage of nursing or gestational age of the infant; and even within the timing of a single nursing session.[58] Donated human milk is typically from mothers of infants who are born at term gestation and are older than 1 month of age. As described earlier, due to the individual variability in DHM, human milk banks will batch DHM among multiple donors prior to the pasteurization and freezing process. Perrin and colleagues conducted a large systematic review to quantify reports of energy and macronutrient content in DHM from nonprofit and commercial milk banks in the United States. Overall, the group found a twofold difference in fat, protein, and energy content of DHM among the relatively small studies. Furthermore, most values for mean energy and fat content were below the AAP reference ranges for DHM.[59] In an effort to provide guidance toward optimizing DHM protocols, a few groups have investigated the impact of the number of milk donors in a batch and changes in macronutrient concentration, as donor pools vary greatly from 1 to 10 donors commonly in nonprofit milk banks compared to 250 donors in for-profit milk banks. Both studies found that DHM batches with fewer than five milk donors may be deficient in levels of fat and protein.[60,61] The largest and most comprehensive study on pooling practices also found evidence that mixing technique and even the material type of the mixing container resulted in heterogeneity of macronutrient content.[62] Optimal practices for these processes have yet to be defined.[37]

COST OF DONOR HUMAN MILK

In 2017, the AAP released a policy statement recommending the use of DHM for very-low-birth-weight infants, citing the cost and variation in reimbursement among states as a major limitation for access in NICUs across the United States.[63] The burden of cost of DHM compared to its alternatives, MM and formula, is a universal concern. A survey on DHM use in NICUs in the United Kingdom cited cost as the leading limitation in its broader use.[64] The first prospective economic analysis on the cost-effectiveness of very-low-birth-weight infants randomized to receive DHM versus formula was conducted in 2018 in four Canadian hospitals by Trang and colleagues.[65] The cost analysis evaluated the societal costs for each group, which included all formal and informal costs and health effects. Consistent with other reports throughout the literature, the formula-fed group had a significantly higher incidence of NEC than the DHM group, ultimately resulting in no difference in cost between the two groups due to saved costs in the DHM group from decreased incidence of NEC.[65] In a postdischarge analysis, there was a decreased cost in the DHM group due to more productivity losses for family members in the formula-fed group, suggesting a potential financial advantage of DHM compared to formula for the very-low-birth-weight infant population due to reduction of NEC.[65]

A retrospective cost-effective analysis was conducted by Johnson et al. in 2020 to determine the economic effects of DHM in a tertiary care center in the United States. This study compared infants born <32 weeks gestation before and after the initiation of a DHM program and adjusted cost for inflation based on the 2016 US dollar.[66] While the median feeding cost of DHM was estimated at $381 more per patient than MM or formula, this was comparably much lower than the total cost of the NICU stay. The adjusted model found that the use of DHM resulted in a 7% reduction in NICU cost due to decreased incidence of NEC by 4.2%. The use of DHM was also associated with shortened duration to full feeds and decreased days on parental nutrition, likely accounting for the added reductions in cost in this study compared to the Canadian study.

Evidence suggests that the use of DHM might provide financial benefits, not increased burden, for the very-low-birth-weight infant population. These studies are limited in that they are at single centers and the majority are retrospective. There is limited information available on the cost-effectiveness of DHM in older neonatal populations.

INEQUITIES IN ACCESS TO AND USE OF DONOR HUMAN MILK

Based on recent survey data, safety net hospitals that typically care for patients of lower income status have 70% lower odds of having DHM programs than other neonatal care facilities.[67] This patient population is also at higher risk for preterm delivery and therefore is more likely to have infants who would benefit most from implementation of these programs. This finding is likely related to inconsistencies in insurance reimbursements for DHM, as these policies vary statewide, with no national recommendation for universal coverage. A retrospective cohort analysis by Kair and colleagues of healthy term and late preterm infants in a single Midwestern care facility found that non-White women were less likely to use DHM, and the gap was widened in families whose first primary language was not English and who had public over private insurance.[14] These studies highlight factors that are contributing to healthcare inequities among minorities and low-income families leading to lower quality of maternal and infant health. It is imperative to identify these inequities so that providers can work to implement local policy changes and advocate for systemic changes to narrow the gap and improve care for all infants, but particularly those from diverse backgrounds.

Current State of Donor Human Milk Use in the NICU

RECOMMENDED USE BY AAP STANDARDS

The most recent policy statement by the AAP recommends the use of DHM when MM is not available for all preterm infants, but especially for those infants born weighing less than 1500 grams.[63] The policy acknowledges the limitation in supply of DHM and lack of research on benefits for conditions beyond prematurity, including congenital heart disease and congenital gastrointestinal disorders such as omphalocele

and gastroschisis. It concludes based on ample evidence that DHM from HMBANA and commercial milk banks is safe for use due to consistent regulatory policies, including HoP, and recommends against other sources of DHM through informal direct milk sharing or online sources. The policy acknowledges the early studies that have shown reduced growth rates in infants receiving DHM over formula and MM but cites newer retrospective cohort studies that have shown improved growth with optimization of fortification; however, as mentioned earlier, there are no randomized controlled trials to support these findings. Ultimately, the policy concludes that best practices for DHM use are as a bridge before establishment of MM supply, when used in conjunction with mother's milk, and that the superiority of MM over DHM should be emphasized by physicians to their patients.

COMMON DONOR HUMAN MILK PRACTICES ACROSS NICUS

Since 2011, when the US Surgeon General issued a call to action to find barriers preventing the distribution of safe banked DHM for at-risk infants, the prevalence of DHM banks and use in hospitals has increased significantly. The most recent report on DHM use in Level II to IV NICUs in the United States was published in 2020 and is based on survey data of medical directors from randomly selected hospitals nationwide. This study reported a prevalence of DHM programs in 28% of Level II neonatal care facilities and 88% of Levels III and IV centers.[67] A hospital's adoption of DHM use was found to vary based on a number of factors, including geography, breastfeeding rates, proximity to milk banks, and Baby Friendly Status.[68] In the past 15 years, the availability of DHM has increased due to an expansion in human milk banks across the United States and growing distribution to include a larger number of hospitals. A recent paper cited a 12% increase in DHM distribution from 2017 to 2018 and a total of 7.4 million ounces of DHM distributed in the United States and Canada in the year 2019.[69] The population of patients eligible for DHM is expanding, with many hospitals in the Northeast now considering use of DHM for healthy term newborns, which has led to higher rates of exclusive breastfeeding at hospital discharge.[15] Of those that responded, 32% of Level I nurseries surveyed in the

Northeast reported DHM use for infants >35 weeks gestational age, with the majority citing eligibility criteria. Eligibility criteria varied but most frequently included specific infant health conditions such as hypoglycemia, hyperbilirubinemia, and weight loss/dehydration. It was uncommon for policies to contain eligibility criteria listing maternal conditions that led to a contraindication to breastfeeding. Many of the policies required plans for exclusive breastfeeding, using DHM as a bridge prior to the establishment of a reliable milk supply.[70]

Hospital policies and practices of use of DHM in Level III and IV NICUs are also highly variable and not standardized due to lack of national recommendations, including eligibility criteria. The majority of DHM programs list birth weight and gestational age cutoffs in their DHM protocols; however, these are often varied and flexible.[71] Neonatal clinical illness, certain maternal conditions, and even parental preference are often also included as qualifying criteria for an infant to receive DHM, according to survey data of medical directors.[71] Table 9.2 references four different pasteurized DHM hospital policies for Level III and IV NICUs in the New England area. Not one policy had the same eligibility criteria, criteria for discontinuation, or plan for transition to formula.

TABLE 9.2   Pasteurized Donor Human Milk Policies of Four Level III/IV NICUs in the New England Area

Hospital	Eligibility Criteria	Additional Qualifying Criteria	Criteria for Discontinuing	Transition to Formula Plan
Hospital A	<30 WGA or <1500 g	Nutrition post NEC treatment, siblings of infants who are eligible	>34 WGA and >1500 g	¼ formula, ¾ DHM × 24 h ½ formula, ½ DHM × 24 h
Hospital B	<34 WGA or <1500 g	Nutrition post NEC treatment, postsurgical nutrition, siblings of infants who are eligible, or 5-day bridge for any infant to establish exclusive mother's milk feeding	34 weeks PMA and minimum of 4 days old Or if <1500 g, until on full enteral feedings Or when 100% mother's milk is available	2 formula feedings × 24 h 4 formula feedings × 24 h 6 formula feedings × 24 h
Hospital C	<32 WGA or <1500 g	Nutrition post NEC treatment, congenital heart disease or congenital anomalies that increase risk of developing ischemic bowel, term hospitalized neonates as a 7-day bridge to establish exclusive human milk feeding	Once the infant reaches full volume enteral feeds and if preterm, >32 WGA and >1500 g Up to 7 days to establish exclusive mother's milk feeding	Formula for 1 of every 4 feedings × 24 h Formula for 2 of every 4 feedings × 24 h Formula for 3 of every 4 feedings × 24 h No transitional plan for bridge milk therapy
Hospital D	<37 WGA	Nutrition post NEC treatment or other gastrointestinal surgeries, hypoxia, any patient the medical team thinks would benefit, supporting mother's choice for exclusive breastfeeding, parental request	Once infant is tolerating full feeds or at discretion of medical team	¼ formula, ¾ DHM × 12 h ½ formula, ½ DHM × 12 h ¾ formula, ¼ DHM × 12 h
Hospital E	<32 WGA or <1500 g	None	34 WGA	¼ formula, ¾ DHM × 24 h ½ formula, ½ DHM × 24 h ¼ formula, ¾ DHM × 24 h

DHM, Donor human milk; *g*, grams; *h*, hours; *NEC*, necrotizing enterocolitis; *PMA*, postmenstrual age; *WGA*, weeks gestational age.

PRACTICE KNOWLEDGE GAPS IN TIMING AND METHODOLOGY FOR TRANSITIONING OFF DONOR HUMAN MILK

Due to the increased cost of DHM, limited supply in the outpatient setting, and concerns for growth delays without maternal supplementation, many centers will transition to formula, discontinuing DHM for preterm infants whose mothers lack a reliable milk supply once they reach a certain gestational age considered at lower risk for NEC. Survey data from medical directors of Level III and IV NICUs in the United States showed a wide variety of methods for transitioning from DHM to formula. Some reported transitioning to formula all at once, while others reported gradual introduction, either through whole formula feeds with increasing frequency or partial formula feeds with increasing ratio of formula to milk.[71] This study also revealed a wide variability among DHM programs in duration of use, with the majority discontinuing based on an infant's gestational age (with a mode of 34 weeks gestation) and others discontinuing based on weight (mode of 1500 grams), age of life (mode of 30 days), or feeding tolerance.[71] Current practices may also be guided by protocols in established clinical trials that have supported use of DHM over preterm infant formula to prevent NEC. Of the four randomized controlled trials that were conducted since 2000, three continued DHM if MM was not available for up to 90 days of life or at discharge, whichever occurred first.[24,27,72] The fourth study only assessed use of DHM in the first 10 days of life, and then infants were fed preterm formula if MM was not available.[26] Table 9.2 demonstrates the wide variability in transition plans of five Level III and IV NICUs located in the greater New England area (Hospitals A-E).

Ample evidence of the beneficial roles of MM in immunologic protection and promotion of gut development is demonstrated in the literature. Compared with formula, maternal human milk has been shown to lead to shorter gastric emptying times,[73] increased intestinal permeability and gut maturation,[74] increased gut microbial diversity,[75] and preservation of splanchnic oxygenation of the gut (which is decreased after formula use).[76] DHM provides some of these benefits, particularly through the preservation of HMOs after the pasteurization process.[77] There is a lack of research investigating the effect of transition from MM or DHM to formula and the impact this transition has on these well-established benefits, including the timing of transition and the percentage of MM feeds necessary to establish these effects. The lack of foundational studies on the abrupt transition from MM to formula has led to the wide variation in practice described earlier.

While anecdotally there are concerns for increased risk of NEC during the time of discontinuation of DHM, there are no case reports describing this association in the literature. Concerns for adverse events related to rapid weaning of breastfeeding for replacement with formula were reported in comparison to two separate populations of infants enrolled in randomized controlled trials to identify factors associated with increased mortality of infants exposed to but not infected with HIV in Malawi. While these studies represent different patient populations, transition from MM (not DHM), and environments than infants in neonatal tertiary care hospitals in developed nations, these findings provide supportive evidence of the potential risks in gut health with the rapid cessation and transition to formula. These two studies were the nevirapine/AZT trial (NVAZ) conducted from 2000 to 2003, in which infants received prolonged breastfeeding;[78] and the Postexposure Prophylaxis to the Infant (PEPI) trial, from 2004 to 2007, in which recommendations were to discontinue breastfeeding by 6 months of age.[79] The infants in the PEPI trial had a higher incidence of severe gastrointestinal illness and mortality over those in the NVAZ trial.[80] Furthermore, with each age interval, cessation of breastfeeding was associated with increased mortality, increased rates of illness, and increased hospital admission.[81] Similar findings were reported in a population of infants with HIV exposure in Africa, with early cessation of breastfeeding being associated with increased mortality through the second year of life.[82]

Due to a paucity of studies in the literature regarding best timing for discontinuation of DHM in the preterm population and method for transition, to date there are no established guidelines or literature to support best practices for transition from DHM to formula.

PUBLIC KNOWLEDGE GAPS

Qualitative studies reveal a knowledge gap among mothers surveyed in the NICU regarding safety practices and use of DHM banks. Mothers who chose formula over DHM cited concerns over the use of human milk other than their own (88%), risk of disease transmission with DHM (78%), and cost concerns (30%) as the main factors that contributed to their decision-making. Mothers less likely to choose DHM also were less likely to be aware of DHM banks and cited limited support and uncertainty from medical providers.[83] Results from another study found that history of a sick infant or a prior breastfeeding experience of more than 3 months were factors associated with positive attitudes toward DHM and its safety.[84] While these studies provide a start, more research is needed to identify patient and provider knowledge gaps related to DHM and best educational practices for healthcare workers and families.

Summary

DHM remains an important mainstay of neonatal care for preterm infants, and while over the past decade its use has expanded to populations of hospitalized neonates beyond those with prematurity, more research is necessary to understand the specific benefits it may provide to these groups. With these benefits unsupported by research and the limitations as described in this chapter, it is imperative for providers to continue to present the use of DHM ideally as a bridge toward the establishment of MM supply, and to simultaneously supply lactation support and education for mothers in addition to access to DHM. Investment in research to continue to optimize DHM processing and pasteurization is necessary to better preserve important biological and macronutrient components that are reduced using techniques implemented today. This includes promising novel techniques such as inoculation with MM to reestablish the microbiota of donor breast milk.[85] Further development for evidence-based consensus statements for processing as well as establishment of guidelines for inclusion criteria and weaning off DHM would reduce the heterogeneity existing in current practice. Finally, providers need to advocate for government support for broadened insurance coverage and reimbursement for DHM use, improve DHM education practices for families and colleagues, and work toward reducing the current inequities among DHM use and access that exist today.

REFERENCES

1. American Academy of Pediatrics. Breastfeeding and the use of human milk. *Pediatrics*. 2012;129(3):e827-e841. doi:10.1542/peds.2011-3552.
2. World Health Organization. *Maternal, Newborn, Child and Adolescent Health; Guidelines on Optimal Feeding of Low Birth-Weight Infants in Low- and Middle-Income Countries.* 2011. Available at: https://www.who.int/publications/i/item/9789241548366.
3. Cassidy TM. Historical research: more than milk: the origins of human milk banking social relations. *J Hum Lact*. 2022;38(2):344-350. doi:10.1177/08903344221082674.
4. Arslanoglu S, Moro GE. Quality standards for human milk banks. *World Rev Nutr Diet*. 2021;122:248-264. doi:10.1159/000514750.
5. Aceti A, Cavallarin L, Martini S, et al. Effect of alternative pasteurization techniques on human milk's bioactive proteins. *J Pediatr Gastroenterol Nutr*. 2020;70(4):508-512. doi:10.1097/MPG.0000000000002598.
6. Billeaud C. High hydrostatic pressure treatment ensures the microbiological safety of human milk including Bacillus cereus and preservation of bioactive proteins including lipase and immuno-proteins: a narrative review. *Foods*. 2021;10(6):1327. doi:10.3390/foods10061327.
7. Christen L, Lai CT, Hartmann B, Hartmann PE, Geddes DT. The effect of UV-C pasteurization on bacteriostatic properties and immunological proteins of donor human milk. *PLoS One*. 2013;8(12):e85867. doi:10.1371/journal.pone.0085867.
8. Meredith-Dennis L, Xu G, Goonatilleke E, Lebrilla CB, Underwood MA, Smilowitz JT. Composition and variation of macronutrients, immune proteins, and human milk oligosaccharides in human milk from nonprofit and commercial milk banks. *J Hum Lact*. 2018;34(1):120-129. doi:10.1177/0890334417710635.
9. Lima H, Vogel K, Wagner-Gillespie M, Wimer C, Dean L, Fogleman A. Nutritional comparison of raw, holder pasteurized, and shelf-stable human milk products. *J Pediatr Gastroenterol Nutr*. 2018;67(5):649-653. doi:10.1097/MPG.0000000000002094.
10. Lima HK, Wagner-Gillespie M, Perrin MT, Fogleman AD. Bacteria and bioactivity in Holder pasteurized and shelf-stable human milk products. *Curr Dev Nutr*. 2017;1(8):e001438. doi:10.3945/cdn.117.001438.
11. Daniels B, Coutsoudis A, Autran C, Amundson Mansen K, Israel-Ballard K, Bode L. The effect of simulated flash heating pasteurisation and Holder pasteurisation on human milk oligosaccharides. *Paediatr Int Child Health*. 2017;37(3):204-209. doi:10.1080/20469047.2017.1293869.
12. Tyebally Fang M, Chatzixiros E, Grummer-Strawn L, et al. Developing global guidance on human milk banking. *Bull World Health Organ*. 2021;99(12):892-900. doi:10.2471/BLT.21.286943.
13. Parker MG, Stellwagen LM, Noble L, Kim JH, Poindexter BB, Puopolo KM. Promoting human milk and breastfeeding for the very low birth weight infant. *Pediatrics*. 2021;148(5):e2021054272. doi:10.1542/peds.2021-054272.
14. Kair LR, Nidey NL, Marks JE, et al. Disparities in donor human milk supplementation among well newborns. *J Hum Lact*. 2020;36(1):74-80. doi:10.1177/0890334419888163.
15. Belfort MB, Drouin K, Riley JF, et al. Prevalence and trends in donor milk use in the well-baby nursery: a survey of Northeast United States birth hospitals. *Breastfeed Med*. 2018;13(1):34-41. doi:10.1089/bfm.2017.0147.
16. Lucas A, Cole TJ. Breast milk and neonatal necrotising enterocolitis. *Lancet*. 1990;336(8730):1519-1523. doi:10.1016/0140-6736(90)93304-8.

17. Schanler RJ, Shulman RJ, Lau C. Feeding strategies for premature infants: beneficial outcomes of feeding fortified human milk versus preterm formula. *Pediatrics.* 1999;103(6 Pt 1): 1150-1157. doi:10.1542/peds.103.6.1150.

18. Furman L, Taylor G, Minich N, Hack M. The effect of maternal milk on neonatal morbidity of very low-birth-weight infants. *Arch Pediatr Adolesc Med.* 2003;157(1):66-71. doi:10.1001/archpedi.157.1.66.

19. Sisk PM, Lovelady CA, Dillard RG, Gruber KJ, O'Shea TM. Early human milk feeding is associated with a lower risk of necrotizing enterocolitis in very low birth weight infants. *J Perinatol.* 2007;27(7):428-433. doi:10.1038/sj.jp.7211758.

20. Quigley M, Embleton ND, McGuire W. Formula versus donor breast milk for feeding preterm or low birth weight infants. *Cochrane Database Syst Rev.* 2019;7(7):CD002971. doi:10.1002/14651858.CD002971.pub5.

21. Lucas A, Gore SM, Cole TJ, et al. Multicentre trial on feeding low birthweight infants: effects of diet on early growth. *Arch Dis Child.* 1984;59(8):722-730. doi:10.1136/adc.59.8.722.

22. Gross SJ. Growth and biochemical response of preterm infants fed human milk or modified infant formula. *N Engl J Med.* 1983;308(5):237-241. doi:10.1056/NEJM198302033080501.

23. Tyson JE, Lasky RE, Mize CE, et al. Growth, metabolic response, and development in very-low-birth-weight infants fed banked human milk or enriched formula. I. Neonatal findings. *J Pediatr.* 1983;103(1):95-104. doi:10.1016/s0022-3476(83)80790-2.

24. Schanler RJ, Lau C, Hurst NM, Smith EO. Randomized trial of donor human milk versus preterm formula as substitutes for mothers' own milk in the feeding of extremely premature infants. *Pediatrics.* 2005;116(2):400-406. doi:10.1542/peds.2004-1974.

25. O'Connor DL, Gibbins S, Kiss A, et al. Effect of supplemental donor human milk compared with preterm formula on neurodevelopment of very-low-birth-weight infants at 18 months: a randomized clinical trial. *JAMA.* 2016;316(18):1897-1905. doi:10.1001/jama.2016.16144.

26. Corpeleijn WE, de Waard M, Christmann V, et al. Effect of donor milk on severe infections and mortality in very low-birth-weight infants: The Early Nutrition Study randomized clinical trial. *JAMA Pediatr.* 2016;170(7):654-661. doi:10.1001/jamapediatrics.2016.0183.

27. Cristofalo EA, Schanler RJ, Blanco CL, et al. Randomized trial of exclusive human milk versus preterm formula diets in extremely premature infants. *J Pediatr.* 2013;163(6): 1592-1595.e1. doi:10.1016/j.jpeds.2013.07.011.

28. Costa S, Maggio L, Alighieri G, Barone G, Cota F, Vento G. Tolerance of preterm formula versus pasteurized donor human milk in very preterm infants: a randomized non-inferiority trial. *Ital J Pediatr.* 2018;44(1):96. doi:10.1186/s13052-018-0532-7.

29. Silano M, Milani GP, Fattore G, Agostoni C. Donor human milk and risk of surgical necrotizing enterocolitis: a meta-analysis. *Clin Nutr.* 2019;38(3):1061-1066. doi:10.1016/j.clnu.2018.03.004.

30. Taylor SN, Fenton TR, Groh-Wargo S, et al. Exclusive maternal milk compared with exclusive formula on growth and health outcomes in very-low-birthweight preterm infants: phase II of the Pre-B Project and an Evidence Analysis Center systematic review. *Front Pediatr.* 2021;9:793311. doi:10.3389/fped.2021.793311.

31. Miller J, Tonkin E, Damarell RA, et al. A systematic review and meta-analysis of human milk feeding and morbidity in very low birth weight infants. *Nutrients.* 2018;10(6):707. doi:10.3390/nu10060707.

32. Hoban R, Khatri S, Patel A, Unger SL. Supplementation of mother's own milk with donor milk in infants with gastroschisis or intestinal atresia: a retrospective study. *Nutrients.* 2020;12(2):589. doi:10.3390/nu12020589.

33. Colaizy TT, Saftlas AF, Morriss Jr FH. Maternal intention to breast-feed and breast-feeding outcomes in term and preterm infants: Pregnancy Risk Assessment Monitoring System (PRAMS), 2000-2003. *Public Health Nutr.* 2012;15(4):702-710. doi:10.1017/S1368980011002229.

34. Rochow N, Fusch G, Choi A, et al. Target fortification of breast milk with fat, protein, and carbohydrates for preterm infants. *J Pediatr.* 2013;163(4):1001-1007. doi:10.1016/j.jpeds.2013.04.052.

35. Hair AB, Hawthorne KM, Chetta KE, Abrams SA. Human milk feeding supports adequate growth in infants ≤ 1250 grams birth weight. *BMC Res Notes.* 2013;6:459. doi:10.1186/1756-0500-6-459.

36. Ford SL, Lohmann P, Preidis GA, et al. Improved feeding tolerance and growth are linked to increased gut microbial community diversity in very-low-birth-weight infants fed mother's own milk compared with donor breast milk. *Am J Clin Nutr.* 2019;109(4):1088-1097. doi:10.1093/ajcn/nqz006.

37. Colaizy TT. Effects of milk banking procedures on nutritional and bioactive components of donor human milk. *Semin Perinatol.* 2021;45(2):151382. doi:10.1016/j.semperi.2020.151382.

38. Ahrabi AF, Handa D, Codipilly CN, et al. Effects of extended freezer storage on the integrity of human milk. *J Pediatr.* 2016;177:140-143. doi:10.1016/j.jpeds.2016.06.024.

39. Garcia-Lara NR, Vieco DE, De la Cruz-Bertolo J, Lora-Pablos D, Velasco NU, Pallas-Alonso CR. Effect of Holder pasteurization and frozen storage on macronutrients and energy content of breast milk. *J Pediatr Gastroenterol Nutr.* 2013;57(3):377-382. doi:10.1097/MPG.0b013e31829d4f82.

40. Ley SH, Hanley AJ, Stone D, O'Connor DL. Effects of pasteurization on adiponectin and insulin concentrations in donor human milk. *Pediatr Res.* 2011;70(3):278-281. doi:10.1203/PDR.0b013e318224287a.

41. Adhisivam B, Vishnu Bhat B, Rao K, Kingsley SM, Plakkal N, Palanivel C. Effect of Holder pasteurization on macronutrients and immunoglobulin profile of pooled donor human milk. *J Matern Fetal Neonatal Med.* 2019;32(18):3016-3019. doi:10.1080/14767058.2018.1455089.

42. Vieira AA, Soares FV, Pimenta HP, Abranches AD, Moreira ME. Analysis of the influence of pasteurization, freezing/thawing, and offer processes on human milk's macronutrient concentrations. *Early Hum Dev.* 2011;87(8):577-580. doi:10.1016/j.earlhumdev.2011.04.016.

43. Piemontese P, Mallardi D, Liotto N, et al. Macronutrient content of pooled donor human milk before and after Holder pasteurization. *BMC Pediatr.* 2019;19(1):58. doi:10.1186/s12887-019-1427-5.

44. Peila C, Coscia A, Bertino E, et al. Effects of Holder pasteurization on the protein profile of human milk. *Ital J Pediatr.* 2016;42:36. doi:10.1186/s13052-016-0248-5.

45. Arroyo G, Ortiz Barrientos KA, Lange K, et al. Effect of the various steps in the processing of human milk in the concentrations of IgA, IgM, and lactoferrin. *Breastfeed Med.* 2017; 12(7):443-445. doi:10.1089/bfm.2016.0154.

46. Granger CL, Lamb CA, Embleton ND, et al. Secretory immunoglobulin A in preterm infants: determination of normal values in breast milk and stool. *Pediatr Res.* 2022;92(4):979-986. doi:10.1038/s41390-021-01930-8.

47. Kell DB, Heyden EL, Pretorius E. The biology of lactoferrin, an iron-binding protein that can help defend against viruses and bacteria. *Front Immunol.* 2020;11:1221. doi:10.3389/fimmu.2020.01221.

48. Sousa SG, Delgadillo I, Saraiva JA. Effect of thermal pasteurisation and high-pressure processing on immunoglobulin content and lysozyme and lactoperoxidase activity in human colostrum. *Food Chem.* 2014;151:79-85. doi:10.1016/j.foodchem.2013.11.024.

49. Wesolowska A, Brys J, Barbarska O, et al. Lipid profile, lipase bioactivity, and lipophilic antioxidant content in high pressure processed donor human milk. *Nutrients.* 2019;11(9):1972. doi:10.3390/nu11091972.

50. Henderson TR, Fay TN, Hamosh M. Effect of pasteurization on long chain polyunsaturated fatty acid levels and enzyme activities of human milk. *J Pediatr.* 1998;132(5):876-878. doi:10.1016/s0022-3476(98)70323-3.

51. Koh J, Victor AF, Howell ML, et al. Bile salt-stimulated lipase activity in donor breast milk influenced by pasteurization techniques. *Front Nutr.* 2020;7:552362. doi:10.3389/fnut.2020.552362.

52. de Oliveira SC, Bellanger A, Menard O, et al. Impact of human milk pasteurization on gastric digestion in preterm infants: a randomized controlled trial. *Am J Clin Nutr.* 2017;105(2):379-390. doi:10.3945/ajcn.116.142539.

53. Ewaschuk JB, Unger S, O'Connor DL, et al. Effect of pasteurization on selected immune components of donated human breast milk. *J Perinatol.* 2011;31(9):593-598. doi:10.1038/jp.2010.209.

54. Newburg DS. Glycobiology of human milk. *Biochemistry (Mosc).* 2013;78(7):771-785. doi:10.1134/S0006297913070092.

55. Bertino E, Coppa GV, Giuliani F, et al. Effects of Holder pasteurization on human milk oligosaccharides. *Int J Immunopathol Pharmacol.* 2008;21(2):381-385. doi:10.1177/039463200802100216.

56. Coscia A, Peila C, Bertino E, et al. Effect of holder pasteurisation on human milk glycosaminoglycans. *J Pediatr Gastroenterol Nutr.* 2015;60(1):127-130. doi:10.1097/MPG.0000000000000570.

57. Schnabl KL, Larsen B, Van Aerde JE, et al. Gangliosides protect bowel in an infant model of necrotizing enterocolitis by suppressing proinflammatory signals. *J Pediatr Gastroenterol Nutr.* 2009;49(4):382-392. doi:10.1097/MPG.0b013e3181b6456d.

58. Martin CR, Ling PR, Blackburn GL. Review of infant feeding: key features of breast milk and infant formula. *Nutrients.* 2016;8(5):279. doi:10.3390/nu8050279.

59. Perrin MT, Belfort MB, Hagadorn JI, et al. The nutritional composition and energy content of donor human milk: a systematic review. *Adv Nutr.* 2020;11(4):960-970. doi:10.1093/advances/nmaa014.

60. Young BE, Borman LL, Heinrich R, et al. Effect of pooling practices and time postpartum of milk donations on the energy, macronutrient, and zinc concentrations of resultant donor human milk pools. *J Pediatr.* 2019;214:54-59. doi:10.1016/j.jpeds.2019.07.042.

61. John A, Sun R, Maillart L, Schaefer A, Hamilton Spence E, Perrin MT. Macronutrient variability in human milk from donors to a milk bank: implications for feeding preterm infants. *PLoS One.* 2019;14(1):e0210610. doi:10.1371/journal.pone.0210610.

62. Friend LL, Perrin MT. Fat and protein variability in donor human milk and associations with milk banking processes. *Breastfeed Med.* 2020;15(6):370-376. doi:10.1089/bfm.2020.0046.

63. Abrams Steven, Landers Susan, Noble Lawrence, et al. Donor human milk for the high-risk infant: preparation, safety, and usage options in the United States. *Pediatrics.* 2017;139(1). doi:10.1542/peds.2016-3440.

64. Zipitis CS, Ward J, Bajaj R. Use of donor breast milk in neonatal units in the UK. *Arch Dis Child Fetal Neonatal Ed.* 2015;100(3):F279-F281. doi:10.1136/archdischild-2014-307606.

65. Trang S, Zupancic JAF, Unger S, et al. Cost-effectiveness of supplemental donor milk versus formula for very low birth weight infants. *Pediatrics.* 2018;141(3):e20170737. doi:10.1542/peds.2017-0737.

66. Johnson TJ, Berenz A, Wicks J, et al. The economic impact of donor milk in the neonatal intensive care unit. *J Pediatr.* 2020;224:57-65.e4. doi:10.1016/j.jpeds.2020.04.044.

67. Parker MG, Burnham LA, Kerr S, et al. Prevalence and predictors of donor milk programs among U.S. advanced neonatal care facilities. *J Perinatol.* 2020;40(4):672-680. doi:10.1038/s41372-020-0620-6.

68. Perrin MT. Donor human milk and fortifier use in United States Level 2, 3, and 4 neonatal care hospitals. *J Pediatr Gastroenterol Nutr.* 2018;66(4):664-669. doi:10.1097/MPG.0000000000001790.

69. Bai Y, Kuscin J. The current state of donor human milk use and practice. *J Midwifery Womens Health.* 2021;66(4):478-485. doi:10.1111/jmwh.13244.

70. Drouin KH, Riley JF, Benjamin C, Gregory KE, Sen S, Belfort MB. Donor milk policies for Level 1 newborn care: a descriptive analysis. *Breastfeed Med.* 2019;14(8):592-596. doi:10.1089/bfm.2019.0094.

71. Hagadorn JI, Brownell EA, Lussier MM, Parker MG, Herson VC. Variability of criteria for pasteurized donor human milk use: a survey of U.S. neonatal intensive care unit medical directors. *JPEN J Parenter Enteral Nutr.* 2016;40(3):326-333. doi:10.1177/0148607114550832.

72. O'Connor DL, Gibbins S, Kiss A, et al. Effect of supplemental donor human milk compared with preterm formula on neurodevelopment of very low-birth-weight infants at 18 months: a randomized clinical trial. *JAMA.* 2016;316(18):1897-1905. doi:10.1001/jama.2016.16144.

73. Cavell B. Gastric emptying in preterm infants. *Acta Paediatr Scand.* 1979;68(5):725-730. doi:10.1111/j.1651-2227.1979.tb18446.x.

74. Taylor SN, Basile LA, Ebeling M, Wagner CL. Intestinal permeability in preterm infants by feeding type: mother's milk versus formula. *Breastfeed Med.* 2009;4(1):11-15. doi:10.1089/bfm.2008.0114.

75. Cong X, Judge M, Xu W, et al. Influence of feeding type on gut microbiome development in hospitalized preterm infants. *Nurs Res.* 2017;66(2):123-133. doi:10.1097/NNR.0000000000000208.

76. Dani C, Coviello C, Montano S, et al. Effect on splanchnic oxygenation of breast milk, fortified breast milk, and formula milk in preterm infants. *Pediatr Res.* 2021;89(1):171-174. doi:10.1038/s41390-020-0935-1.

77. Carr LE, Virmani MD, Rosa F, et al. Role of human milk bioactives on infants' gut and immune health. *Front Immunol.* 2021;12:604080. doi:10.3389/fimmu.2021.604080.

78. Taha TE, Kumwenda NI, Gibbons A, et al. Short postexposure prophylaxis in newborn babies to reduce mother-to-child transmission of HIV-1: NVAZ randomised clinical trial. *Lancet.* 2003;362(9391):1171-1177. doi:10.1016/S0140-6736(03)14538-2.

79. Taha TE, Li Q, Hoover DR, et al. Postexposure prophylaxis of breastfeeding HIV-exposed infants with antiretroviral drugs to age 14 weeks: updated efficacy results of the PEPI-Malawi trial. *J Acquir Immune Defic Syndr.* 2011;57(4):319-325. doi:10.1097/QAI.0b013e318217877a.

80. Kafulafula G, Hoover DR, Taha TE, et al. Frequency of gastroenteritis and gastroenteritis-associated mortality with early weaning in HIV-1-uninfected children born to HIV-infected women in Malawi. *J Acquir Immune Defic Syndr.* 2010;53(1):6-13. doi:10.1097/QAI.0b013e3181bd5a47.

81. Taha TE, Hoover DR, Chen S, et al. Effects of cessation of breastfeeding in HIV-1-exposed, uninfected children in Malawi. *Clin Infect Dis.* 2011;53(4):388-395. doi:10.1093/cid/cir413.

82. Kuhn L, Sinkala M, Semrau K, et al. Elevations in mortality associated with weaning persist into the second year of life among uninfected children born to HIV-infected mothers. *Clin Infect Dis.* 2010;50(3):437-444. doi:10.1086/649886.

83. Rabinowitz MR, Kair LR, Sipsma HL, Phillipi CA, Larson IA. Human donor milk or formula: a qualitative study of maternal perspectives on supplementation. *Breastfeed Med.* 2018;13(3):195-203. doi:10.1089/bfm.2017.0114.

84. Pal A, Soontarapornchai K, Noble L, Hand I. Attitudes towards donor breast milk in an inner city population. *Int J Pediatr.* 2019;2019:3847283. doi:10.1155/2019/3847283.

85. Torrez Lamberti MF, Harrison NA, Bendixen MM, et al. Frozen mother's own milk can be used effectively to personalize donor human milk. *Front Microbiol.* 2021;12:656889. doi:10.3389/fmicb.2021.656889.

Chapter 10

Different Forms of Intestinal Injury: Moving Beyond NEC

Diomel de la Cruz and Daniel R. Gipson

Chapter Outline

Key Points

1. Necrotizing enterocolitis (NEC) is a poorly defined umbrella diagnosis for what is more likely a heterogenous group of acquired neonatal intestinal injuries.
2. Multiple criteria exist for NEC, of varying sensitivities and specificities. However, much of the research is clouded by inaccurate definitions and diagnoses.
3. Classic preterm NEC likely has a multifactorial pathophysiology with intestinal immaturity, immune immaturity, and microbial dysbiosis all contributing toward a reduced intestinal barrier and resultant inflammatory response.
4. Feeding with human milk is a protective factor against the development of NEC.
5. Spontaneous intestinal perforation (SIP) tends to occur at a younger postnatal age and in smaller infants compared to classic preterm NEC. SIP presents as isolated pneumoperitoneum resulting from focal perforation of the intestinal muscularis propria layer without intestinal necrosis.
6. Cardiac-induced mesenteric hypoperfusion syndrome associated with insufficient systemic blood flow to the intestines can result in necrotizing intestinal injury. It more commonly involves the large intestine, which is more prone to watershed injury.
7. Preterm infants often demonstrate slow gastrointestinal motility that can present with similar signs to other serious acquired intestinal injuries.
8. More research is needed to better define different types of acquired neonatal intestinal injuries and to develop tailored diagnostic and treatment strategies.

Introduction

Despite decades of hypotheses and research, there has been a recognized stagnation surrounding advancements in diagnosing and treating necrotizing enterocolitis (NEC). This is partly attributable to an overly inclusive diagnosis that amalgamates a host of disease processes under a single label. While NEC has previously been described as a heterogeneous disease with various presentations, it is time for the field to go beyond adherence to an outdated umbrella diagnosis and move toward reclassifying and redefining distinctly different types of acquired intestinal injuries, each of which requires a unique treatment approach.[1,2] To that end, we herein describe a myriad of neonatal intestinal pathologies that are increasingly recognized as unique entities rather than points along a single disease spectrum.

Necrotizing Enterocolitis Background

NEC, as per our current understanding, is one of the most critical clinical encounters neonatologists experience in the NICU, with an overall mortality rate of 32%.[3] Unfortunately, it is also one of the most prevalent, with an incidence of 5% to 12% in very-low-birth-weight infants (born <1500 g).[4] It is a very costly disease that significantly increases length of stay and hospitalization charges.[5] First classified by Mizrahi and colleagues in 1964–1965, NEC has for decades perniciously remained a single diagnosis for a heterogeneous group of diseases with heterogeneous pathophysiologies.[6,7] Martin Bell proposed the first widely used staging system for NEC in 1978, a laudable attempt at describing a diverse disease process.[8] Bell's staging classified NEC into three stages of increasing severity: stage I consisted of suspected NEC, stage II was indicative of "definite" NEC, and stage III was indicative of advanced NEC requiring surgical attention. However, Bell's staging had significant limitations. The original paper cited concerns that stage I criteria were overly inclusive and likely contributing to incorrect diagnoses of NEC that were not genuinely present.[8]

In 1986, Walsh and Kliegman introduced a modified version of Bell's staging criteria, subdividing each of the original stages into two subcategories classified as A and B.[9] With these subdivisions, more specific criteria were included and organized by systemic signs, intestinal signs, and radiographic signs, and the recommended treatment was outlined for each stage (Table 10.1). However, growing experience with an evolving patient population of younger neonates with a diverse range of neonatal intestinal injuries has created a greater emphasis on improving the definition of what we are labeling as necrotizing enterocolitis. Multiple attempts at improved diagnostic criteria were developed over recent years including VON (Vermont Oxford Network), CDC (Centers for Disease Control and Prevention), Stanford in 2014, UK (United Kingdom Neonatal Collaborative) in 2017, 2of3 Rule in 2018, and INC (International Neonatal Consortium) criteria in 2019 (Table 10.2).[10–16] Though it remains unclear which set of criteria may be superior in sensitivity and specificity, no single set of criteria has yet emerged as the gold standard across the field. Many sets of criteria continue to include nonspecific signs such as abdominal distension and thrombocytopenia that occur with other illnesses and could contribute to the overdiagnosis of NEC.

Meanwhile, Bell's staging continues to be most frequently utilized in research, with studies often including only Bell's stage II and stage III in their definitions of NEC. However, it is increasingly clear that what has previously been called "NEC" represents more than one disease process. A lack of consensus and an inability to establish effective and exclusive criteria have contributed to nonspecific datasets inclusive of pathologies other than necrotizing intestinal injuries. In the absence of clear definitions, it has proved challenging to develop precise predictive and diagnostic biomarkers and has hindered advancement in preventive and therapeutic strategies. Future research into better defining distinct types of neonatal intestinal injuries and their corresponding markers is needed. Nevertheless, to discuss pathologies that are not necrotizing intestinal injuries, we will first review what is generally considered "classic NEC."

Classic Preterm Enterocolitis

CLINICAL PRESENTATION AND DIAGNOSIS

Despite shortcomings in specific diagnostic criteria, there is a severe and fulminant form of necrotizing

TABLE 10.1	Walsh and Kliegman's Modified Bell's Staging			
Stage	Systemic Signs	Intestinal Signs	Radiologic Signs	Treatment
IA – Suspected NEC	Temperature instability, apnea, bradycardia, lethargy	Elevated pre-gavage residuals, mild abdominal distention, emesis, guaiac-positive stool	Normal or intestinal dilation, mild ileus	NPO, antibiotics × 3d pending culture
IB – Suspected NEC	Same as above	Bright red blood from rectum	Same as above	Same as above
IIA – Definite NEC Mildly ill	Same as above	Same as above, *plus* absent bowel sounds, ± abdominal tenderness	Intestinal dilation, ileus, pneumatosis intestinalis	NPO, antibiotics × 7–10 d if exam is normal in 24–48 h
IIB – Definite NEC Moderately ill	Same as above, *plus* mild metabolic acidosis, mild thrombocytopenia	Same as above, *plus* absent bowel sounds, definite abdominal tenderness, ± abdominal cellulitis or RLQ mass	Same as IIA, *plus* portal vein gas, ± ascites	NPO, antibiotics × 14 d, NaHCO$_3$ for acidosis
IIIA – Advanced NEC Severely ill, bowel intact	Same as IIB, *plus* hypotension, bradycardia, severe apnea, combined respiratory and metabolic acidosis, DIC, neutropenia	Same as above, *plus* signs of generalized peritonitis, marked tenderness, and distension of abdomen	Same as IIB, *plus* definite ascites	Same as above, *plus* 200 + mL/kg fluids, inotropic agents, ventilation, therapy, paracentesis
IIIB – Advanced NEC Severely ill, bowel perforated	Same as IIIA	Same as IIIA	Same as IIB, *plus* pneumoperitoneum	Same as above, *plus* surgical intervention

d, Days; *DIC*, disseminated intravascular coagulation; *h*, hours; *NEC*, necrotizing enterocolitis; *NPO*, nil per os; *RLQ*, right lower quadrant..

neonatal intestinal injury, herein described as classic preterm NEC. Affected infants may present with several nonspecific signs including abdominal distension, feeding intolerance, bilious emesis, and bloody stools while receiving enteral feeds. However, differentiating these signs from signs seen with other types of intestinal injuries remains a diagnostic hurdle. Radiographic evidence of pneumatosis intestinalis and portal venous gas are prominent features that likely represent fermentation by bacteria translocated through the intestinal wall (Fig. 10.1).[17] Unfortunately, identifying pneumatosis intestinalis remains subjective and challenging for accurate diagnosis, especially considering pneumatosis may occasionally be present with other pathology.[18,19] Overdiagnosis of NEC is likely to accompany frequent X-rays obtained for signs of feeding intolerance and abdominal distension that may be secondary to other causes such as continuous positive airway pressure (CPAP). Presentation is often abrupt and rapidly progressive to intestinal perforation, severe shock, and death. If surgery is performed, necrosis of the bowel is visualized, and this is currently the only indisputable method of diagnosis.

PATHOPHYSIOLOGY

While NEC has been reported across the gamut from extremely preterm infants to full-term infants, its incidence peaks around 30 weeks corrected gestational age.[20] The pathophysiology is likely multifactorial with interplaying factors of intestinal immaturity, immune immaturity, and microbial dysbiosis all contributing.[21] The intestinal mucosal lining provides a vital barrier of protection against pathogens, but it is underdeveloped in the preterm infant and is significantly impacted by the developing microbiome.[22] A symbiotic microbiome, including *Bifidobacterium*, aids in establishing a healthy mucosal lining and immune tolerance.[22]

However, a relative shift in the fecal microbiome prior to the development of NEC has been demonstrated, with

TABLE 10.2 Comparison Criteria for Necrotizing Enterocolitis						
	UK	**VON**	**CDC**	**2of3**	**Stanford**	**INC**
Risk Grouping						
Gestational age	+			+		+
Postnatal age				+	+	+
Gender					+	
Ethnicity					+	
Exclusion Criteria						
SIP	+	+		+		+
Congenital anomaly				+		+
Fed <80 mL/kg/d				+		
GA ≥36 weeks				+		+
Systemic Signs						
Thrombocytopenia				+	+	+
Acidosis					+	
DIC						+
Ventilated					+	
Intestinal Signs						
Poor feeding					+	
Emesis		+	+			
Pre-gavage residuals	+					
Bilious aspirates	+	+	+			
Abdominal distension	+	+	+	+		+
Rectal bleeding	+	+	+	+		+
Abdominal tenderness	+					
Abdominal discoloration	+				+	
Radiographic Signs						
Ileus					+	
Pneumatosis intestinalis	+	+	+	+	+	+
Portal venous gas	+	+	+	+	+	+
Pneumoperitoneum	+	+	+			
Fixed bowel loop	+					

2of3, 2of3 Rule in 2018; *CDC*, Centers for Disease Control and Prevention; *DIC*, disseminated intravascular coagulation; *GA*, gestational age; *INC*, International Neonatal Consortium; *SIP*, spontaneous intestinal perforation; *VON*, Vermont Oxford Network; *UK*, United Kingdom Neonatal Collaborative.

Adapted from Patel RM, Ferguson J, McElroy SJ, Khashu M, Caplan MS. Defining necrotizing enterocolitis: current difficulties and future opportunities. *Pediatr Res*. 2020;88(suppl 1):10-15. doi:10.1038/S41390-020-1074-4.

gram-positive *Firmicutes* and gram-negative *Bacteroidetes* becoming notably less abundant and gram-negative *Proteobacteria* becoming more abundant.[20] This shift also occurs around 30 weeks corrected gestational age (similar to the peak incidence of NEC) and is impacted by perinatal antibiotic exposure.[20,23] This is significant as *Firmicutes* contribute to increased butyrate, which is essential for maintaining tight junctions and intestinal mucosal integrity.[24,25] Conversely, *Proteobacteria* have significant lipopolysaccharide in the cell wall that is recognized by toll-like receptor 4 (TLR4), which is increased in the preterm intestinal tract.[17,20] This suggests that a proinflammatory effect of *Proteobacteria* in addition to a compromised intestinal mucosal layer (affected by a decrease in *Firmicutes*) could contribute to the pathogenesis of NEC. Furthermore, bacteria from the vaginally derived *Bacteroidetes* phylum have been shown to contribute to immune tolerance, suggesting that a reduction in these bacteria may also contribute to a proinflammatory state involved in the pathogenesis of the disease.[22]

As with many disease states, it is also reasonable to hypothesize that there may be an underlying genetic predisposition. While some genetic variants have been identified as areas of interest, confirming their role in

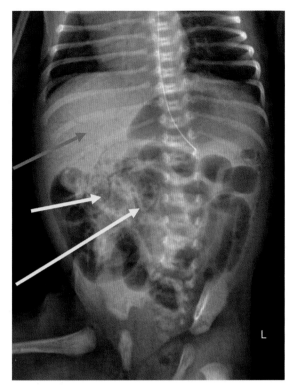

Fig. 10.1 Radiographic evidence of pneumatosis intestinalis *(yellow arrows)* and portal venous gas *(blue arrow)*.

the pathogenesis of NEC requires continued research as none have been definitively implicated.[26]

PREVENTION

There are recognized protective factors and risk factors for the development of disease. In many years of research, only a handful have had evidence to support the decreased risk of NEC including increasing the delivery of mother's own milk, standardization of feeding regimens, antenatal steroids, and delayed cord clamping.[27–30]

Human milk, including both mother's expressed breast milk and donor milk, is an important protective factor that is readily accessible in most modern NICUs.[31–33] Human milk contains antioxidants essential in reducing oxidative stress and avoiding increased intestinal barrier permeability that is induced by bovine-based formulas.[31,34] However, whether human milk–based fortification of breast milk helps reduce NEC compared with bovine-based fortification is less

clear, as the data do not consistently support the routine use of one over the other.[35,36] Slow progression of incremental feeding volume has been a traditional approach to feeding advancement in the NICU. While this strategy may still be helpful for general feeding intolerance associated with prematurity, it has not been shown to reduce the rate of NEC.[37] Furthermore, early fortification does not seem to significantly impact NEC incidence compared to late fortification.[38,39] Delaying the introduction of feeds has also not proven to prevent NEC.[40,41]

Routine surveillance of gastric residuals was a previously widespread practice, with large residuals raising concern for early signs of NEC. However, monitoring gastric residuals has no impact on reducing the incidence of NEC,[42] and many NICUs have largely abandoned this long-held practice due to the potential associated risks of prolonging time to full feeds and increasing the duration of hospitalization.

There have been numerous studies focused on the use of probiotics for the reduction of NEC, and a review of multiple meta-analyses supports a consensus that probiotics, precisely a combination of *Lactobacillus* and *Bifidobacteria*, likely reduce the incidence of NEC and death.[43] However, there remain significant obstacles into implementing routine probiotic use in the NICU. There are clinically impactful differences between unique bacterial strains among the same genus, and identifying the optimal combination of strains deserves more study.[43] Furthermore, probiotics are classified as dietary supplements, which do not undergo the same rigorous review by the US Food and Drug Administration (FDA) as pharmaceuticals for safety and efficacy.[44] The American Academy of Pediatrics (AAP) Committee on the Fetus and Newborn has examined this issue closely and raised concerns. The consistency of probiotics is decidedly variable among manufacturers and ensuring a quality probiotic for our patient population remains a challenge. As such, any use of probiotics to reduce NEC remains off-label and should be used with caution.[43,44] Furthermore, according to AAP recommendations, "current evidence does not support the routine universal administration of probiotics to preterm infants, particularly those with a birth weight of less than 1000 g." Therefore probiotic administration for the reduction of NEC remains controversial.

MANAGEMENT

When true necrotizing intestinal injury is suspected, patients should immediately be made nil per os (NPO) to avoid any additional metabolic demand on the intestine in crisis, and parenteral nutrition (PN) should be initiated. A large bore orogastric tube (Replogle) should be placed to permit gastric decompression. Antibiotics such as metronidazole or piperacillin/tazobactam are often used to cover enteric anaerobic organisms, and though thought to be beneficial, this practice is currently not evidence based. Surgical consultation should be sought as soon as possible in case the disease progresses to warrant surgical attention, which can occur precipitously. Serial X-rays may be performed to monitor for evolution of the bowel gas pattern, which may help distinguish an "NEC scare" from feeding intolerance. Serial X-rays may also be helpful to differentiate true pneumatosis intestinalis from simply stool that will later pass, previously described as "poopatosis."[1]

Surgery is often pursued for patients who fail to improve with conservative therapy. There are primarily two surgical treatment approaches to NEC: placement of a peritoneal drain versus exploratory laparotomy with resection of necrotic bowel. Identifying the superior treatment approach has long been a topic of debate, with previous evidence showing no statistically significant difference in mortality, dependence on PN, and duration of hospitalization between the two.[45–47] However, the most glaring limitation of previous studies is that these surgical approaches were evaluated concurrently for diagnoses of both NEC and spontaneous intestinal perforation (SIP), which are two distinctly different diseases that would benefit from tailored approaches. This alludes to the substantial difficulty in accurate diagnosis preoperatively. This is supported by evidence that 9% to 74% of infants initially receiving peritoneal drain later require a laparotomy.[46–48] More recent evidence suggests that laparotomy is likely more beneficial than peritoneal drain for initial operative management of suspected true necrotizing intestinal injury.[48] Considering the significant research obstacles in definitively proving a superior surgical approach in a relatively rare disease state that occurs during a surgical emergency, a shift in practice toward initial laparotomy for NEC based on this recent

evidence arguably may be the best approach to improving patient outcomes in the near future.[48]

Spontaneous Intestinal Perforation

Case reports and case series of SIP isolated from any surgical or pathologic evidence of necrotizing bowel injury first emerged in the 1980s.[49,50] With the widespread availability of surfactant in the 1990s, the neonatal population treated in the NICU evolved to include a sizable proportion of younger, smaller neonates.[2] Similar to the rapid evolution of pathologies and development seen throughout pediatrics as a child grows, these age-specific differences are magnified even greater in the neonatal population, where a week of life has vast effects on the viability and development of an infant. Thus SIP has become increasingly common with this shift in the neonatal population and has evolved to be recognized as a distinct clinical entity.[2,51]

CLINICAL PRESENTATION AND DIAGNOSIS

Although there is considerable overlap in the timing and presentation of SIP and classic preterm NEC, the illness tends to present at an earlier postnatal age than NEC, with most cases occurring during the first one to two weeks of life, with an incidence of 3.9% to 7.4% in very-low-birth-weight infants.[1,48,51–54] It also occurs in smaller infants with a younger corrected gestational age than NEC.[51,53] Infants typically present with abdominal distension and bluish discoloration of the abdomen.[50,51] X-rays will often show *isolated* pneumoperitoneum without the typical accompanying radiographic signs of NEC such as thickening of the intestinal wall, pneumatosis intestinalis, and portal venous gas.[51] While abdominal free air is also commonly seen in classic preterm NEC with bowel perforation, identifying isolated pneumoperitoneum can be essential in accurately diagnosing SIP preoperatively. An absence of abdominal gas is another concerning X-ray pattern seen with SIP.[50,51] It should also be noted that an absence of pneumoperitoneum on X-ray does not exclude SIP.[51] If surgery is performed, a single 5–10 mm perforation with surrounding hemorrhagic changes is usually visualized.[51] Though this has often been seen along the antimesenteric border of the distal ileum,[51] perforations may also occur elsewhere along the intestine.[55] The extensive necrosis seen in classic preterm NEC is absent.[50,51]

PATHOPHYSIOLOGY

The pathophysiology of SIP is not fully understood. Pathology of surgical specimens reveals thinned submucosa with focal perforation of the muscularis propria layer, which has led to hypotheses that either a congenital or acquired defect in the intestinal muscularis propria predisposes infants to SIP.[2,55] The intestinal muscle layer has been shown to increase in thickness with increasing corrected gestational age while the incidence of SIP decreases with increasing gestational age.[55] In addition, adjacent areas of normal-appearing bowel in patients with SIP demonstrate standard thickness of the muscularis layer, which further supports the theory that a defect in the intestinal muscle layer plays a role in pathogenesis.[55]

Indomethacin was first associated with SIP from the initial case reports that identified SIP as a separate disease.[49,50] Indomethacin and postnatal dexamethasone have both been identified as independent risk factors for SIP.[52,56] However, when indomethacin is combined with postnatal glucocorticoids, there is a synergistic effect that substantially increases the risk for SIP.[52,57,58] Therefore this combination is usually avoided if possible. Recently, the co-exposure of indomethacin and antenatal steroids has been associated with an increase in the risk of SIP.[59] It should be noted that SIP can occur in the absence of these risk factors,[55] so they do not seem essential to the pathogenesis of disease but rather augment the effects of disease through unclear mechanisms.

MANAGEMENT

Management for SIP is currently like management of classic preterm NEC. When SIP is suspected, patients should be made NPO, a large bore orogastric tube should be placed to provide abdominal decompression, and surgical consultation should be sought. As previously discussed, optimal surgical management for SIP remains unclear due to past research evaluating surgical outcomes in tandem with NEC, which showed no superior treatment between peritoneal drain and exploratory laparotomy.[45–47] However, the diagnosis of SIP versus intestinal necrosis is unclear with peritoneal drain, and definitive diagnosis can

only be confirmed with direct visualization during exploratory laparotomy. The preoperative diagnosis does influence the outcome of surgery,[48] making accurate preoperative diagnosis critical to improving patient outcomes. A recent study has identified machine learning as a potential for improving preoperative diagnosis that could hopefully contribute to improved patient outcomes in the future.[53]

Cardiac-Induced Mesenteric Hypoperfusion Syndrome

NEC has been reported in term neonates, echoing of the heterogeneity of what has previously been deemed "NEC."[60] Notably, congenital heart disease has been identified as a significant risk factor for an ischemic intestinal injury resulting in necrosis that was previously classified under the NEC umbrella, but herein is described as cardiac-induced mesenteric hypoperfusion syndrome (MHS).

CLINICAL PRESENTATION AND DIAGNOSIS

While classic preterm NEC is usually seen around 30 weeks, MHS is primarily seen in term infants with an average gestational age of 38.6 weeks.[20,61] Signs at presentation are very similar to those seen in classic preterm NEC with abdominal distension and feeding intolerance. However, congenital heart disease prior to surgical correction is the distinguishing feature for diagnosis.[61] While the syndrome has been seen across multiple cardiac pathologies, a shared feature is decreased perfusion to the lower body (including the gastrointestinal tract) through either pulmonary steal or obstruction of systemic circulation.[61] Surgery is indicated as commonly for MHS as for classic preterm NEC.[61] However, if surgery is performed, the necrotic bowel is more likely to be focal and involve the large intestine. In contrast, classic NEC in preterm infants is more likely to involve the small intestine and ileocecal region.[61]

PATHOPHYSIOLOGY

Like many other intestinal injuries previously classified as NEC, the pathophysiology of cardiac-induced MHS is not fully understood. However, cardiac-induced intestinal ischemia is thought to be the major driving factor in pathogenesis leading to necrotic bowel injury.[61] This is supported by increased acidosis seen in MHS compared to classic preterm NEC and increased frequency of colonic involvement seen with MHS, as the colon is more susceptible to watershed injury than the small intestine.[61] Persistent retrograde diastolic flow is associated with a considerably increased risk of cardiac-associated necrotizing bowel injury: 47% compared to 15% in one case-control study.[62] As blood flow will follow the path of least resistance, this supports the hypothesis that pulmonary steal is a common mechanism for the cardiac-induced ischemia seen with MHS.[61] In a study by Bubberman et al., classic preterm NEC tended to have higher C-reactive protein (CRP) concentrations at presentation than MHS, supporting the concept that classic preterm NEC is likely a primarily inflammatory disorder with subsequent necrosis while MHS is likely a primarily ischemic disorder with secondary inflammation.[61]

MANAGEMENT

Cardiac-induced MHS is managed similarly to the more commonly seen preterm necrotizing intestinal injury: by halting of any enteral feeds, abdominal decompression, and prompt surgical consultation. Prevention is best achieved through a multidisciplinary team involving both neonatology and cardiology expertise. Abdominal near-infrared spectroscopy (NIRS), which has been shown to be useful for monitoring postoperative cardiac output, is one area among many for future study.[63] Future research should focus on MHS as a unique entity to best implement successful strategies for early intervention and to minimize the morbidity and mortality of MHS.

Food Protein–Induced Enterocolitis Syndrome

Food protein–induced enterocolitis syndrome (FPIES) is a well-recognized diagnosis in older infants typically seen after exposure to cow's milk or soy protein.[64] Though reports of enterocolitis in the infant population date back to 1976,[65,66] this condition is likely underdiagnosed in the preterm population due to a significant overlap in clinical presentation with classic preterm NEC signs.[18] However, FPIES is now increasingly being added to the differential diagnosis of neonatal abdominal complications.[18,19]

CLINICAL PRESENTATION AND DIAGNOSIS

FPIES has a range of presentations that can vary from mild to quite severe, and the incidence of the disorder among preterm infants is unknown.[18] Signs of emesis, diarrhea, and bloody or hemoccult positive stools are typical, but poor feeding, abdominal distension, and severe dehydration leading to shock may develop.[18,19,64,66] Although the mechanism is unclear, pneumatosis intestinalis has been reported on abdominal X-rays associated with FPIES, though pneumoperitoneum is not expected.[18,19] There are no radiographic signs specific to FPIES diagnosis.[64] Labs show evidence of predominantly neutrophilic leukocytosis and thrombocytosis, and a higher percentage of eosinophils can be a clue.[18,64] Accurate diagnosis requires strong clinical suspicion, and FPIES should be considered on the differential diagnosis when signs typically associated with NEC develop in infants outside of the usual age range expected for classic preterm NEC. No biomarkers have been identified to aid in diagnosing FPIES, making differentiation from other intestinal pathologies based on presentation alone challenging.

PATHOPHYSIOLOGY

FPIES is a non-IgE hypersensitivity that can develop following exposure to various food allergens, most commonly cow's milk protein or soy protein in the infant population.[64] It is suspected to be a T cell–mediated hypersensitivity leading to increased intestinal permeability, fluid shift, and inflammation.[64] Although it is not primarily an IgE-mediated process, it is associated with a higher rate of atopy than the general population.[64]

MANAGEMENT

Treatment for FPIES entails removing the causal agent, which is usually a cow's milk or soy protein in formula for infants, and transitioning to an extensively hydrolyzed or elemental formula.[18,19] For infants who are breastfeeding or exclusively receiving unfortified breast milk, elimination of maternal exposure to dietary cow's milk or soy protein should be considered.[18] For infants in the NICU, removal of cow's milk–based fortifier in breast milk may be required for symptom resolution. Resolution of symptoms after dietary modifications confirms the diagnosis, and endoscopy is not recommended.[64] Tolerance to the causative agent usually develops, but the age at which tolerance develops is highly variable between individuals.[64] Tolerance usually occurs around 3 years of age for cow's milk, and it usually occurs around 12 months for soy protein.[64] However, these ages should not be deemed classic, as tolerance has been reported at much younger as well as significantly older ages.[64]

General Feeding Intolerance

While not an actual neonatal intestinal injury, generalized feeding intolerance attributable to slow motility of the gastrointestinal tract in the preterm infant can present with similar signs to other serious acquired intestinal injuries previously described. Feeding intolerance is also poorly defined, especially when criteria such as abdominal circumference and gastric residuals are used, which may fluctuate for a variety of reasons. X-rays will show gaseous distension or evidence of an ileus, and radiographs may raise concern for pneumatosis that in actuality is a bubbly appearance of stool mixed with bowel gas.[1] Differentiating which infant with abdominal distension and emesis has classic preterm NEC versus slow motility can be difficult and is becoming increasingly necessary with the shift in the NICU population toward younger infants who consistently demonstrate motility issues. Approaches to feeding intolerance will be discussed separately in this book, but it should be emphasized that although many of these infants meet Bell's criteria for "stage 1 NEC," most of these infants likely do not have a necrotizing intestinal injury. Furthermore, there is no evidence that these infants are at risk to progress to genuine necrotizing intestinal injury.[1]

Summary

A host of distinctly different neonatal intestinal injuries are being recognized, each with their own unique pathophysiology and need for a tailored treatment approach. While this collection of intestinal diseases has historically fallen under the umbrella of "NEC," this catch-all diagnosis is inaccurate, imprecise, and no longer appropriate. To continue to diagnose a variety of conditions under a single label supports a fallacy

and has hindered the field from moving forward. For example, despite first recognition of SIP as a distinct entity in the 1980s,[49,50] there continues to be no specific international classification of disease code for the disorder, markedly impacting research with the use of electronic health records. Without clear identification of distinct diseases, we are encumbered from making progress. The challenge lies ahead in continuing to better define what constitutes the various types of intestinal injuries and what contributes to their underlying pathophysiologies so that precise and predictive diagnostic and therapeutic strategies can be implemented. Fortunately, artificial intelligence, machine learning, and identification of biomarkers and metabolomics are showing promising contributions to more accurate distinction and prognostication and could be integral to advancing the field.[67–70]

REFERENCES

1. Neu J, Modi N, Caplan M. Necrotizing enterocolitis comes in different forms: historical perspectives and defining the disease. *Semin Fetal Neonatal Med.* 2018;23(6):370-373. doi:10.1016/J.SINY.2018.07.004.
2. Gordon PV, Swanson JR, Attridge JT, Clark R. Emerging trends in acquired neonatal intestinal disease: is it time to abandon Bell's criteria? *J Perinatol.* 2007;27(11):661-671. doi:10.1038/SJ.JP.7211782.
3. Thyoka M, de Coppi P, Eaton S, et al. Advanced necrotizing enterocolitis part 1: mortality. *Eur J Pediatr Surg.* 2012;22(1):8-12. doi:10.1055/S-0032-1306263.
4. Meister AL, Doheny KK, Travagli RA. Necrotizing enterocolitis: it's not all in the gut. *Exp Biol Med (Maywood).* 2020;245(2):85. doi:10.1177/1535370219891971.
5. Bisquera JA, Cooper TR, Berseth CL. Impact of necrotizing enterocolitis on length of stay and hospital charges in very low birth weight infants. *Pediatrics.* 2002;109(3):423-428. doi:10.1542/PEDS.109.3.423.
6. Berdon WE, Grossman H, Baker DH, Mizrahi A, Barlow O, Blanc WA. Necrotizing enterocolitis in the premature infant. *Radiology.* 1964;83:879-887. doi:10.1148/83.5.879.
7. Mizrahi A, Barlow O, Berdon W, Blanc WA, Silverman WA. Necrotizing enterocolitis in premature infants. *J Pediatr.* 1965;66(4):697-706. doi:10.1016/S0022-3476(65)80003-8.
8. Bell MJ, Ternberg JL, Feigin RD, et al. Neonatal necrotizing enterocolitis. Therapeutic decisions based upon clinical staging. *Ann Surg.* 1978;187(1):1-7. doi:10.1097/00000658-197801000-00001.
9. Walsh MC, Kliegman RM. Necrotizing enterocolitis: treatment based on staging criteria. *Pediatr Clin North Am.* 1986;33(1):179-201. doi:10.1016/S0031-3955(16)34975-6.
10. Vermont Oxford Network. *2022 Manual of Operations, Part 2, Release 26.1 (PDF) – Help Center.* Available at: https://vtoxford.zendesk.com/hc/en-us/articles/4405064008467-2022-Manual-of-Operations-Part-2-Release-26-1-PDF-. Accessed January 26, 2022.

11. CDC, Ncezid, DHQP. *CDC/NHSN Surveillance Definitions for Specific Types of Infections*. Published Online 2023.

12. Ji J, Ling XB, Zhao Y, et al. A data-driven algorithm integrating clinical and laboratory features for the diagnosis and prognosis of necrotizing enterocolitis. *PLoS One*. 2014;9(2):e89860. doi:10.1371/JOURNAL.PONE.0089860.

13. Battersby C, Longford N, Costeloe K, Modi N. Development of a gestational age-specific case definition for neonatal necrotizing enterocolitis. *JAMA Pediatr*. 2017;171(3):256-263. doi:10.1001/JAMAPEDIATRICS.2016.3633.

14. Gephart SM, Gordon PV, Penn AH, et al. Changing the paradigm of defining, detecting, and diagnosing NEC: perspectives on Bell's stages and biomarkers for NEC. *Semin Pediatr Surg*. 2018;27(1):3-10. doi:10.1053/J.SEMPEDSURG.2017.11.002.

15. Caplan MS, Underwood MA, Modi N, et al. Necrotizing enterocolitis: using regulatory science and drug development to improve outcomes. *J Pediatr*. 2019;212:208-215.e1. doi:10.1016/J.JPEDS.2019.05.032.

16. Patel RM, Ferguson J, McElroy SJ, Khashu M, Caplan MS. Defining necrotizing enterocolitis: current difficulties and future opportunities. *Pediatr Res*. 2020;88(suppl 1):10-15. doi:10.1038/S41390-020-1074-4.

17. Morowitz MJ, Poroyko V, Caplan M, Alverdy J, Liu DC. Redefining the role of intestinal microbes in the pathogenesis of necrotizing enterocolitis. *Pediatrics*. 2010;125(4):777-785. doi:10.1542/PEDS.2009-3149.

18. Kim YI, Joo JY, Jung YH, Choi CW, Kim BI, Yang HR. Differentiation of food protein-induced enterocolitis syndrome misleading to necrotizing enterocolitis. *Ann Allergy Asthma Immunol*. 2022;128(2):193-198. doi:10.1016/j.anai.2021.09.024.

19. Lenfestey MW, de la Cruz D, Neu J. Food protein-induced enterocolitis instead of necrotizing enterocolitis? A neonatal intensive care unit case series. *J Pediatr*. 2018;200:270-273. doi:10.1016/J.JPEDS.2018.04.048.

20. Pammi M, Cope J, Tarr PI, et al. Intestinal dysbiosis in preterm infants preceding necrotizing enterocolitis: a systematic review and meta-analysis. *Microbiome*. 2017;5(1):31. doi:10.1186/S40168-017-0248-8.

21. Neu J, Walker WA. Necrotizing enterocolitis. *N Engl J Med*. 2011;364(3):255. doi:10.1056/NEJMRA1005408.

22. van Belkum M, Mendoza Alvarez L, Neu J. Preterm neonatal immunology at the intestinal interface. *Cell Mol Life Sci*. 2020;77(7):1209-1227. doi:10.1007/S00018-019-03316-W.

23. Mai V, Young CM, Ukhanova M, et al. Fecal microbiota in premature infants prior to necrotizing enterocolitis. *PLoS One*. 2011;6(6):e20647. doi:10.1371/JOURNAL.PONE.0020647.

24. Louis P, Flint HJ. Formation of propionate and butyrate by the human colonic microbiota. *Environ Microbiol*. 2017;19(1):29-41. doi:10.1111/1462-2920.13589.

25. Peng L, Li ZR, Green RS, Holzman IR, Lin J. Butyrate enhances the intestinal barrier by facilitating tight junction assembly via activation of AMP-activated protein kinase in Caco-2 cell monolayers. *J Nutr*. 2009;139(9):1619-1625. doi:10.3945/JN.109.104638.

26. Cuna A, George L, Sampath V. Genetic predisposition to necrotizing enterocolitis in premature infants: current knowledge, challenges, and future directions. *Semin Fetal Neonatal Med*. 2018;23(6):387-393. doi:10.1016/J.SINY.2018.08.006.

27. Patole SK, de Klerk N. Impact of standardised feeding regimens on incidence of neonatal necrotising enterocolitis: a systematic review and meta-analysis of observational studies. *Arch Dis Child Fetal Neonatal Ed*. 2005;90(2):F147-F151. doi:10.1136/ADC.2004.059741.

28. Jasani B, Patole S. Standardized feeding regimen for reducing necrotizing enterocolitis in preterm infants: an updated systematic review. *J Perinatol*. 2017;37(7):827-833. doi:10.1038/JP.2017.37.

29. Travers CP, Clark RH, Spitzer AR, Das A, Garite TJ, Carlo WA. Exposure to any antenatal corticosteroids and outcomes in preterm infants by gestational age: prospective cohort study. *BMJ*. 2017;356:1039. doi:10.1136/BMJ.J1039.

30. Garg BD, Kabra NS, Bansal A. Role of delayed cord clamping in prevention of necrotizing enterocolitis in preterm neonates: a systematic review. *J Matern Fetal Neonatal Med*. 2019;32(1):164-172. doi:10.1080/14767058.2017.1370704.

31. Patel AL, Kim JH. Human milk and necrotizing enterocolitis. *Semin Pediatr Surg*. 2018;27(1):34-38. doi:10.1053/J.SEMPEDSURG.2017.11.007.

32. Boyd CA, Quigley MA, Brocklehurst P. Donor breast milk versus infant formula for preterm infants: systematic review and meta-analysis. *Arch Dis Child Fetal Neonatal Ed*. 2007;92(3):F169-F175. doi:10.1136/ADC.2005.089490.

33. Quigley M, Embleton ND, Mcguire W. Formula versus donor breast milk for feeding preterm or low birth weight infants. *Cochrane Database Syst Rev*. 2018;6(6):CD002971. doi:10.1002/14651858.CD002971.PUB4.

34. Shoji H, Shimizu T, Shinohara K, Oguchi S, Shiga S, Yamashiro Y. Suppressive effects of breast milk on oxidative DNA damage in very low birthweight infants. *Arch Dis Child Fetal Neonatal Ed*. 2004;89(2):F136-F138. doi:10.1136/ADC.2002.018390.

35. Parker MG, Stellwagen LM, Noble L, Kim JH, Poindexter BB, Puopolo KM. Promoting human milk and breastfeeding for the very low birth weight infant. *Pediatrics*. 2021;148(5):e2021054272. doi:10.1542/PEDS.2021-054272.

36. O'Connor DL, Kiss A, Tomlinson C, et al. Nutrient enrichment of human milk with human and bovine milk-based fortifiers for infants born weighing. *Am J Clin Nutr*. 2018;108(1):108-116. doi:10.1093/AJCN/NQY067.

37. Dorling J, Abbott J, Berrington J, et al. Controlled trial of two incremental milk-feeding rates in preterm infants. *N Engl J Med*. 2019;381(15):1434-1443. doi:10.1056/NEJMOA1816654.

38. Sullivan S, Schanler RJ, Kim JH, et al. An exclusively human milk-based diet is associated with a lower rate of necrotizing enterocolitis than a diet of human milk and bovine milk-based products. *J Pediatr*. 2010;156(4):562-567.e1. doi:10.1016/J.JPEDS.2009.10.040.

39. Oddie SJ, Young L, McGuire W. Slow advancement of enteral feed volumes to prevent necrotizing enterocolitis in very low birth weight infants. *Cochrane Database Syst Rev*. 2021;8(8):CD001241. doi:10.1002/14651858.CD001241.pub8.

40. Morgan J, Young L, Mcguire W. Delayed introduction of progressive enteral feeds to prevent necrotising enterocolitis in very low birth weight infants. *Cochrane Database Syst Rev*. 2014;2014(12):CD001970. doi: 10.1002/14651858.CD001970.pub5.

41. Salas AA, Li P, Parks K, Lal CV, Martin CR, Carlo WA. Early progressive feeding in extremely preterm infants: a randomized trial. *Am J Clin Nutr*. 2018;107(3):365-370. doi:10.1093/AJCN/NQY012.

42. Parker LA, Weaver M, Murgas Torrazza RJ, et al. Effect of gastric residual evaluation on enteral intake in extremely preterm infants: a randomized clinical trial. *JAMA Pediatr*. 2019;173(6):534-543. doi:10.1001/JAMAPEDIATRICS.2019.0800.

43. Underwood MA. Probiotics and the prevention of necrotizing enterocolitis. *J Pediatr Surg*. 2019;54(3):405-412. doi:10.1016/J.JPEDSURG.2018.08.055.

44. Poindexter B, Cummings J, Hand I, et al. Use of probiotics in preterm infants. *Pediatrics*. 2021;147(6):e2021051485. doi:10.1542/peds.2021-051485.

45. Rao SC, Basani L, Simmer K, Samnakay N, Deshpande G. Peritoneal drainage versus laparotomy as initial surgical treatment for perforated necrotizing enterocolitis or spontaneous intestinal perforation in preterm low birth weight infants. *Cochrane Database System Rev*. 2011;(6):CD006182. doi:10.1002/14651858.CD006182.PUB2.

46. Moss RL, Dimmitt RA, Barnhart DC, et al. Laparotomy versus peritoneal drainage for necrotizing enterocolitis and perforation. *N Engl J Med*. 2006;354(21):2225-2234. doi:10.1056/NEJMOA054605.

47. Rees CM, Eaton S, Kiely EM, Wade AM, McHugh K, Pierro A. Peritoneal drainage or laparotomy for neonatal bowel perforation? A randomized controlled trial. *Ann Surg*. 2008;248(1):44-51. doi:10.1097/SLA.0B013E318176BF81.

48. Blakely ML, Tyson JE, Lally KP, et al. Initial laparotomy versus peritoneal drainage in extremely low birthweight infants with surgical necrotizing enterocolitis or isolated intestinal perforation: a multicenter randomized clinical trial. *Ann Surg*. 2021;274(4):e370-e380. doi:10.1097/SLA.0000000000005099.

49. Nagaraj HS, Sandhu AS, Cook LN, Buchino JJ, Groff DB. Gastrointestinal perforation following indomethacin therapy in very low birth weight infants. *J Pediatr Surg*. 1981;16(6):1003-1007. doi:10.1016/S0022-3468(81)80865-2.

50. Aschner JL, Deluga KS, Metlay LA, Emmens RW, Hendricks-Munoz KD. Spontaneous focal gastrointestinal perforation in very low birth weight infants. *J Pediatr*. 1988;113(2):364-367. doi:10.1016/S0022-3476(88)80285-3.

51. Pumberger W, Mayr M, Kohlhauser C, Weninger M. Spontaneous localized intestinal perforation in very-low-birth-weight infants: a distinct clinical entity different from necrotizing enterocolitis. *J Am Coll Surg*. 2002;195(6):796-803. doi:10.1016/S1072-7515(02)01344-3.

52. Attridge JT, Clark R, Walker MW, Gordon PV. New insights into spontaneous intestinal perforation using a national data set: (1) SIP is associated with early indomethacin exposure. *J Perinatol*. 2006;26(2):93-99. doi:10.1038/SJ.JP.7211429.

53. Lure AC, Du X, Black EW, et al. Using machine learning analysis to assist in differentiating between necrotizing enterocolitis and spontaneous intestinal perforation: a novel predictive analytic tool. *J Pediatr Surg*. 2021;56(10):1703-1710. doi:10.1016/J.JPEDSURG.2020.11.008.

54. Berrington J, Embleton ND. Discriminating necrotising enterocolitis and focal intestinal perforation. *Arch Dis Child Fetal Neonatal Ed*. 2022;107(3):336-339. doi:10.1136/ARCHDISCHILD-2020-321429.

55. Lai S, Yu W, Wallace L, Sigalet D. Intestinal muscularis propria increases in thickness with corrected gestational age and is focally attenuated in patients with isolated intestinal perforations. *J Pediatr Surg*. 2014;49(1):114-119. doi:10.1016/J.JPEDSURG.2013.09.045.

56. Gordon P, Rutledge J, Sawin R, Thomas S, Woodrum D. Early postnatal dexamethasone increases the risk of focal small bowel perforation in extremely low birth weight infants. *J Perinatol*. 1999;19(8 Pt 1):573-577. doi:10.1038/SJ.JP.7200269.

57. Stark AR, Carlo WA, Tyson JE, et al. Adverse effects of early dexamethasone treatment in extremely-low-birth-weight infants.

National Institute of Child Health and Human Development Neonatal Research Network. *N Engl J Med*. 2001;344(2):163-164. doi:10.1056/NEJM200101113440203.

58. Watterberg KL, Gerdes JS, Cole CH, et al. Prophylaxis of early adrenal insufficiency to prevent bronchopulmonary dysplasia: a multicenter trial. *Pediatrics*. 2004;114(6):1649-1657. doi:10.1542/PEDS.2004-1159.

59. Kandraju H, Kanungo J, Lee KS, et al. Association of co-exposure of antenatal steroid and prophylactic indomethacin with spontaneous intestinal perforation. *J Pediatr*. 2021;235:34-41.e1. doi:10.1016/J.JPEDS.2021.03.012.

60. Short SS, Papillon S, Berel D, Ford HR, Frykman PK, Kawaguchi A. Late onset of necrotizing enterocolitis in the full-term infant is associated with increased mortality: results from a two-center analysis. *J Pediatr Surg*. 2014;49(6):950-953. doi:10.1016/J.JPEDSURG.2014.01.028.

61. Bubberman JM, van Zoonen A, Bruggink JLM, et al. Necrotizing enterocolitis associated with congenital heart disease: a different entity? *J Pediatr Surg*. 2019;54(9):1755-1760. doi:10.1016/J.JPEDSURG.2018.11.012.

62. Carlo WF, Kimball TR, Michelfelder EC, Border WL. Persistent diastolic flow reversal in abdominal aortic Doppler-flow profiles is associated with an increased risk of necrotizing enterocolitis in term infants with congenital heart disease. *Pediatrics*. 2007;119(2):330-335. doi:10.1542/PEDS.2006-2640.

63. Hickok RL, Spaeder MC, Berger JT, Schuette JJ, Klugman D. Postoperative abdominal NIRS values predict low cardiac output syndrome in neonates. *World J Pediatr Congenit Heart Surg*. 2016;7(2):180-184. doi:10.1177/2150135115618939.

64. Nowak-Węgrzyn A, Chehade M, Groetch ME, et al. International consensus guidelines for the diagnosis and management of food protein-induced enterocolitis syndrome: executive summary—workgroup report of the Adverse Reactions to Foods Committee, American Academy of Allergy, Asthma & Immunology. *J Allergy Clin Immunol*. 2017;139(4):1111-1126.e4. doi:10.1016/J.JACI.2016.12.966.

65. Powell GK. Enterocolitis in low-birth-weight infants associated with milk and soy protein intolerance. *J Pediatr*. 1976;88(5):840-844. doi:10.1016/S0022-3476(76)81128-6.

66. Powell GK. Milk- and soy-induced enterocolitis of infancy. Clinical features and standardization of challenge. *J Pediatr*. 1978;93(4):553-560. doi:10.1016/S0022-3476(78)80887-7.

67. Ji J, Ling XB, Zhao Y, et al. A data-driven algorithm integrating clinical and laboratory features for the diagnosis and prognosis of necrotizing enterocolitis. *PLoS One*. 2014;9(2):e89860. doi:10.1371/JOURNAL.PONE.0089860.

68. Irles C, González-Pérez G, Muiños SC, et al. Estimation of neonatal intestinal perforation associated with necrotizing enterocolitis by machine learning reveals new key factors. *Int J Environ Res Public Health*. 2018;15(11):2509. doi:10.3390/IJERPH15112509.

69. Ng PC. An update on biomarkers of necrotizing enterocolitis. *Semin Fetal Neonatal Med*. 2018;23(6):380-386. doi:10.1016/J.SINY.2018.07.006.

70. Agakidou E, Agakidis C, Gika H, Sarafidis K. Emerging biomarkers for prediction and early diagnosis of necrotizing enterocolitis in the era of metabolomics and proteomics. *Fronts Pediatr*. 2020;8:602255. doi:10.3389/FPED.2020.602255.

Chapter 11

Science-Based Strategies for Providing Nutrition for High-Risk Neonates

Diomel de la Cruz

Chapter Outline

Key Points

1. Optimization of the delivery of nutrition to the high-risk infant is essential for ideal growth and development.

2. Standardizing nutrition guidelines based on the current best evidence leads to reduced risk of infection and necrotizing enterocolitis (NEC), fewer parenteral nutrition–associated morbidities, improved postnatal growth, and earlier attainment of full enteral feeds.

3. Mother's own milk (MoM) is considered the preferred enteral dietary choice for the preterm infant. Provision of MoM has been associated with fewer morbidities, such as sepsis, NEC, and retinopathy of prematurity, in the high-risk infant.

4. Human donor milk (HDM) is the preferred alternative to MoM when MoM is unavailable. However, the pasteurization process results in decreased protein and immunomodulatory factors.

5. Prolonged fasting is detrimental to the high-risk infant. The current evidence suggests that volume increases of up to 30 mL/kg/d of enteral feeds may be safe and beneficial to the neonate. Delaying the advancement of enteral nutrition does not decrease the risk for NEC.

6. Fortification of feeds is imperative in the optimization of neonatal nutrition. Unfortified feeds increase the risk of osteopenia, poor growth, and nutrient deficiency. Earlier initiation of fortification increases protein intake and has not been shown to increase the risk for feeding intolerance and intestinal catastrophes.

7. More studies are needed to determine the superiority of human milk–based fortification versus bovine milk–based fortification. The routine use of human milk–based fortification is still controversial and comes with concerns of poor growth and high costs.

8. Both standardized and individualized fortification are methods to add multicomponent fortifiers to MoM and HDM.

9. The routine evaluation of gastric residuals is not beneficial in preventing NEC and may lead to delays in achieving complete enteral nutrition.

10. Parenteral nutrition (PN) is needed to provide adequate nutrients until the neonate's gastrointestinal tract can accept sufficient enteral load. However, PN has potential complications such as central line–associated bloodstream infections, parenteral nutrition–associated liver disease (PNALD), and other metabolic disturbances.

11. Glucose, lipids, and proteins are carefully titrated to optimize PN delivery.

Introduction

Providing adequate and appropriate nutrition is vital for ideal development and growth of preterm infants. The nutrition goal for a premature infant is to approximate the rate of growth and body composition of the average healthy fetus of the same age.[1,2] Clinicians often target growth velocities of approximately 15 g/kg/d or 10 to 30 g/d for weight and 1 cm/week for head circumference and length.[3-5] Correlations between anthropometric measurements and improved outcomes later in life have been reported. However, they do not fully account for body composition.[6] Most infants fail to keep up with this intrauterine growth rate and are relatively growth restricted.[7] Growth failure ensues when there is a failure to provide adequate amounts of essential nutrients to the infant. Neurodevelopmental limitations and increased morbidity also accompany this.[8,9]

Delivering nutrition to a very premature infant is compounded by issues unrelated to nutritional support. Many premature infants are critically ill with pathologic stresses such as necrotizing enterocolitis (NEC), bronchopulmonary dysplasia (BPD), hypoxic-ischemic conditions, sepsis, and anemia of prematurity

that reduce the infant's capacity for growth.[10-12] Growth is also negatively affected by common medications used in the NICU, such as corticosteroids, diuretics, and catecholamines.

The premature infant's intestinal tract is predisposed to vulnerabilities and difficulties in providing suitable enteral nutrition. Gastric acid production is limited in this population, impairing host defenses against harmful organisms predisposing to NEC.[13] The developing premature infant has increased gut permeability, reduced immunoglobulins, immature intestinal epithelia, and a decreased mucin barrier. These infants are widely known to have issues with dysmotility and decreased gastric emptying.[14] All these factors play a role in the undernutrition of the premature infant, which has been shown to have cumulative protein and energy deficits.[15] This leads to delays in providing adequate enteral nutrition; interruptions in initiating, advancing, and fortifying enteral feeds; and regular withholding of feeds.

If provided in adequate quantity, nutrition via parenteral and enteral routes promotes positive energy and protein balance, resulting in improved outcomes. Stephens et al. showed that first-week protein and caloric intake was associated with an improved 18-month mental developmental index.[16] Appropriate premature infant growth is also associated with fewer morbidities, such as severe retinopathy of prematurity and chronic diseases.[17,18] Evidence-based standardization of care and optimization of nutritional intervention is an essential component of the medical management of the premature infant. Standardization of feeding protocols minimizes variation in nutritional practices and has been shown to improve postnatal growth, shorten the time to attain full feeds, and decrease days on PN.[19] Moreover, standardized feeding regimens are a method to reduce the incidence of NEC.[20]

Enteral Nutrition

MOTHER'S OWN MILK AND HUMAN DONOR MILK

Mother's own milk (MoM) is the preferred dietary choice for preterm infants due to its protective benefits.[21,22] These benefits are related to the composition of human milk, which contains many growth factors, micro- and macronutrients, hormones, antimicrobial agents, oligosaccharides, enzymes, hormones, and stem cells.[23] For more than 30 years breast milk has been accepted as superior to preterm formula in preventing NEC.[24] Provision of human milk to the premature infant has been associated with reduced rates of sepsis, NEC, and retinopathy of prematurity.[25-28] Analysis by Miller et al. of 6 randomized trials and 43 observational studies in very-low-birth-weight (<1500 g) infants, or those <28 weeks gestational age, revealed a 5% reduction in late-onset sepsis (LOS) and a 7.6% reduction in retinopathy of prematurity.[29] Sisk et al. showed that MoM is dose dependent with an 83% reduction in NEC if infant feeds comprise more than 50% MoM in the first 14 days.[30] The likelihood of NEC or death decreased by a factor of 0.83 for each 10% increase in the proportion of MoM of the total intake.[31] In the event the mother does not produce sufficient amounts of MoM, human donor milk (HDM) has emerged as an accepted alternative.[32] The recent Cochrane database review concluded that HDM conferred a protective effect for NEC compared to infants who were fed formula; however, HDM does not affect LOS incidence.[33] Yet, as with most meta-analyses, the conclusions can be misleading because they are only as good as the review studies. There is still a need for large prospective studies on this issue. Human milk also seems to confer a more appropriate intestinal microbiome with greater diversity and is better tolerated by the infant.[34,35] Compared to formula-fed infants, those fed with MoM have improved neurodevelopmental outcomes, although the influence of pasteurized HDM on neurodevelopment is controversial.[36,37] The Donor Milk for Improved Neurodevelopmental Outcomes (DoMINO) study analyzed neurodevelopmental outcomes of infants randomized to HDM versus preterm formula and did not find a significant benefit at 18 months.[38] HDM is pooled and pasteurized from donors who undergo medical screening. The pasteurization process affects some milk components, resulting in lower protein and lipase content, diminished immunomodulatory factors such as lactoferrin and IgA, and removal of potentially beneficial bacteria.[39,40] Studies comparing an exclusive human milk–based diet versus those with some bovine components (bovine formula, bovine fortifier) have revealed mixed results in NEC prevention.[41] One of the most extensive recently conducted randomized trials did not find a significant advantage in morbidity, mortality, growth, or 18-month neurodevelopmental outcomes.[42,43]

INITIATION AND ADVANCEMENT OF FEEDS

The initiation and advancement of enteral feeding has been a challenge in preterm infants where there is vulnerability and susceptibility of the immature gastrointestinal tract to injury and insult. Therefore enteral feeding has been met with resistance due to fear of a catastrophic gastrointestinal insult. However, human and animal studies have shown that both withholding enteral feeds and prolonged fasting are detrimental to the premature tract. Prolonged fasting has been shown to increase proinflammatory cytokines, resulting in villus atrophy, decreased mesenteric blood flow, enzyme activity digestive capability, and functional adaptation of the immature gastrointestinal tract.[44-46] Furthermore, delayed introduction of enteral nutrition has been linked with fewer days on full feeds and increased morbidities such as retinopathy of prematurity, BPD, and intestinal inflammation.[47-49] A meta-analysis of 14 randomized trials of 1551 infants found no evidence that delaying initiation of enteral feeds beyond 4 days of life affects the risk of NEC development.[50] The provision of early and minimal enteral nutrition is now widely accepted in clinical practice.

The optimal enteral feed volume advancement rate remains controversial and is variable among clinicians. Raban et al. compared daily feeding advancements of 36 mL/kg/d versus 24 mL/kg/d and found that rapid advancement was well tolerated and improved weight gain.[51] The recent Cochrane review of 13 randomized trials analyzed the slow advancement of enteral feeds in NEC prevention. *Slow advancement* was defined as a daily increment of 15 to 20 mL/kg of enteral feeding volume and faster advancement as a daily increment of 30 to 40 mL/kg. No difference in NEC risk or all-cause mortality was found between the groups. Advancing at a slower rate may slightly increase the risk for infection.[52] The Speed of Increasing milk Feeds Trial (SIFT) randomized more than 2800 infants to 18 mL/kg/d versus 30 mL/kg/d volume advancement until reaching full feeding volumes. There was no significant difference in survival or morbidity between the groups at 24 months.[53,54] Extremely premature infants may tolerate faster (30–40 mL/kg/d) feeding advancement to optimize their enteral nutrition. Some caution should be heeded for unstable infants and high-risk infants, where slower advancement may initially be needed. Slower rates of feeding advancement and delays in attaining full feeds are associated with neurodevelopmental impairment and complications related to prolonged PN and central line–associated bloodstream infections.[8,52]

FORTIFICATION OF HUMAN MILK

Unfortified human milk provision at full enteral volumes of 130 to 160 mL/kg/d will result in nutrient deficiency, poor growth, and increased risk for osteopenia.[55] Human milk is deficient in some critical nutrients such as phosphorous and protein relative to the high needs of the premature infant.[56-60] Calcium and phosphorous delivery will still be suboptimal at higher volumes of 250 to 300 mL/kg/d, which premature infants do not generally tolerate.[61] Fortification of human milk products (MoM and HDM) is necessary to meet the nutritional needs of the preterm infant by increasing the caloric density of feeds and supplying vitamins and minerals, such as sodium, phosphorus, calcium, and iron.[55,62] However, postnatal growth failure persists in this population even after fortification. Variability of human milk composition and variability of the needs of each infant have been proposed as the reason for this phenomenon.[58,59,63,64] Although the benefits of fortification have been well established, reluctance to fortify human milk remains. Often, clinicians cite fear of feeding intolerance or increased rates of NEC due to increased osmolality of feeds after fortification. However, there is no evidence that increased osmolality of feeds causes NEC or feeding intolerance.[55,65,66]

Initiation of Fortification

Once feeding tolerance is determined, a multicomponent human milk fortifier (HMF) is added to human milk, but this definition varies among NICUs and clinical trials. A randomized trial of 100 infants comparing early fortification with bovine milk–based HMF at 20 mL/kg/d of human milk with delayed fortification at 100 mL/kg/d did not demonstrate greater feeding intolerance or morbidities such as NEC. Increased protein intake was found in the early-fortification group.[67] Sullivan et al. allowed for early fortification with human milk–based HMF at 40 mL/kg/d with a control group fortified at 100 mL/kg/d. They found no significant difference in feeding tolerance or morbidity.[27] Early fortification (at <60 mL/kg/d) revealed improved growth outcomes compared to late fortification (at >60 mL/kg/d) when using human milk–based fortification.[68] Available evidence is insufficient to refute or support early fortification in preterm infants.[69]

Human Milk–Based Versus Bovine Milk–Based Standard Fortification

The effect of an exclusive human milk–based diet using human milk–based fortification was studied by Sullivan and colleagues and revealed a reduction in NEC rates.[27] However, the control group also received preterm infant formula instead of HDM when MoM was unavailable. This puts into doubt the establishment of causality, which is further complicated by the high rate of NEC (16%) in the control group. In a retrospective study, an exclusive human milk diet (MoM and HDM + human milk–based fortifier) significantly reduced NEC incidence, LOS, retinopathy of prematurity, BPD, and mortality when compared with a bovine-based diet.[41] Cristofalo et al. showed that infants fed an exclusive human milk diet had decreased incidence of NEC when compared to those fed with preterm formula (3% vs. 21%).[25] In a retrospective observational study, an exclusive human milk diet was reported to be neuroprotective against intraventricular hemorrhage (IVH) and periventricular leukomalacia.[70] In a recent, well-designed, large randomized study from the OptiMoM Feeding group, premature infants <1250 g were randomized to human milk–based fortifier versus bovine milk–based fortifier. Importantly, the use of a human milk–based fortifier had no statistically significant advantage in morbidity, mortality, growth, or 18-month neurodevelopmental outcomes.[42,71] The most recent Cochrane review comparing human-based fortifiers versus bovine-based fortifiers revealed insufficient data to conclude that human milk–based fortifiers reduce morbidity, mortality, or feeding intolerance or that they improve growth.[72]

Using a human milk–based fortifier comes with potential disadvantages. In a recent observational study, Eibensteiner et al. reported poor weight gain, longer duration of PN, and delayed achievement of full enteral feeds.[73] In a review of six randomized studies, human milk–based fortification was associated with lower weight gain than bovine milk–derived fortification.[74] Human milk–based fortification must be added at a 1:1 ratio to reach a caloric density of 100 kcal/100 mL, which results in a dilution of MoM and may diminish its dose-dependent protective effect. Lastly, the high cost of human milk–based fortification can be prohibitive when there are insufficient data to justify its routine recommendation. A randomized controlled trial is ongoing to further compare human milk–based fortifiers and bovine milk fortifiers (NCT03797517). More data are needed to routinely recommend using human milk–based fortification over the less expensive bovine milk–based fortification.

Standardized Versus Individualized Fortification

Standard fortification is the most-used method of milk fortification in NICUs.[75] A fixed amount of fortifier is added to a fixed composition of human milk to reach recommended nutrient intakes. Standard fortification improves postnatal growth compared to unfortified human milk.[55] However, postnatal growth failure persists even after standard fortification. Hypoproteinemia is a common problem following this method, mainly when using pasteurized HDM, and additional strategies must be implemented to correct it.[75] This is attributed to the variability in protein content of native human milk and the variability of protein needs of

each critically ill infant in the NICU. Although standard fortification improves postnatal growth and bone mineralization, this approach does not provide adequate nutrition for every infant. Strategies are needed to compensate for calories, vitamins and minerals, and protein.

Individualized fortification is the addition of variable amounts of products to reach a target human milk composition or to adjust to the individual's protein status. It is typically used when standard fortification is not meeting the nutritional demands of an infant. In comparison to standard fortification, individualized fortification significantly improves postnatal growth.[76] The two methods of individualized fortification being studied are targeted and adjustable fortification. The Cochrane review comparing individualized fortification with standard fortification revealed improvement in growth parameters when individualized fortification was used.[77]

Targeted fortification aims to evaluate the components of human milk using a milk analyzer and then tailoring macronutrient content with the addition of fortifiers. Spectroscopy is used to evaluate the macronutrient components of human milk, allowing for targeted protein replacement with modifiers. This method has been shown to decrease variability in the composition of human milk.[78] Several studies have shown a benefit of targeted fortification compared to standard fortification (Table 11.1).[79-81] However, some limitations remain. Targeted fortification does not address the variability of individual infant protein requirements. Moreover, targeted fortification requires a significant volume of human milk used for analysis

TABLE 11.1 Targeted Versus Standard Fortification		
Author	**Intervention for Targeted Fortification Group**	**Results**
de Halleux et al., 2007[79]	Addition of modular fat and multicomponent fortifier to reach target fat content of 4 g/100 mL and protein of 4.3 g/kg/d	Improved weight gain compared to standard fortification
Hair et al., 2014[80]	Human milk–derived cream added in addition to human milk–based fortifier if energy density <67 kcal/100 mL	Infants in the human milk–derived cream group with greater weight and length
Rochow et al., 2021[81]	Standard fortification and then targeted fortification to target ESPGHAN-recommended nutrient intake	Greater weight gain, fat-free mass, and macronutrient intake

ESPGHAN, The European Society for Paediatric Gastroenterology Hepatology and Nutrition.

TABLE 11.2	Adjustable Versus Standard Fortification	
Author	**Intervention Adjustable Fortification Group**	**Results**
Arslanoglu et al., 2019[62]	At 150 mL/kg/d, twice weekly BUN measurements and adjusted with protein supplementation	Infants in intervention group showed significantly greater gain in weight (17.5 ± 3.0 vs. 14.4 ± 3.0 g/kg/d, $P < 0.01$) and greater gain in head circumference (1.4 ± 0.3 vs. 1.0 ± 0.3; $P < 0.05$) than infants in control group
Alan et al., 2013[86]	Additional protein supplementation adjusted according to BUN levels weekly in intervention group	Protein intake and daily growth indexes (weight, length, head circumference) were significantly higher in intervention group
Picaud et al., 2016[85]	Additional protein fortification done based on growth fortification and BUN	Significant increase in weight for age, length for age, and head circumference z-scores after additional protein fortification

BUN, Blood urea nitrogen.

and significant workload and expenses for the analysis of human milk.[81,82]

Adjustable fortification evaluates the infant's metabolic response to a feeding regimen, and adjustments to protein intake are made based on blood urea nitrogen (BUN).[83] BUN is monitored as a measure of protein intake, and if considered low (e.g., <9–10 mg/dL), fortification is increased or additional protein is supplemented. If BUN is high (e.g., >14–16 mg/dL), fortification is decreased.[62,75,84] The benefits of adjustable fortification have been reported in several studies (Table 11.2).[84-86] The utility of using BUN as an index for protein intake may be impacted by acute changes in hydration status and renal function or critically unstable infants with organ dysfunction secondary to sepsis or congenital heart disease. Drugs such as diuretics and corticosteroids may also influence BUN levels.

Two randomized studies compared protein-targeted fortification with adjustable fortification. Simsek et al. did not find any significant differences in growth parameters between the two, but both were significantly superior to standard fortification.[76] Meanwhile, in a study by Bulut et al., protein-targeted fortification resulted in higher weight and head circumference gains than adjustable fortification.[87]

CONTINUOUS OR BOLUS ENTERAL NUTRITION

Continuous enteral nutrition (feeding via pump over 24 hours) is believed to reduce feeding intolerance, improve energy efficiency, and stimulate enteric motor function. Clinicians also suppose that continuous feeding can diminish the occurrence of reflux events. However, there is concern about decreasing fat, phosphorous, and calcium delivery with continuous feeding.[88-90] In animal studies, continuous feeding results in less insulin and amino acid level signaling in skeletal muscle.[91-93] *Bolus feeding*, defined as intermittent feeding through a gastric tube over 10 to 30 minutes every three to four hours, may mimic a cyclical surge of hormones seen in healthy term infants.[94] This may also explain increasing protein synthesis in neonatal mice studies.[95] The Cochrane review comparing intermittent and continuous feeding in very-low-birth-weight infants concluded that there was insufficient evidence to recommend one strategy over the other.[90] In a recent meta-analysis of eight studies totaling 707 infants, continuous-feeding infants took longer to reach full enteral feeding volumes than intermittent-feeding infants.[88]

TRANSPYLORIC FEEDING VERSUS NASO/OROGASTRIC FEEDING

Enteral feeding of the premature neonate usually commences via a nasogastric or orogastric tube until the infant develops proper oral motor and coordination skills to feed by mouth successfully. It is vital to initiate and advance enteral feeding early to avoid the deleterious effects of prolonged fasting and the risks associated with a prolonged course of PN and central vascular access. There is a historical belief that nasogastric tubes may impair respiration. Studies have shown no advantage between nasogastric and orogastric feeding tubes in apnea, bradycardia, or hypoxic episodes.[96-98]

Transpyloric feeding is performed on the assumption that it prevents the occurrence of aspiration or reflux. Some data from observational studies suggest transpyloric feeding is linked with less frequent apnea and bradycardia.[99-101] However, the most recent Cochrane review concluded insufficient evidence of any benefit for transpyloric feeds versus gastric feeding. Some evidence of harm, such as gastrointestinal disturbance (e.g., diarrhea and feeding intolerance) and increased mortality, were noted but should be viewed with caution given the methodological weaknesses of the studies analyzed.[102]

GASTRIC RESIDUALS

Aspiration of residual gastric fluid has long been the standard of care in the NICU to gauge feeding tolerance or an early sign of NEC.[103,104] Routine gastric residual monitoring is one of the most documented reasons for slow feeding advancement. Residuals are evaluated based on color (green, yellow, white), quality (digested vs. undigested), and volume, but provider response to this information can vary significantly. Several studies have shown that omitting routine evaluation of gastric residuals is safe and leads to improved nutritional outcomes, shorter duration of hospitalization, and quicker time to achieve complete enteral nutrition and regain birth weight.[105-107] The most recent meta-analysis did not reveal an increased risk for NEC, death, ventilator-associated pneumonia, or sepsis.[108] Overall, it appears safe to omit routine evaluation of gastric residuals while considering their ad hoc use if clinical concerns arise.

Parenteral Nutrition

The immaturity of the preterm gastrointestinal tract limits its ability to accept large volumes of adequate enteral nutrition during the early postnatal days. Preterm infants also experience conditions that may increase metabolic demand and are exposed to medications that may impair growth.[109] Smaller infants have lower body stores of protein, fat, and glycogen to provide sources of energy. Hence the provision, immediately after birth, of PN containing amino acids, lipids, and electrolytes is now considered the nutritional standard of care for severely premature infants. PN ultimately serves as a bridge to deliver adequate nutrients until the infant advances and tolerates full fortified enteral nutrition. It can also provide nutrition to unstable infants or those suffering from gastrointestinal catastrophes that do not allow for enteral feeds, such as NEC, spontaneous intestinal perforations, and congenital gastrointestinal malformations. PN does not come without potential complications, among them central venous catheter–related complications, parenteral nutrition–associated liver disease (PNALD), extravasations, and metabolic complications such as hyperglycemia and hypertriglyceridemia.[110]

CARBOHYDRATES

Glucose is the primary source of energy in the body. The preterm infant has similar or higher glucose demands as a fetus of the same gestational age and requires glucose supplementation or production via gluconeogenesis or glycogenolysis. The normal glucose utilization rate is about 6 to 7 mg/kg/min in premature infants at birth, which increases to 12–13 mg/kg/min for full intravenous nutrition.[111,112] Glycogenolysis and gluconeogenesis of preterm infants develop and are maintained at 2 to 3 mg/kg/min.[113] Glucose production is also supplemented by lipid delivery leading to gluconeogenesis.[114] Therefore, to avoid hyperglycemia, glucose infusion rates should typically be started at ~4 mg/kg/min to keep glucose delivery within infants' maximal utilization rates. Glucose infusion rates should then be titrated to keep glucose below hyperglycemia levels of >200 mg/dL. At higher rates, fat synthesis occurs after glucose synthesis is maximized.[115]

Excessive infusion of intravenous glucose is the leading cause of hyperglycemia in the preterm neonate. Other risk factors include insulin resistance, decreased enteral feeds and increased catecholamine, and glucocorticoid release due to stress.[116,117] Hyperglycemia is linked to cellular injury and higher mortality.[117,118] Complications of hyperglycemia include increased fat deposition, increased oxygen consumption, hyperosmolarity, and reduced neuronal development. Hyperosmolarity results in polyuria, electrolyte abnormalities, and dehydration. Excessive fat deposition can also result in fatty infiltration of the heart and liver.[116]

LIPIDS

Lipids make up a significant portion of the energy delivery from parenteral and enteral nutrition required for the infant's growth. Providing adequate amounts of lipids is essential to the growth of the extremely premature infant as a noncarbohydrate source delivered in a low volume. Lipids also help with the delivery of fat-soluble vitamins A, D, E, and K. Intrauterine lipid deposition remains at about 2 g/kg/d from 25 weeks onward.[119] Deficiency of lipases and carnitine palmitoyl-transferase in extremely preterm infants makes them vulnerable to suboptimal clearance of plasma lipids. However, carnitine and lipases found in MoM facilitate lipid oxidation, making the advancement of enteral feeding more vital. Intravenous lipids are given to prevent fatty acid deficiency. Arachidonic acid (ARA) and docosahexaenoic acid (DHA) are long-chain polyunsaturated fatty acids (LC-PUFAs) actively transferred across the placenta and accumulated in the fetal brain. The current premature infant enteral diet of lipids (~150 mL/kg/d) does not provide *in utero* accretion rates of DHA.[120] Preterm infants supplemented with DHA have higher Bayley developmental scores and visual acuity.[121,122] LC-PUFAs are indispensable substrates early in life, and supplementation leads to superior growth, improved developmental outcomes, and immune modulation.[123]

Intravenous lipid emulsions (ILEs) are integral in the PN of the preterm infant and should be started no later than day 2 of life. Current intravenous preparations for lipids include soybean-based products, fish oil–based emulsions, and a composite of these. The maximum recommended dose of ILE is 3 to 4 g/kg/d.[124,125] A dose of 0.25 g/kg/d of linoleic acid prevents essential fatty acid deficiency (EFAD).

Soybean-based lipid preparations, used for decades in the adult and pediatric populations due to their low concentrations of antiinflammatory alpha-tocopherols, high levels of phytosterols, and low DHA, are associated with liver disease (PNALD). They have high concentrations of essential fatty acids but lack adequate amounts of long-chain polyunsaturated fats.[126] On the other hand, fish-oil products contain high levels of DHA as well as alpha-tocopherols, the latter of which are used to improve fatty acid status and reverse cholestasis.[127] However, concerns remain regarding fish oil emulsions, including decreased delivery of the linoleic and alpha-linolenic essential fatty acids, and therefore they are not recommended for routine use.[124] Composite emulsions composed of a mixture of soybean oil, fish oil, medium-chain triglycerides, and olive oil contain higher amounts of vitamin E and phytosterols. Non-pure soybean-based lipids were shown to decrease the risk of sepsis compared to pure soybean oil lipids.[128] These composite lipid emulsions have been associated with a hepatoprotective effect and less PNALD, making them preferred over soybean oil emulsions.[124,129-131] However, some meta-analyses report that there is no evidence of benefit for infants requiring a short duration of PN.[132,133]

Tolerance of lipid administration is generally done by checking biochemical markers such as serum triglycerides and hepatic function panels. There is no association found between hypertriglyceridemia and infection.[134] There is also no current consensus as to acceptable triglyceride levels with gestational age or how frequently to check after lipid administration. Normal triglyceride levels may not reflect optimal lipid oxidation. On the other hand, EFAD may quickly result with limited lipid delivery and increased demands. Triene to tetraene ratios of more than 0.2 suggest that more Mead acid than ARA is produced and are indicative of EFAD.[135]

AMINO ACIDS

Protein accounts for 80% to 90% of non-water growth over the last one-third of gestation.[116] Providing adequate amounts of amino acids is essential for promoting growth in the preterm neonate. Preterm infants require 4 g/kg/d for normal protein balance and growth at 24 to 28 weeks gestation. This gradually decreases to 2.5 to 3.5 g/kg/d for late preterm infants and then to 1.5 to 2.0 g/kg/d for infants at term gestation.[136] This should be accompanied by non-protein intakes of ~65 kcal/kg/d to guarantee amino acid utilization.[137] Early administration of intravenous amino acid leads to increased protein synthesis without decreased proteolysis.[138] Poindexter et al. found significant improvements in growth parameters at 36 weeks for those given early amino acids.[139] First-week protein and energy intakes in extremely low-birth-weight infants were associated with improved neurodevelopmental indexes at 18 months.[140] Higher amino acid intake may reduce the incidence of postnatal growth failure and retinopathy of prematurity.[141]

Recent randomized studies did not show long- or short-term benefits to increased amino acid intake.[142,143]

There has been some concern regarding the metabolic effects of intravenous amino acid administration; however, no detrimental effects have been consistently reported.[144,145] The Cochrane database review shows that higher amino acid intake does not affect mortality.[141] Uthaya and colleagues, in a propensity-matched retrospective study of more than 65,000 preterm infants, compared early versus later initiation of PN and found increased survival in the early-PN group.[146] Further studies need to be done to address intravenous amino acid delivery concerns.

Summary

The long-term outcomes and survival of preterm infants are better with the provision of adequate nutrition. Therefore NICUs must ensure safe and effective nutrition via the development of standardized guidelines based on the most robust scientific evidence available. Evidence shows that implementing standardized feeding guidelines leads to more rapid attainment of full enteral feeds, reduced PN–associated morbidities, reduced risk of infection, a reduction in NEC, and better growth velocity.[147–150] However, execution of the guidelines mentioned in this chapter depends on the efficient work of a complex multidisciplinary team that ideally includes the infant's parents. Multidisciplinary team implementation improves nutrient intake and growth, reduces duration of PN, and reduces length of NICU stay.[151]

In the future, large datasets can help guide nutrition delivery to a more precise and individualized method making use of machine learning and artificial intelligence. These technologies will integrate prenatal and postnatal factors and biomarkers as well as multiomic information to personalize nutrition delivery and tailor it to each infant.

REFRENCES

1. Kleinman RE, Greer RE, Frank R. *Pediatric Nutrition*. Vol 8. 2014. Accessed March 15, 2022. Available at: https://www.vasiliadis-books.gr/Vasiliadis-books/wp-content/uploads/2015/06/PEDIATRIC-NUTRITION-LOOK-INSIDE.pdf.
2. Cordova EG, Cherkerzian S, Bell K, et al. Association of poor postnatal growth with neurodevelopmental impairment in infancy and childhood: comparing the fetus and the healthy preterm infant references. *J Pediatr*. 2020;225:37-43.e5. doi:10.1016/J.JPEDS.2020.05.063.
3. Fenton TR, Nasser R, Eliasziw M, Kim JH, Bilan D, Sauve R. Validating the weight gain of preterm infants between the reference growth curve of the fetus and the term infant. *BMC Pediatr*. 2013;13:92. doi:10.1186/1471-2431-13-92.
4. Griffin I. Nutritional assessment in preterm infants. *Nestle Nutr Workshop Ser Pediatr Program*. 2007;59:177-188. doi:10.1159/000098535.
5. Anderson DM. Nutritional assessment and therapeutic interventions for the preterm infant. *Clin Perinatol*. 2002;29(2):313-326. doi:10.1016/S0095-5108(02)00008-8.
6. Kiger JR, Taylor SN, Wagner CL, Finch C, Katikaneni L. Preterm infant body composition cannot be accurately determined by weight and length. *J Neonatal Perinatal Med*. 2016;9(3):285-290. doi:10.3233/NPM-16915125.
7. Horbar JD, Ehrenkranz RA, Badger GJ, et al. Weight growth velocity and postnatal growth failure in infants 501 to 1500 grams: 2000-2013. *Pediatrics*. 2015;136(1):e84-e92. doi:10.1542/PEDS.2015-0129.
8. Ehrenkranz RA, Dusick AM, Vohr BR, Wright LL, Wrage LA, Poole WK. Growth in the neonatal intensive care unit influences neurodevelopmental and growth outcomes of extremely low birth weight infants. *Pediatrics*. 2006;117(4):1253-1261. doi:10.1542/PEDS.2005-1368.
9. Bouyssi-Kobar M, du Plessis AJ, McCarter R, et al. Third trimester brain growth in preterm infants compared with in utero healthy fetuses. *Pediatrics*. 2016;138(5):e20161640. doi:10.1542/PEDS.2016-1640.
10. Wahlig TM, Georgieff MK. The effects of illness on neonatal metabolism and nutritional management. *Clin Perinatol*. 1995;22(1):77-96. doi:10.1016/S0095-5108(18)30302-6.
11. Wahlig TM, Gatto CW, Boros SJ, Mammel MC, Mills MM, Georgieff MK. Metabolic response of preterm infants to variable degrees of respiratory illness. *J Pediatr*. 1994;124(2):283-288. doi:10.1016/S0022-3476(94)70321-3.
12. Stockman JA, Clark DA. Weight gain: a response to transfusion in selected preterm infants. *Am J Dis Child*. 1984;138(9):828-830. doi:10.1001/ARCHPEDI.1984.02140470028009.
13. Hyman PE, Clarke DD, Everett SL, et al. Gastric acid secretory function in preterm infants. *J Pediatr*. 1985;106(3):467-471. doi:10.1016/S0022-3476(85)80682-X.
14. Kim JH. Necrotizing enterocolitis: the road to zero. *Semin Fetal Neonatal Med*. 2014;19(1):39-44. doi:10.1016/j.siny.2013.10.001.
15. Dinerstein A, Nieto RM, Solana CL, Perez GP, Otheguy LE, Larguia AM. Early and aggressive nutritional strategy (parenteral and enteral) decreases postnatal growth failure in very low birth weight infants. *J Perinatol*. 2006;26(7):436-442. doi:10.1038/SJ.JP.7211539.
16. Stephens BE, Walden RV, Gargus RA, et al. First-week protein and energy intakes are associated with 18-month developmental outcomes in extremely low birth weight infants. *Pediatrics*. 2009;123(5):1337-1343. doi:10.1542/PEDS.2008-0211.
17. Binenbaum G, Tomlinson LA, de Alba Campomanes AG, et al. Validation of the postnatal growth and retinopathy of prematurity screening criteria. *JAMA Ophthalmol*. 2020;138(1):31-37. doi:10.1001/JAMAOPHTHALMOL.2019.4517.
18. Matinolli HM, Hovi P, Levälahti E, et al. Neonatal nutrition predicts energy balance in young adults born preterm at very low birth weight. *Nutrients*. 2017;9(12):1282. doi:10.3390/NU9121282.

19. Patole SK, de Klerk N. Impact of standardised feeding regimens on incidence of neonatal necrotising enterocolitis: a systematic review and meta-analysis of observational studies. *Arch Dis Child Fetal Neonatal Ed.* 2005;90(2):F147-F151. doi:10.1136/adc.2004.059741.

20. Jasani B, Patole S. Standardized feeding regimen for reducing necrotizing enterocolitis in preterm infants: an updated systematic review. *J Perinatol.* 2017;37(7):827-833. doi:10.1038/JP.2017.37.

21. Arslanoglu S, Corpeleijn W, Moro G, et al. Donor human milk for preterm infants: current evidence and research directions. *J Pediatr Gastroenterol Nutr.* 2013;57(4):535-542. doi:10.1097/MPG.0B013E3182A3AF0A.

22. Parker MG, Stellwagen LM, Noble L, Kim JH, Poindexter BB, Puopolo KM. Promoting human milk and breastfeeding for the very low birth weight infant. *Pediatrics.* 2021;148(5):2021054272. doi:10.1542/PEDS.2021-054272/181366.

23. Ballard O, Morrow AL. Human milk composition: nutrients and bioactive factors. *Pediatr Clin.* 2013;60(1):P49-P74. Accessed March 17, 2022. Available at: https://www.pediatric.theclinics.com/article/S0031-3955(12)00167-8/abstract.

24. Lucas A, Cole TJ. Breast milk and neonatal necrotising enterocolitis. *Lancet.* 1990;336(8730):1519-1523. doi:10.1016/0140-6736(90)93304-8.

25. Cristofalo EA, Schanler RJ, Blanco CL, et al. Randomized trial of exclusive human milk versus preterm formula diets in extremely premature infants. *J Pediatr.* 2013;163(6):1592-1595.e1. doi:10.1016/J.JPEDS.2013.07.011.

26. Schanler RJ, Lau C, Hurst NM, Smith EO. Randomized trial of donor human milk versus preterm formula as substitutes for mothers' own milk in the feeding of extremely premature infants. *Pediatrics.* 2005;116(2):400-406. doi:10.1542/peds.2004-1974.

27. Sullivan S, Schanler RJ, Kim JH, et al. An exclusively human milk-based diet is associated with a lower rate of necrotizing enterocolitis than a diet of human milk and bovine milk-based products. *J Pediatr.* 2010;156(4):562-567.e1. doi:10.1016/j.jpeds.2009.10.040.

28. Abrams SA, Schanler RJ, Lee ML, Rechtman DJ. Greater mortality and morbidity in extremely preterm infants fed a diet containing cow milk protein products. *Breastfeed Med.* 2014;9(6):281-285. doi:10.1089/BFM.2014.0024.

29. Miller J, Tonkin E, Damarell RA, et al. A systematic review and meta-analysis of human milk feeding and morbidity in very low birth weight infants. *Nutrients.* 2018;10(6):707. doi:10.3390/NU10060707.

30. Sisk PM, Lovelady CA, Dillard RG, Gruber KJ, O'Shea TM. Early human milk feeding is associated with a lower risk of necrotizing enterocolitis in very low birth weight infants. *J Perinatol.* 2007;27(7):428-433. doi:10.1038/SJ.JP.7211758.

31. Meinzen-Derr J, Poindexter B, Wrage L, Morrow AL, Stoll B, Donovan EF. Role of human milk in extremely low birth weight infants' risk of necrotizing enterocolitis or death. *J Perinatol.* 2009;29(1):57-62. doi:10.1038/jp.2008.117.

32. Abrams SA, Landers S, Noble LM, Poindexter BB. Donor human milk for the high- risk infant: Preparation, safety, and usage options in the United States. *Pediatrics.* 2017;139(1):e20163440. doi:10.1542/PEDS.2016-3440/52000.

33. Quigley M, Embleton ND, McGuire W. Formula versus donor breast milk for feeding preterm or low birth weight infants. *Cochrane Database Syst Rev.* 2019;2019(7):CD002971. doi:10.1002/14651858.CD002971.PUB5/EPDF/ABSTRACT.

34. Zanella A, Silveira RC, Roesch LFW, et al. Influence of own mother's milk and different proportions of formula on intestinal microbiota of very preterm newborns. *PLoS One.* 2019;14(5):e0217296. doi:10.1371/JOURNAL.PONE.0217296.

35. Xu W, Judge MP, Maas K, et al. Systematic review of the effect of enteral feeding on gut microbiota in preterm infants. *J Obstet Gynecol Neonatal Nurs.* 2018;47(3):451-463. doi:10.1016/J.JOGN.2017.08.009.

36. Lechner BE, Vohr BR. Neurodevelopmental outcomes of preterm infants fed human milk: a systematic review. *Clin Perinatol.* 2017;44(1):69-83. doi:10.1016/J.CLP.2016.11.004.

37. Rozé JC, Darmaun D, Boquien CY, et al. The apparent breast-feeding paradox in very preterm infants: relationship between breast feeding, early weight gain and neurodevelopment based on results from two cohorts, EPIPAGE and LIFT. *BMJ Open.* 2012;2(2):e000834. doi:10.1136/BMJOPEN-2012-000834.

38. O'Connor DL, Gibbins S, Kiss A, et al. Effect of supplemental donor human milk compared with preterm formula on neurodevelopment of very low-birth-weight infants at 18 months. *JAMA.* 2016;316(18):1897. doi:10.1001/jama.2016.16144.

39. Colaizy TT. Effects of milk banking procedures on nutritional and bioactive components of donor human milk. *Semin Perinatol.* 2021;45(2):151382. doi:10.1016/J.SEMPERI.2020.151382.

40. Perrin M, Belfort MB, Hagadorn JI, et al. The nutritional composition and energy content of donor human milk: a systematic review. *Adv Nutr.* 2020;11(4):960-970. Accessed March 17, 2022. Available at: https://academic.oup.com/advances/article-abstract/11/4/960/5771483.

41. Hair AB, Rechtman DJ, Lee ML, Niklas V. Beyond necrotizing enterocolitis: other clinical advantages of an exclusive human milk diet. *Breastfeed Med.* 2018;13(6):408-411. doi:10.1089/BFM.2017.0192.

42. O'Connor DL, Kiss A, Tomlinson C, et al. Nutrient enrichment of human milk with human and bovine milk-based fortifiers for infants born weighing <1250 g: a randomized clinical trial. *Am J Clin Nutr.* 2018;108(1):108-116. doi:10.1093/ajcn/nqy067.

43. Hopperton KE, O'Connor DL, Bando N, et al. Nutrient enrichment of human milk with human and bovine milk-based fortifiers for infants born. *Curr Dev Nutr.* 2019;3(12):nzz129. doi:10.1093/CDN/NZZ129.

44. Niinikoski H, Stoll B, Guan X, et al. Onset of small intestinal atrophy is associated with reduced intestinal blood flow in TPN-fed neonatal piglets. *J Nutr.* 2004;134(6):1467-1474. doi:10.1093/JN/134.6.1467.

45. Wildhaber BE, Yang H, Spencer AU, Drongowski RA, Teitelbaum DH. Lack of enteral nutrition—effects on the intestinal immune system. *J Surg Res.* 2005;123(1):8-16. doi:10.1016/J.JSS.2004.06.015.

46. Kudsk KA. Current aspects of mucosal immunology and its influence by nutrition. *Am J Surg.* 2002;183(4):390-398. doi:10.1016/S0002-9610(02)00821-8.

47. Salas AA, Li P, Parks K, Lal CV, Martin CR, Carlo WA. Early progressive feeding in extremely preterm infants: a randomized trial. *Am J Clin Nutr.* 2018;107(3):365-370. doi:10.1093/AJCN/NQY012.

48. Konnikova Y, Zaman MM, Makda M, D'Onofrio D, Freedman SD, Martin CR. Late enteral feedings are associated with intestinal inflammation and adverse neonatal outcomes. *PLoS One.* 2015;10(7):e0132924. doi:10.1371/JOURNAL.PONE.0132924.

49. Morgan J, Bombell S, Mcguire W. Early trophic feeding versus enteral fasting for very preterm or very low birth weight infants. *Cochrane Database Syst Rev.* 2013;(3):CD000504. doi:10.1002/14651858.CD000504.pub4.

50. Young L, Oddie SJ, McGuire W. Delayed introduction of progressive enteral feeds to prevent necrotising enterocolitis in very low birth weight infants. *Cochrane Database Syst Rev.* 2022;1(1):CD001970. doi:10.1002/14651858.CD001970.pub6.

51. Raban S, Santhakumaran S, Keraan Q, et al. A randomised controlled trial of high vs low volume initiation and rapid vs slow advancement of milk feeds in infants with birthweights ≤ 1000 g in a resource-limited setting. *Paediatr Int Child Health.* 2016;36(4):288-295. doi:10.1179/20469055 15Y.0000000056.

52. Oddie SJ, Young L, McGuire W. Slow advancement of enteral feed volumes to prevent necrotising enterocolitis in very low birth weight infants. *Cochrane Database Syst Rev.* 2021;8(8):CD001241. doi:10.1002/14651858.CD001241.PUB8.

53. Dorling J, Hewer O, Hurd M, et al. Two speeds of increasing milk feeds for very preterm or very low-birthweight infants: the SIFT RCT. *Health Technol Assess (Rockv).* 2020;24(18):1-94. doi:10.3310/hta24180.

54. Dorling J, Abbott J, Berrington J, et al. Controlled trial of two incremental milk-feeding rates in preterm infants. *N Engl J Med.* 2019;381(15):1434-1443. doi:10.1056/NEJMOA1816654.

55. Brown JVE, Lin L, Embleton ND, Harding JE, McGuire W. Multi-nutrient fortification of human milk for preterm infants. *Cochrane Database Syst Rev.* 2020;2020(6):CD000343. doi:10.1002/14651858.CD000343.PUB4.

56. Koletzko B, Poindexter B, Uauy R. Recommended nutrient intake levels for stable, fully enterally fed very low birth weight infants. *World Rev Nutr Diet.* 2014;110:297-299. doi:10.1159/000360195.

57. Koletzko B, Wieczorek S, Domellöf M, Poindexter BB. Defining nutritional needs of preterm infants. *World Rev Nutr Diet.* 2021;122:5-11. doi:10.1159/000514739.

58. Gidrewicz DA, Fenton TR. A systematic review and meta-analysis of the nutrient content of preterm and term breast milk. *BMC Pediatr.* 2014;14:216. doi:10.1186/1471-2431-14-216.

59. Bauer J, Gerss J. Longitudinal analysis of macronutrients and minerals in human milk produced by mothers of preterm infants. *Clin Nutr.* 2011;30(2):215-220. doi:10.1016/J.CLNU.2010.08.003.

60. Ziegler EE. 3.14 Preterm and low-birth-weight infants. *World Rev Nutr Diet.* 2015;113:214-217. doi:10.1159/000360342.

61. Agostoni C, Buonocore G, Carnielli VP, et al. Enteral nutrient supply for preterm infants: commentary from the European Society of Paediatric Gastroenterology, Hepatology and Nutrition Committee on Nutrition. *J Pediatr Gastroenterol Nutr.* 2010;50(1):85-91. doi:10.1097/MPG.0B013E3181ADAEE0.

62. Arslanoglu S, Boquien CY, King C, et al. Fortification of human milk for preterm infants: Update and recommendations of the European milk bank association (EMBA) working group on human milk fortification. *Front Pediatr.* 2019;7:76. doi:10.3389/FPED.2019.00076/BIBTEX.

63. de Halleux V, Rigo J. Variability in human milk composition: benefit of individualized fortification in very-low-birth-weight infants. *Am J Clin Nutr.* 2013;98(2):529S-535S. doi:10.3945/AJCN.112.042689.

64. Anderson GH. Human milk feeding. *Pediatr Clin North Am.* 1985;32(2):335-353. doi:10.1016/S0031-3955(16)34790-3.

65. Yigit S, Akgoz A, Memisoglu A, Akata D, Ziegler EE. Breast milk fortification: effect on gastric emptying. *J Matern Fetal Neonatal Med.* 2008;21(11):843-846. doi:10.1080/14767050802287176.

66. Pearson F, Johnson MJ, Leaf AA. Milk osmolality: does it matter? *Arch Dis Child Fetal Neonatal Ed.* 2013;98(2):F166-F169. doi:10.1136/ADC.2011.300492.

67. Shah SD, Dereddy N, Jones TL, Dhanireddy R, Talati AJ. Early versus delayed human milk fortification in very low birth weight infants-a randomized controlled trial. *J Pediatr.* 2016;174:126-131.e1. doi:10.1016/j.jpeds.2016.03.056.

68. Huston R, Lee M, Rider E, et al. Early fortification of enteral feedings for infants. *J Neonatal Perinatal Med.* 2020;13(2):215-221. doi:10.3233/NPM-190300.

69. Thanigainathan S, Abiramalatha T. Early fortification of human milk versus late fortification to promote growth in preterm infants. *Cochrane Database Syst Rev.* 2020;7(7):CD013392. doi:10.1002/14651858.CD013392.PUB2.

70. Carome K, Rahman A, Parvez B. Exclusive human milk diet reduces incidence of severe intraventricular hemorrhage in extremely low birth weight infants. *J Perinatol.* 2020;41(3):535-543. doi:10.1038/s41372-020-00834-5.

71. O'Connor DL, Gibbins S, Kiss A, et al. Effect of supplemental donor human milk compared with preterm formula on neurodevelopment of very-low-birth-weight infants at 18 months: a randomized clinical trial. *JAMA.* 2016;316(18):1897-1905. doi:10.1001/JAMA.2016.16144.

72. Premkumar MH, Pammi M, Suresh G. Human milk-derived fortifier versus bovine milk-derived fortifier for prevention of mortality and morbidity in preterm neonates. *Cochrane Database Syst Rev.* 2019;2019(11):CD013145. doi:10.1002/14651858.CD013145.PUB2.

73. Eibensteiner F, Auer-Hackenberg L, Jilma B, Thanhaeuser M, Wald M, Haiden N. Growth, feeding tolerance and metabolism in extreme preterm infants under an exclusive human milk diet. *Nutrients.* 2019;11(7):1443. doi:10.3390/NU11071443.

74. Ananthan A, Balasubramanian H, Rao S, Patole S. Human milk-derived fortifiers compared with bovine milk-derived fortifiers in preterm infants: a systematic review and meta-analysis. *Adv Nutr.* 2020;11(5):1325-1333. doi:10.1093/ADVANCES/NMAA039.

75. Radmacher PG, Adamkin DH. Fortification of human milk for preterm infants. *Semin Fetal Neonatal Med.* 2017;22(1):30-35. doi:10.1016/J.SINY.2016.08.004.

76. Simsek GK, Alyamaç Dizdar E, Araylcl S, et al. Comparison of the effect of three different fortification methods on growth of very low birth weight infants. *Breastfeed Med.* 2019;14(1):63-68. doi:10.1089/bfm.2018.0093.

77. Fabrizio V, Trzaski JM, Brownell EA, et al. Individualized versus standard diet fortification for growth and development in preterm infants receiving human milk. *Cochrane Database Syst Rev.* 2020;(11)11:CD013465. doi:10.1002/14651858.CD013465.PUB2.

78. de Halleux V, Rigo J. Variability in human milk composition: benefit of individualized fortification in very-low-birth-weight infants. *Am J Clin Nutr.* 2013;98(2):529S-535S. doi:10.3945/AJCN.112.042689.

79. de Halleux V, Close A, Stalport S, Studzinski F, Habibi F, Rigo J. Advantages of individualized fortification of human milk for preterm infants. *Arch Pediatr.* 2007;14(suppl 1):S5-S10. doi:10.1016/S0929-693X(07)80004-2.

80. Hair AB, Blanco CL, Moreira AG, et al. Randomized trial of human milk cream as a supplement to standard fortification of an exclusive human milk-based diet in infants 750-1250 g birth weight. *J Pediatr.* 2014;165(5):915-920. doi:10.1016/J.JPEDS.2014.07.005.

81. Rochow N, Fusch G, Ali A, et al. Individualized target fortification of breast milk with protein, carbohydrates, and fat for preterm infants: a double-blind randomized controlled trial. *Clin Nutr.* 2021;40(1):54-63. doi:10.1016/J.CLNU.2020.04.031.

82. McLeod G, Sherriff J, Hartmann PE, Nathan E, Geddes D, Simmer K. Comparing different methods of human breast milk fortification using measured v. assumed macronutrient composition to target reference growth: a randomised controlled trial. *Br J Nutr.* 2016;115(3):431-439. doi:10.1017/S0007114515004614.

83. Polberger S, Räihä NCR, Juvonen P, Moro GE, Minoli I, Warm A. Individualized protein fortification of human milk for preterm infants: comparison of ultrafiltrated human milk protein and a bovine whey fortifier. *J Pediatr Gastroenterol Nutr.* 1999;29(3):332-338. doi:10.1097/00005176-199909000-00017.

84. Arslanoglu S, Moro GE, Ziegler EE. Adjustable fortification of human milk fed to preterm infants: does it make a difference? *J Perinatol.* 2006;26(10):614-621. doi:10.1038/sj.jp.7211571.

85. Picaud JC, Houeto N, Buffin R, Loys CM, Godbert I, Haÿs S. Additional protein fortification is necessary in extremely low-birth-weight infants fed human milk. *J Pediatr Gastroenterol Nutr.* 2016;63(1):103-105. doi:10.1097/MPG.0000000000001142.

86. Alan S, Atasay B, Cakir U, et al. An intention to achieve better postnatal in-hospital-growth for preterm infants: adjustable protein fortification of human milk. *Early Hum Dev.* 2013;89(12):1017-1023. doi:10.1016/J.EARLHUMDEV.2013.08.015.

87. Bulut O, Coban A, Uzunhan O, Ince Z. Effects of targeted versus adjustable protein fortification of breast milk on early growth in very-low-birth-weight preterm infants: a randomized clinical trial. *Nutr Clin Pract.* 2020;35(2):335-343. doi:10.1002/NCP.10307.

88. Wang Y, Zhu W, Luo BR. Continuous feeding versus intermittent bolus feeding for premature infants with low birth weight: a meta-analysis of randomized controlled trials. *Eur J Clin Nutr.* 2019;74(5):775-783. doi:10.1038/s41430-019-0522-x.

89. Rogers SP, Hicks PD, Hamzo M, Veit LE, Abrams SA. Continuous feedings of fortified human milk lead to nutrient losses of fat, calcium and phosphorous. *Nutrients.* 2010;2(3):230-240. doi:10.3390/NU2030240.

90. Premji SS, Chessell L. Continuous nasogastric milk feeding versus intermittent bolus milk feeding for premature infants less than 1500 grams. *Cochrane Database Syst Rev.* 2011;2011(11):CD001819. doi:10.1002/14651858.CD001819.PUB2.

91. El-Kadi SW, Boutry C, Suryawan A, et al. Intermittent bolus feeding promotes greater lean growth than continuous feeding in a neonatal piglet model. *Am J Clin Nutr.* 2018;108(4):830-841. doi:10.1093/AJCN/NQY133.

92. El-Kadi SW, Boutry-Regard C, Suryawan A, et al. Intermittent bolus feeding enhances organ growth more than continuous feeding in a neonatal piglet model. *Curr Dev Nutr.* 2020;4(12):nzaa170. doi:10.1093/CDN/NZAA170.

93. El-Kadi SW, Gazzaneo MC, Suryawan A, et al. Viscera and muscle protein synthesis in neonatal pigs is increased more by intermittent bolus than by continuous feeding. *Pediatr Res.* 2013;74(2):154-162. doi:10.1038/PR.2013.89.

94. Bozzetti V, Paterlini G, de Lorenzo P, Gazzolo D, Valsecchi MG, Tagliabue PE. Impact of continuous vs bolus feeding on splanchnic perfusion in very low birth weight infants: a randomized trial. *J Pediatr.* 2016;176:86-92.e2. doi:10.1016/J.JPEDS.2016.05.031.

95. Suryawan A, El-Kadi SW, Nguyen HV, Fiorotto ML, Davis TA. Intermittent bolus compared with continuous feeding enhances insulin and amino acid signaling to translation initiation in skeletal muscle of neonatal pigs. *J Nutr.* 2021;151(9):2636-2645. doi:10.1093/JN/NXAB190.

96. Watson J, Mcguire W, Hawes J. Nasal versus oral route for placing feeding tubes in preterm or low birth weight infants. *Cochrane Database Syst Rev.* 2013;2013(2):CD003952. doi:10.1002/14651858.CD003952.pub3.

97. van Someren V, Linnett SJ, Stothers JK, Sullivan PG. An investigation into the benefits of resiting nasoenteric feeding tubes. *Pediatrics.* 1984;74(3):379-383. doi:10.1542/PEDS.74.3.379.

98. Bohnhorst B, Cech K, Peter C, Doerdelmann M. Oral versus nasal route for placing feeding tubes: No effect on hypoxemia and bradycardia in infants with apnea of prematurity. *Neonatology.* 2010;98(2):143-149. doi:10.1159/000279617.

99. Wallenstein MB, Brooks C, Kline TA, et al. Early transpyloric vs gastric feeding in preterm infants: a retrospective cohort study. *J Perinatol.* 2019;39(6):837-841. doi:10.1038/S41372-019-0372-3.

100. Misra S, Macwan K, Albert V. Transpyloric feeding in gastroesophageal-reflux-associated apnea in premature infants. *Acta Paediatr.* 2007;96(10):1426-1429. doi:10.1111/J.1651-2227.2007.00442.X.

101. Malcolm WF, Smith PB, Mears S, Goldberg RN, Cotten CM. Transpyloric tube feeding in very low birthweight infants with suspected gastroesophageal reflux: impact on apnea and bradycardia. *J Perinatol.* 2009;29(5):372-375. doi:10.1038/jp.2008.234.

102. Watson J, Mcguire W. Transpyloric versus gastric tube feeding for preterm infants. *Cochrane Database Syst Rev.* 2013;2013(2):CD003487. doi:10.1002/14651858.CD003487.PUB3.

103. Bertino E, Giuliani F, Prandi G, Coscia A, Martano C, Fabris C. Necrotizing enterocolitis: risk factor analysis and role of gastric residuals in very low birth weight infants. *J Pediatr Gastroenterol Nutr.* 2009;48(4):437-442. doi:10.1097/MPG.0B013E31817B6DBE.

104. Cobb BA, Carlo WA, Ambalavanan N. Gastric residuals and their relationship to necrotizing enterocolitis in very low birth weight infants. *Pediatrics.* 2004;113(1 Pt 1):50-53. doi:10.1542/PEDS.113.1.50.

105. Riskin A, Cohen K, Kugelman A, Toropine A, Said W, Bader D. The Impact of routine evaluation of gastric residual volumes on the time to achieve full enteral feeding in preterm infants. *J Pediatr.* 2017;189:128-134. doi:10.1016/J.JPEDS.2017.05.054.

106. Parker LA, Weaver M, Murgas Torrazza RJ, et al. Effect of gastric residual evaluation on enteral intake in extremely preterm infants: a randomized clinical trial. *JAMA Pediatr.* 2019;173(6):534-543. doi:10.1001/JAMAPEDIATRICS.2019.0800.

107. Li YF, Lin HC, Torrazza RM, Parker L, Talaga E, Neu J. Gastric residual evaluation in preterm neonates: a useful monitoring technique or a hindrance? *Pediatr Neonatol.* 2014;55(5):335-340. doi:10.1016/J.PEDNEO.2014.02.008.

108. Abiramalatha T, Thanigainathan S, Ninan B. Routine monitoring of gastric residual for prevention of necrotising enterocolitis in preterm infants. *Cochrane Database Syst Rev.* 2019;7(7):CD012937. doi:10.1002/14651858.CD012937.PUB2.

109. Cuestas E, Aguilera B, Cerutti M, Rizzotti A. Sustained neonatal inflammation is associated with poor growth in infants born very preterm during the first year of life. *J Pediatr.* 2019;205:91-97. doi:10.1016/J.JPEDS.2018.09.032.

110. Calkins KL, Venick RS, Devaskar SU. Complications associated with parenteral nutrition in the neonate. *Clin Perinatol.* 2014;41(2):331-345. doi:10.1016/J.CLP.2014.02.006.

111. Sunehag A, Ewald U, Larsson A, Gustafsson J. Glucose production rate in extremely immature neonates. *Pediatr Res.* 1993;33(2):97-100. doi:10.1203/00006450-199302000-00001.

112. Mesotten D, Joosten K, van Kempen A, et al. ESPGHAN/ES-PEN/ESPR/CSPEN guidelines on pediatric parenteral nutrition: carbohydrates. *Clin Nutr.* 2018;37(6):2337-2343. doi:10.1016/j.clnu.2018.06.947.

113. Chacko SK, Sunehag AL. Gluconeogenesis continues in premature infants receiving total parenteral nutrition. *Arch Dis Child Fetal Neonatal Ed.* 2010;95(6):F413-F418. doi:10.1136/ADC.2009.178020.

114. Sunehag AL. The role of parenteral lipids in supporting gluconeogenesis in very premature infants. *Pediatr Res.* 2003;54(4):480-486. doi:10.1203/01.PDR.0000081298.06751.76.

115. Hay WW, Brown LD, Denne SC. Energy requirements, protein-energy metabolism and balance, and carbohydrates in preterm infants.*WorldRevNutrDiet.*2014;110:64-81.doi:10.1159/000358459.

116. Hay Jr WW. Nutritional support strategies for the preterm infant in the neonatal intensive care unit. *Pediatr Gastroenterol Hepatol Nutr.* 2018;21(4):234. doi:10.5223/PGHN.2018.21.4.234.

117. Limesand SW, Rozance PJ. Fetal adaptations in insulin secretion result from high catecholamines during placental insufficiency. *J Physiol.* 2017;595(15):5103-5113. doi:10.1113/JP273324.

118. Picard M, Juster RP, McEwen BS. Mitochondrial allostatic load puts the "gluc" back in glucocorticoids. *Nat Rev Endocrinol.* 2014;10(5):303-310. doi:10.1038/NRENDO.2014.22.

119. Song Z, Xiaoli AM, Yang F. Regulation and metabolic significance of de novo lipogenesis in adipose tissues. *Nutrients.* 2018;10(10):1383. doi:10.3390/NU10101383.

120. Lapillonne A, Eleni Dit Trolli S, Kermorvant-Duchemin E. Postnatal docosahexaenoic acid deficiency is an inevitable consequence of current recommendations and practice in preterm infants.*Neonatology.*2010;98(4):397-403.doi:10.1159/000320159.

121. Carlson SE, Werkman SH, Rhodes PG, Tolley EA. Visual-acuity development in healthy preterm infants: effect of marine-oil supplementation. *Am J Clin Nutr.* 1993;58(1):35-42. doi:10.1093/AJCN/58.1.35.

122. Tam EWY, Chau V, Barkovich AJ, et al. Early postnatal docosahexaenoic acid levels and improved preterm brain development. *Pediatr Res.* 2016;79(5):723-730. doi:10.1038/PR.2016.11.

123. Moon K, Rao SC, Schulzke SM, Patole SK, Simmer K. Long-chain polyunsaturated fatty acid supplementation in preterm infants. *Cochrane Database Syst Rev.* 2016;12(12):CD000375. doi:10.1002/14651858.CD000375.PUB5.

124. Lapillonne A, Fidler Mis N, Goulet O, et al. ESPGHAN/ESPEN/ESPR/CSPEN guidelines on pediatric parenteral nutrition: lipids. *Clin Nutr.* 2018;37(6 Pt B):2324-2336. doi:10.1016/j.clnu.2018.06.946.

125. Cober MP, Gura KM, Mirtallo JM, et al. ASPEN lipid injectable emulsion safety recommendations part 2: neonate and pediatric considerations. *Nutr Clin Pract.* 2021;36(6):1106-1125. doi:10.1002/NCP.10778.

126. Vlaardingerbroek H, van Goudoever JB. Intravenous lipids in preterm infants: impact on laboratory and clinical outcomes and long-term consequences. *World Rev Nutr Diet.* 2015;112:71-80. doi:10.1159/000365459.

127. Anez-Bustillos L, Dao DT, Fell GL, et al. Redefining essential fatty acids in the era of novel intravenous lipid emulsions. *Clin Nutr.* 2018;37(3):784-789. doi:10.1016/J.CLNU.2017.07.004.

128. Vlaardingerbroek H, Veldhorst MAB, Spronk S, van den Akker CHP, van Goudoever JB. Parenteral lipid administration to very-low-birth-weight infants—early introduction of lipids and use of new lipid emulsions: a systematic review and meta-analysis. *Am J Clin Nutr.* 2012;96(2):255-268. doi:10.3945/AJCN.112.040717.

129. Jackson RL, White PZ, Zalla J. SMOFlipid vs Intralipid 20%: effect of mixed-oil vs soybean-oil emulsion on parenteral nutrition-associated cholestasis in the neonatal population. *JPEN J Parenter Enteral Nutr.* 2021;45(2):339-346. doi:10.1002/JPEN.1843.

130. Stramara L, Hernandez L, Bloom BT, Durham C. Development of parenteral nutrition-associated liver disease and other adverse effects in neonates receiving SMOFlipid or Intralipid. *JPEN J Parenter Enteral Nutr.* 2020;44(8):1530-1534. doi:10.1002/JPEN.1774.

131. Vlaardingerbroek H, Ng K, Stoll B, et al. New generation lipid emulsions prevent PNALD in chronic parenterally fed preterm pigs.*J Lipid Res.* 2014;55(3):466-477. doi:10.1194/JLR.M044545.

132. Kapoor V, Malviya MN, Soll R. Lipid emulsions for parenterally fed term and late preterm infants. *Cochrane Database Syst Rev.* 2019;6(6):CD013171. doi:10.1002/14651858.CD013171.PUB2/EPDF/ABSTRACT.

133. Hojsak I, Colomb V, Braegger C, et al. ESPGHAN Committee on nutrition position paper. Intravenous lipid emulsions and risk of hepatotoxicity in infants and children: a systematic review and meta-analysis. *J Pediatr Gastroenterol Nutr.* 2016;62(5):776-792. doi:10.1097/MPG.0000000000001121.

134. Toce SS, Keenan WJ. Lipid intolerance in newborns is associated with hepatic dysfunction but not infection. *Arch Pediatr Adolesc Med.* 1995;149(11):1249-1253. doi:10.1001/ARCH-PEDI.1995.02170240067010.

135. Gura KM, Crowley M. A detailed guide to lipid therapy in intestinal failure. *Semin Pediatr Surg.* 2018;27(4):242-255. doi:10.1053/J.SEMPEDSURG.2018.07.003.

136. Ziegler EE, O'Donnell AM, Nelson SE, Fomon SJ. Body composition of the reference fetus. *Growth.* 1976;40(4):329-341. Accessed March 21, 2022. Available at: https://pubmed.ncbi.nlm.nih.gov/1010389/.

137. van Goudoever JB, Carnielli V, Darmaun D, et al. ESPGHAN/ESPEN/ESPR/CSPEN guidelines on pediatric parenteral nutrition: Amino acids. *Clinical Nutr.* 2018;37(6 Pt B):2315-2323. doi:10.1016/j.clnu.2018.06.945.

138. van den Akker CHP, te Braake FWJ, Wattimena DJL, et al. Effects of early amino acid administration on leucine and glucose kinetics in premature infants. *Pediatr Res* 2006;59(5):732-735. doi:10.1203/01.pdr.0000214990.86879.26.

139. Poindexter BB, Langer JC, Dusick AM, Ehrenkranz RA. Early provision of parenteral amino acids in extremely low birth weight infants: relation to growth and neurodevelopmental outcome. *J Pediatr.* 2006;148(3):300-305. doi:10.1016/J.JPEDS.2005.10.038.

140. Stephens BE, Walden RV, Gargus RA, et al. First-week protein and energy intakes are associated with 18-month developmental outcomes in extremely low birth weight infants. *Pediatrics.* 2009;123(5):1337-1343. doi:10.1542/PEDS.2008-0211.

141. Osborn DA, Schindler T, Jones LJ, Sinn JKH, Bolisetty S. Higher versus lower amino acid intake in parenteral nutrition for newborn infants. *Cochrane Database Syst Rev.* 2018;3(3):CD005949. doi:10.1002/14651858.CD005949.PUB2.

142. Roelants JA, Vlaardingerbroek H, van den Akker CHP, de Jonge RCJ, van Goudoever JB, Vermeulen MJ. Two-year follow-up of a randomized controlled nutrition intervention trial in very low-birth-weight infants. *J Parenter Enteral Nutr.* 2018;42(1):122-131. doi:10.1177/0148607116678196.

143. Uthaya S, Liu X, Babalis D, et al. Nutritional Evaluation and Optimisation in Neonates: a randomized, double-blind controlled trial of amino acid regimen and intravenous lipid

composition in preterm parenteral nutrition. *Am J Clin Nutr.* 2016;103(6):1443-1452. doi:10.3945/AJCN.115.125138.

144. Kotsopoulos K, Benadiba-Torch A, Cuddy A, Shah PS. Safety and efficacy of early amino acids in preterm <28 weeks gestation: prospective observational comparison. *J Perinatol.* 2006;26(12):749-754. doi:10.1038/sj.jp.7211611.

145. te Braake FWJ, van den Akker CHP, Wattimena DJL, Huijmans JGM, van Goudoever JB. Amino acid administration to premature infants directly after birth. *J Pediatr.* 2005;147(4):457-461. doi:10.1016/J.JPEDS.2005.05.038.

146. Uthaya S, Longford N, Battersby C, Oughham K, Lanoue J, Modi N. Early versus later initiation of parenteral nutrition for very preterm infants: a propensity score-matched observational study. *Arch Dis Child Fetal Neonatal Ed.* 2022;107(2):137-142. doi:10.1136/archdischild-2021-322383.

147. Thoene MK, Lyden E, Anderson-Berry A. Improving nutrition outcomes for infants < 1500 grams with a progressive, evidenced-based enteral feeding protocol. *Nutr Clin Pract.* 2018;33(5):647-655. doi:10.1002/ncp.10081.

148. Kaplan HC, Poindexter BB. Standardized feeding protocols: evidence and implementation. *World Rev Nutr Diet.* 2021;122:289-300. doi:10.1159/000514746.

149. Chandran S, Anand AJ, Rajadurai VS, Seyed ES, Khoo PC, Chua MC. Evidence-based practices reduce necrotizing enterocolitis and improve nutrition outcomes in very low-birth-weight infants. *JPEN J Parenter Enteral Nutr.* 2021;45(7):1408-1416. doi:10.1002/JPEN.2058.

150. Jasani B, Patole S. Standardized feeding regimen for reducing necrotizing enterocolitis in preterm infants: an updated systematic review. *J Perinatol.* 2017;37(7):827-833. doi:10.1038/jp.2017.37.

151. Johnson MJ, Leaf AA, Pearson F, et al. Successfully implementing and embedding guidelines to improve the nutrition and growth of preterm infants in neonatal intensive care: a prospective interventional study. *BMJ Open.* 2017;7(12):e017727. doi:10.1136/BMJOPEN-2017-017727.

Chapter 12

International Perspective: Management of Nutrition in Preterm Infants in Settings With Limited Resources

Maria Teresa Murguia-Peniche and Rebecca J. Hill

Chapter Outline

Key Points

1. Globally it is estimated that 15 million infants are born preterm and most of them are delivered in low- and middle-income countries. Nutritional interventions may be costly, increasing the financial burden of their care, or may be unavailable.

2. Kangaroo Mother Care is promoted for reducing morbidity and mortality in preterm/low-birth-weight infants.

3. Mother's own milk is the preferred source of nutrition for preterm infants. Support should be given to mothers to breastfeed (in cases where the preterm infant is of sufficient maturity) or to express their milk.

4. Human milk may need to be pasteurized if the mother is HIV positive; refrigeration is not available and expressed milk needs to be kept at room temperature; or donor milk is being used. Heat-flash pasteurization is an option for limited-resource settings where other methods such as Holder pasteurization are not available.

5. Human milk alone may not meet the nutritional needs of very preterm infants. Options for improving the delivery of nutrients and approaching the recommendations for this population in low-resource settings include fortification (with human milk fortifiers if available or with preterm formula); use of supplements (calcium, phosphate, vitamins, zinc, oils, other); early start and advancement of enteral feeds; or increasing the volume of enteral feeds up to 300 mL/kg/d of expressed human milk. The chosen option may depend on cost and available resources; however, optimal results are

not always achieved with these strategies. Further research is needed for this vulnerable population.

6. During the transitional period from gastro-enteral to oral feeds, the World Health Organization recommends feeding with a cup, palladai, or spoon. The use of palladai has been associated with better weight gain, faster achievement of full feeds, and shorter length of hospital stay versus the use of other cups. Finger feeding is an additional strategy that has been associated with fewer complications and lower milk loss versus cup feeding.

7. Other supplements used in low-resource settings include emollient oils applied on the skin and oral probiotics. More research is needed in this area.

Introduction

Globally it is estimated that 15 million infants are born preterm and most of them are delivered in low- and middle-income countries[1]; in these settings,

32.4 million infants (term and preterm) are born small for gestational age (SGA).[2] Fig. 12.1 shows increasing trends for estimates of preterm birth rates from 2000 to 2014 globally and in nearly all regions. Good nutrition is critical for these infants to improve not only survival but short- and long-term health outcomes. Many challenges are encountered when trying to achieve this goal as preterm infants are immature and need nutritional interventions that may be costly, increasing the financial burden of their care, especially in low-resource settings. It is therefore important to understand different practices used in these settings, which may be based on a limited and low or very low quality of evidence. Research is urgently needed to provide these preterm infants with the best possible nutritional care.

In this chapter we will describe strategies used in some low-resource settings to increase nutrient delivery to preterm infants, feeding interventions to improve the transitional period between gastro-enteral and oral feeds, and a low-cost pasteurization technique.

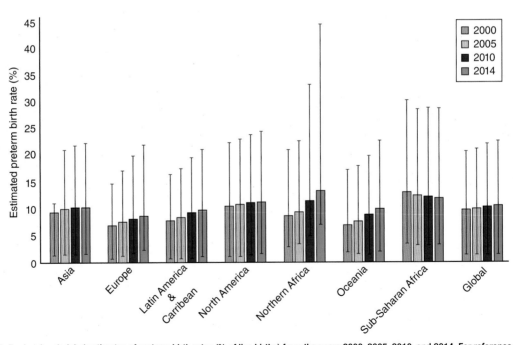

Fig. 12.1 Regional and global estimates of preterm birth rates (% of live births) from the years 2000, 2005, 2010, and 2014. For reference, total live births for each year globally are 129.6 million, 133.2 million, 137.8 million, and 139.9 million for the years 2000, 2005, 2010, and 2014, respectively. From Chawanpaiboon S, Vogel JP, Moller A-B, et al. Global, regional, and national estimates of levels of preterm birth in 2014: a systematic review and modelling analysis. Lancet Glob Health. 2019;7:e37–e46.

Enteral Feeding Strategies to Improve the Nutritional Status of Preterm Infants

Mother's own milk, the preferred source of nutrition for all infants, has multiple benefits including improved survival and immune defense; lower incidence of morbidities, especially necrotizing enterocolitis (NEC); better digestion of nutrients; and better neurodevelopmental outcomes, among others.[3,4] Promoting milk production and maintaining adequate milk supply is an important consideration for mothers who are feeding human milk (HM) to their infants and may be especially so for mothers of preterm infants. Initiation of lactation in mothers of preterm infants may be compromised compared to mothers of term infants and may display greater variability between mothers of preterm infants.[5]

Kangaroo Mother Care (KMC), whereby an infant has skin-to-skin contact with their mother by being held vertically between the breasts and underneath clothing, is associated with frequent and exclusive/near exclusive breastfeeding in preterm and/or low-birth-weight infants.[6] KMC is primarily promoted in resource-limited settings for reducing morbidity and mortality in preterm/low-birth-weight infants; immediate KMC is now recommended, unless the infant is in shock or unable to breathe spontaneously.[6,7]

Research into KMC focuses mainly on initiation and/or exclusivity of feeding at the breast (i.e., breastfeeding) but generally does not consider initiation of lactation per se by the mother when an infant is unable to feed at the breast. The degree of prematurity will influence the ability of an infant to latch and feed at the breast and mothers may need to express their milk.[8] In developed nations, electric breast pumps for expressing HM are readily available, but in resource-limited settings mothers may need to express with a manual breast pump or express manually by hand. A Cochrane review in 2016 indicating effective strategies to support expression of HM included early expression of milk soon after birth, relaxation, massaging and warming the breasts, manual hand expression, and use of low-cost pumps.[9] This review also suggested that some of these measures may influence nutritional content of the expressed HM in addition to influencing volume. For example, the protein content was higher when using hand expression or electric pumping versus manual pumping; higher sodium and lower potassium were reported for hand expression

over either manual or electric pumping; and breast massage while pumping resulted in higher fat/lipid content. Alternatively, no difference in energy content was reported between methods of HM expression. Whichever method is chosen, it is important to consider cost, availability, and preference, and that each mother is taught how to express successfully, with appropriate instruction on hygienic handling and storage of expressed HM to prevent contamination.[10]

HM alone may not meet the nutritional requirements of very preterm infants, and HM should be fortified or enriched to improve the growth and micronutrient status of preterm infants.[11] As HM composition varies between mothers and can be influenced by their dietary intake (particularly for micronutrients),[12–14] published region-specific macro-/micronutrient values for HM should be used wherever possible when calculating fortification needs.

Fortification of HM has been adopted by most countries with high-income economies, but this may not be practical in low-resource settings because of cost, availability, and risk of infection if not handled properly. Explorations of different strategies to increase the nutrient intake of very preterm infants in low-resource settings have been reported. Parenteral nutrition (PN) is not universally available; thus it is critical to start an adequate volume of enteral feeds as soon as medically suitable. It is also important to understand the maximum volume of enteral feeds tolerated by very-low-birth-weight and extremely low-birth-weight infants to deliver nutrients approaching recommend amounts, or at least higher levels of nutrients in conditions where fortification is not possible. Furthermore, it is important to understand the supplements used in low-resource settings to enrich HM when fortifiers are not available. In this section we will discuss some studies that have alluded to these challenges and will focus on:

- Early initiation and advancement of enteral feeds
- Increasing the volume of enteral feeds
- Use of supplements, formulas, or fortifiers to enrich HM

EARLY INITIATION AND ADVANCEMENT OF ENTERAL FEEDS

An unblinded randomized controlled trial conducted in India[15] allocated 180 stable preterm infants (1000–1499 g) to receive either early total enteral feeding (ETEF) from day 1 of life, with 80 mL/kg/d and advancing to 180 mL/kg/d with no intravenous fluids; or conventional enteral feeding (CEF) starting at 20 mL/kg/d on day 1 of life and advancing 20 to 30 mL/kg/d with intravenous fluids (no PN); this group also advanced to 180 mL/kg/d. The ETEF group reached full enteral feeds more quickly (−3.6 days) and had a lower incidence of sepsis (26% vs. 60.6%), less feeding intolerance (15.9% vs. 30.2%), and shorter length of hospital stay (−4.1 days) versus the CEF group. The incidence of NEC was similar. At 1 month of age, infants in the ETEF group were significantly heavier (~100 g) than the CEF group. Results suggest this strategy of ETEF might be safe and may also offer benefits in settings with limited resources. Further research is needed to understand whether these findings could be translated to other populations, especially for unstable or extremely low-birth-weight infants.

INCREASING THE VOLUME OF ENTERAL FEEDS

The intake of enteral feeds up to 200 mL/kg/d may increase the delivery of macro- and micronutrients as well as caloric intake in preterm infants receiving unfortified HM versus those receiving lower enteral intakes (150–160 mL/kg/d). Moreover, volumes up to 300 mL/kg/d may further increase the nutrient intake of preterm infants. A prospective trial conducted in India compared outcomes in 64 very-low-birth-weight infants randomized to receive either 200 or 300 mL/kg/d of expressed HM and followed these infants until they reached 1700 g.[16] Although increased volume of intake resulted in an estimated increase in caloric intake (134 vs. 200 kcal/kg/d), protein (2.2 vs. 3.3 g/kg/d), calcium (68 vs. 102 mg/kg/d), and phosphorus (30 vs. 45 mg/kg/d), values still fell short for some current nutrient recommendations for this population,[17] particularly for micronutrients. Daily weight gain was significantly higher (24.9 vs. 18.7g/kg/d, p < 0.0001) in the group receiving 300 versus 200 mL/kg/d, and importantly, there were no differences in complications or feeding tolerance. Of note, this study was small. In infants assigned to 300 mL/kg/d, 12 of 30 participants received less volume than targeted and 40% of infants had high levels of alkaline phosphatase (expected as the intake of calcium and phosphorus were below recommendations), which

may underscore the importance of not only looking at gain in weight but also bone health and other markers of micronutrient status in these infants. A subgroup analysis of SGA infants in this study showed no effect on weight gain with this high-volume strategy.[16]

Other studies have compared different volume intakes (from 140 to 200 mL/kg/d) in very preterm infants[18,19] and in general, weight gain was increased in the groups with higher volume intakes. One study conducted in the United States[18] included larger but very preterm infants (1001–2500 g) receiving fortified HM. Higher volume intakes were associated with increased length, head circumference, and mid-arm circumference in infants receiving 180 to 200 mL/kg/d versus 140 to 160 mL/kg/d, at 36 weeks gestational age or at discharge; adverse effects were similar between groups.

USE OF SUPPLEMENTS, FORMULAS, OR FORTIFIERS TO ENRICH HUMAN MILK

The World Health Organization (WHO) recommendations for feeding low-birth-weight infants published in 2011 and 2022[7] do not include specific guidance for extremely low-birth-weight or unstable preterm infants.[20,21] In summary, mother's own milk is recommended for very low-birth-weight infants, and if not available, donor milk (if safe and available from affordable HM banks) may be considered.[7,20] Unfortunately, not every country has enough HM banks actively operating, especially in sub-Saharan Africa. Wet nursing and informal milk sharing are used in different regions, but the risks, especially of HIV transmission, have decreased this practice.[21] According to the WHO 2022 guidelines, HM fortification, or enriched preterm formula if HM is not available, may be considered for very-low-birth-weight (<1500g) or very preterm (<32 weeks' gestation) infants.[7]

India is the country with the greatest number of preterm births.[1] In this country, enrichment of HM is recommended for infants <32 to 34 weeks until 40 weeks.[22] Supplements, human milk fortifier (HMF), or preterm formula may be used for this purpose. For infants >1500 to 2500 g, supplementation with iron, vitamin D, and zinc is recommended rather than routine HM fortification. Common supplements used in very-low-birth-weight infants when adequate fortifiers are not available or not used (Box 12.1) are usually

BOX 12.1 COMMONLY USED SUPPLEMENTS FOR VERY-LOW-BIRTH-WEIGHT INFANTS WHEN ROUTINE FORTIFICATION IS NOT AVAILABLE

- Calcium and phosphate
- Vitamin A, vitamin B complex, and zinc supplements; usually in the form of multivitamin drops
- Vitamin D drops
- Folate drops
- Iron drops
- Cod liver oil (used in Ethiopia) as a source of vitamins A and D

given at different feeding times during the day to avoid excessive increase of osmolality. Some of these recommendations are followed in other countries.[23]

Fortification

The Food and Agriculture Organization and the WHO encourage, whenever possible and feasible, use of commercially sterile liquid products for high-risk preterm infants to diminish the risk of infections. The standard marketed commercially sterile liquid HM fortifiers available in countries with high-income economies are not always accessible in many low-resource settings; thus safety guidelines for the use of powder products have been published.[24]

A recent blinded randomized controlled trial from Chile[25] compared growth and adverse events in 146 very-low-birth-weight infants who received mother's milk with either powder or liquid HMF; this multicenter study included NICUs with established feeding protocols. Growth outcomes and adverse events, including sepsis, were not significantly different between groups, suggesting that the use of powder HMF might be a good option in low-resource settings if feeding and safety protocols are followed carefully.

Depending on the fortifiers available, it is important to understand that fortified HM may not meet recommendations for all nutrients. For example, India has on the market two local preparations of powder HMF: Lactodex-HMF and HIJAM-HMF. These HMFs add calories and macro- and micronutrients to HM to increase concentrations of some nutrients and align with selected global recommendations for the nutrition of preterm infants.[26]

However, when compared to ESPGHAN 2010[27] and more recent recommendations,[17] some nutrients are below recommended values.[26] Other commercial powder preparations of HMF are available in India but are not routinely used because they are costlier and not universally available.[22] Further research is needed to understand the impact of these local HMFs on the short- and long-term outcomes of preterm infants as well as their effect on micronutrient status. Additionally, use of local/regional published values for HM composition is important when calculating individual infant nutritional needs, particularly for some micronutrients.

Preterm formula has also been used to fortify HM. A recent review of five studies (four from developing nations) comparing outcomes in hospitalized preterm infants receiving unfortified or fortified HM versus HM enriched with preterm formula demonstrated no difference in the gain in growth parameters between the two study groups. After a sensitivity analysis (very low quality of evidence), infants receiving HM enriched with preterm formula exhibited better growth compared to infants receiving unfortified HM (mean difference in weight +2.03 g/d; gains in head circumference or length were also slightly increased).[28] The trials included in this review were very heterogeneous and included studies with different interventions and populations.

A recent randomized noninferiority trial with 123 preterm infants (<34 weeks postmenstrual age [PMA]) in India compared weight gain between those who received HM fortified with a commercially available fortifier (HMF) versus those receiving HM fortified with preterm formula (HMP).[29] In powder addition, the HMF group received vitamin D as a supplement and the HMP group received calcium, phosphate, and iron. Weight gain at 40 weeks PMA or discharge (whichever occurred first) was similar between both groups (15.7 vs. 16.3 g/kg/d, HMP vs. HMF, respectively); however, the incidence of feeding intolerance was lower in the HMP group compared to the HMF group (1.4 vs. 6.8 per 1000 patient days). At 40 weeks PMA, the prevalence of infants with weight below the 10th percentile was very high in both groups (73% and 81%, HMP and HMF, respectively), suggesting that both strategies need to be revised to achieve better outcomes.

Nutritional Interventions to Facilitate the Transitional Period

CUP, PALLADAI, SPOON OR FINGER FEEDING

Very preterm infants with immature swallowing and sucking reflexes are unable to breastfeed; in these circumstances the WHO recommends expression of breast milk (discussed previously) and cup feeding (cup, palladia, or spoon) for the transition from gastro-enteral to oral feeds while the infants improve their oral motor skills.[20] Naso- or orogastric tubes may also be used if needed.

The use of cups is safe and effective and has some advantages over bottle-feeding; however, it has been associated with some difficulties such as spillage and long feeding times. A review of 12 studies (randomized controlled trials and observational)[30] concluded that cup feeding was associated with better success for breastfeeding up to 6 months postdischarge and better physiologic stability versus bottle-feeding. In addition, cups are washed easily as compared with bottles.

In some countries in Africa and Asia, the palladai is used for this transitional period. The *palladai* is a spouted cup made of metal (Fig. 12.2) that pours about 10 mL of milk. A study by Marofi et al. compared the use of the palladai versus another cup in 69 preterm infants (29–32 weeks gestation). The first feeding was administrated by either cup or palladai in each shift within 7 sequential days. The palladai use was associated with better weight gain, faster achievement of full enteral feeds, and shorter length of hospital stay.[31] In another study conducted in India, with 86 term infants appropriate for gestational age (AGA) or SGA and 14 preterm infants, palladai use was associated with greater intake and better acceptability versus the other cup.[32]

Finger feeding is another strategy to support the transitional period. With this technique the milk is supplied by suction through a tube connected to a syringe and attached to a caregiver's gloved finger. A prospective randomized study performed in Brazil with 53 preterm infants (32–36 weeks gestation) concluded that finger feeding was associated with fewer complications and lower milk loss versus cup feeding.[33] More research is needed to understand the benefits of this technique, especially on breastfeeding rates.

Also, note that these techniques require training and understanding to achieve optimal results.

Pasteurization Methods

Pasteurization of HM may be used in low-resource settings in the following conditions:
- HIV-positive mother providing HM to feed her baby
- Need to preserve expressed HM at room temperature in settings where no refrigerator is available
- Use of donor milk

HEAT-FLASH INACTIVATION

Holder pasteurization is not always available in low-resource settings. An alternative method to pasteurize HM is *heat-flash inactivation*, which is an easy and affordable method demonstrated to effectively inactivate HIV and other viral agents and bacteria[34,35]; this method of pasteurization can be performed in hospital settings or at home.

The nursing staff must demonstrate the technique to the mothers, and the mothers should always be supervised when pasteurizing their breast milk for the first time. The equipment needed for heat-flash pasteurization is shown in Box 12.2.

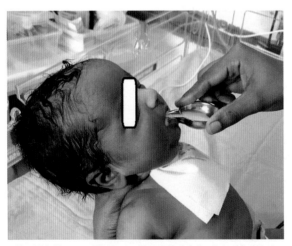

Fig. 12.2 Human milk given with a palladai. Courtesy of Dr. Laleet.

BOX 12.2 EQUIPMENT REQUIRED TO HEAT-FLASH-PASTEURIZE HUMAN MILK

- Pot with approximately 1 L capacity
- Sterilized glass jar with approximately 400 mL capacity (e.g., empty glass peanut butter jar)
- A weight to hold down the jar of milk in the water (e.g., another jar with water)
- Electric/gas stove or hot plate
- Insulation boards on which to place the hot pot
- Patient stickers
- A colored sticker to identify pasteurized HIV-positive expressed breast milk (EBM)
- Pen to write the date on the patient sticker

From Murguia-Peniche T, Kirsten GF. Meeting the challenge of providing neonatal nutritional care to very- or extremely low-birth-weight infants in low-resource settings. *World Rev Nutr Diet.* 2014;110:278-296. doi:10.1159/000358476.

The procedure is as follows[35]:

1. From 50 to 150 mL of HM is expressed into a sterile glass jar and the lid is closed.
2. The jar with expressed HM is placed in a pot that is then placed on the stove, and a weight is placed on the jar.
3. Approximately 450 mL of tap water is poured into the pot; the water level should be two fingers (2 cm) above the level of the expressed milk.
4. The water and milk are heated together on a high heat setting until the water is at a rolling boil.
5. The pot is immediately removed from the stove and the jar with expressed HM is removed from the hot water.
6. The pasteurized expressed HM is allowed to cool at room temperature.

Once pasteurized, the cooled expressed HM can be used immediately or stored in the designated milk refrigerator for up to 96 hours[37]; when stored for longer periods, it should be frozen. There is evidence to suggest that pasteurized expressed HM may be stored at room temperature for up to 24 hours, especially if kept in the pasteurization container and not handled.[38] More research is needed in this area. Strict protocols must be followed to ensure that the correct HM is administered to an infant.

Pasteurized donor HM can be used if the mother does not produce enough breast milk, if the mother is too sick to express, or if the mother dies.

Other Supplements Used in Low-Resource Settings

EMOLLIENT OILS

Emollient oil applied on the skin of infants has been used in low-resource settings as a possible source of essential fatty acids and saturated fat, especially in settings where no intravenous lipids are available. A randomized controlled trial conducted in India showed an increase (pre-intervention to 5 days post-intervention) of serum fat in infants (preterm and term) who were massaged with safflower (increase in linoleic and arachidonic acid) or coconut (increase of saturated fat) oil.[39] Participants in the control group (no oil) also had a gain in fat, but the observed increment of these fats was significantly lower versus the groups receiving the oils. The impact of this intervention to prevent essential fatty acid deficiency in preterm infants remains to be proven. Other studies using different emollient oils applied on the skin of infants have associated this intervention with better growth and lower incidence of sepsis in preterm infants; however, the level of certainty is low.[40,41] More research is needed to understand the benefits and safety of this practice.

PROBIOTICS

A recent meta-analysis reviewed several studies (up to 29) from low- and middle-income countries to explore the role of probiotics on neonatal sepsis, mortality, and NEC. The use of probiotics was associated with a significantly lower risk of these three outcomes (0.78:0.70–0.86; 0.80:0.66–0.96; and 0.46:0.35–0.61, respectively).[42] A large study (n = 4556) was conducted in community settings and included infants who were at least 35 weeks gestation and 2000 g. The use of probiotics (*Lactobacillus plantarum*) and fructo-oligosaccharide was associated with a significant decrease in the combined outcome of sepsis and death up to 60 days versus control (relative risk [RR]: 0.60, 95% confidence interval [CI]: 0.48–0.74).[43]

The analyzed studies used different strains, interventions, and dosages. Results from these studies appear promising, but the debate on probiotic use in preterm infants remains until safety and long-term outcomes are understood.

Summary

Mother's own milk is the preferred source of nutrition for preterm infants, especially in low-resource settings. Support should be given to mothers to breastfeed (where the preterm infant is of sufficient maturity) or to express their milk.

Human milk may need to be pasteurized if the mother is HIV positive; refrigeration is not available and expressed milk needs to be kept at room temperature for a short time; or donor milk is being used. Heat-flash pasteurization is an option for limited-resource settings.

It is important to recognize that human milk alone may not meet the nutritional needs of very preterm infants. Options for improving the delivery of nutrients and approaching the recommendations for this population include fortification (with HMFs or preterm formula); use of supplements; early start and advancement of enteral feeds; or increasing the volume of enteral feeds. The chosen option may depend on cost and available resources.

There are critical feeding periods that need special attention. For example, the WHO recommends during the transitional period from gastro-enteral to oral feeds feeding with a cup, palladia, or spoon. Finger feeding is an additional strategy.

REFERENCES

1. Blencowe H, Cousens S, Chou D, et al. Born too soon: the global epidemiology of 15 million preterm births. *Reprod Health.* 2013;10 Suppl 1(suppl 1):S2. doi:10.1186/1742-4755-10-s1-s2.
2. Lee AC, Katz J, Blencowe H, et al. National and regional estimates of term and preterm babies born small for gestational age in 138 low-income and middle-income countries in 2010. *Lancet Glob Health.* 2013;1(1):e26-e36. doi:10.1016/s2214-109x(13)70006-8.
3. Gertosio C, Meazza C, Pagani S, Bozzola M. Breastfeeding and its gamut of benefits. *Minerva Pediatr.* 2016;68(3):201-212.
4. Patel AL, Kim JH. Human milk and necrotizing enterocolitis. *Semin Pediatr Surg.* 2018;27(1):34-38. doi:10.1053/j.sempedsurg.2017.11.007.
5. Cregan MD, De Mello TR, Kershaw D, McDougall K, Hartmann PE. Initiation of lactation in women after preterm delivery. *Acta Obstet Gynecol Scand.* 2002;81(9):870-877. doi:10.1034/j.1600-0412.2002.810913.x.
6. Conde-Agudelo A, Díaz-Rossello JL. Kangaroo mother care to reduce morbidity and mortality in low birthweight infants. *Cochrane Database Syst Rev.* 2014;22;(4):CD002771. doi:10.1002/14651858.CD002771.pub3.
7. World Health Organization. *WHO recommendations for care of the preterm or low birth weight infant.* Geneva: World Health Organization; 2022. https://www.who.int/publications/i/item/9789240058262, 2022. Accessed July 8, 2023.
8. Dodrill P. Feeding difficulties in preterm infants. *Infant Child Adolesc Nutr.* 2011;3(6):324-331. doi:10.1177/1941406411421003.
9. Becker GE, Smith HA, Cooney F. Methods of milk expression for lactating women. *Cochrane Database Syst Rev.* 2016;9(9):CD006170. doi:10.1002/14651858.CD006170.pub5.
10. Cheah FC, Tan TL. Practical implementation of quality nutritional care to preterm infants in developing countries. *World Rev Nutr Diet.* 2021;122:340-356. doi:10.1159/000514761.
11. Fusch S, Fusch G, Yousuf EI, et al. Individualized target fortification of breast milk: optimizing macronutrient content using different fortifiers and approaches. *Front Nutr.* 2021;8:652641. doi:10.3389/fnut.2021.652641.
12. Innis SM. Impact of maternal diet on human milk composition and neurological development of infants. *Am J Clin Nutr.* 2014;99(3):734s-741s. doi:10.3945/ajcn.113.072595.
13. de Halleux V, Rigo J. Variability in human milk composition: benefit of individualized fortification in very-low-birth-weight infants. *Am J Clin Nutr.* 2013;98(2):529s-535s. doi:10.3945/ajcn.112.042689.
14. Samuel TM, Zhou Q, Giuffrida F, Munblit D, Verhasselt V, Thakkar SK. Nutritional and non-nutritional composition of human milk is modulated by maternal, infant, and methodological factors. *Front Nutr.* 2020;7:576133. doi:10.3389/fnut.2020.576133.
15. Nangia S, Vadivel V, Thukral A, Saili A. Early total enteral feeding versus conventional enteral feeding in stable very-low-birth-weight infants: a randomised controlled trial. *Neonatology.* 2019;115(3):256-262. doi:10.1159/000496015.
16. Thomas N, Cherian A, Santhanam S, Jana AK. A randomized control trial comparing two enteral feeding volumes in very low birth weight babies. *J Trop Pediatr.* 2012;58(1):55-58. doi:10.1093/tropej/fmr011.
17. Travers CP, Wang T, Salas AA, et al. Higher- or usual-volume feedings in infants born very preterm: a randomized clinical trial. *J Pediatr.* 2020;224:66-71.e1. doi:10.1016/j.jpeds.2020.05.033.
18. Kuschel CA, Evans N, Askie L, Bredemeyer S, Nash J, Polverino J. A randomized trial of enteral feeding volumes in infants born before 30 weeks' gestation. *J Paediatr Child Health.* 2000;36(6):581-586. doi:10.1046/j.1440-1754.2000.00577.x.
19. WHO Guidelines Review Committee, Maternal, Newborn, Child & Adolescent Health & Healthy Ageing. Guidelines on Optimal Feeding of Low Birth-Weight Infants in Low- and Middle-Income Countries. Geneva, Switzerland: World Health Organization; 2011.
20. Akindolire A, Talbert A, Sinha I, Embleton N, Allen S. Evidence that informs feeding practices in very low birthweight and very preterm infants in sub-Saharan Africa: an overview of systematic reviews. *BMJ Paediatr Open.* 2020;4(1):e000724. doi:10.1136/bmjpo-2020-000724.
21. Agarwal R, Deorari A, Paul V. Feeding of low birth weight infants. In: Argarwal R, Deorari A, Paul V, Sankar MJ, Sachdeva A, eds. AIIMS Protocols in Neonatology. Delhi: Noble Vision; 2019:234–257. 2nd ed.. [chapter 19].
22. Torabi Z, Moemeni N, Ahmadiafshar A, Mazloomzadeh S. The effect of calcium and phosphorus supplementation on metabolic bone disorders in premature infants. *J Pak Med Assoc.* 2014;64(6):635-639.
23. WHO, Nutrition and Food Safety Standards & Scientific Advice on Food Nutrition. Safe Preparation, Storage and Handling of Powdered Infant Formula: Guidelines. Geneva, Switzerland: World Health Organization; 2007.

24. Masoli D, Mena P, Dominguez A, et al. Growth of very low birth weight infants who received a liquid human milk fortifier: a randomized, controlled multicenter trial. *J Pediatr Gastroenterol Nutr.* 2022;74(3):424-430. doi:10.1097/mpg.0000000000003321.

25. Kler N, Thakur A, Modi M, et al. Human milk fortification in India. *Nestle Nutr Inst Workshop Ser.* 2015;81:145-151. doi:10.1159/000365904.

26. Agostoni C, Buonocore G, Carnielli VP, et al. Enteral nutrient supply for preterm infants: commentary from the European Society of Paediatric Gastroenterology, Hepatology and Nutrition Committee on Nutrition. *J Pediatr Gastroenterol Nutr.* 2010;50(1):85-91. doi:10.1097/MPG.0b013e3181adaee0.

27. Koletzko B, Wieczorek S, Cheah FC, et al. Recommended nutrient intake levels for preterm infants. *World Rev Nutr Diet.* 2021;122:191-197. doi:10.1159/000514772.

28. Kumar M, Upadhyay J, Basu S. Fortification of human milk with infant formula for very low birth weight preterm infants: a systematic review. *Indian Pediatr.* 2021;58(3):253-258.

29. Chinnappan A, Sharma A, Agarwal R, Thukral A, Deorari A, Sankar MJ. Fortification of breast milk with preterm formula powder vs human milk fortifier in preterm neonates: a randomized noninferiority trial. *JAMA Pediatr.* 2021;175(8):790-796. doi:10.1001/jamapediatrics.2021.0678.

30. Penny F, Judge M, Brownell E, McGrath JM. Cup feeding as a supplemental, alternative feeding method for preterm breastfed infants: an integrative review. *Matern Child Health J.* 2018;22(11):1568-1579. doi:10.1007/s10995-018-2632-9.

31. Marofi M, Abedini F, Mohammadizadeh M, Talakoub S. Effect of paladay and cup feeding on premature neonates' weight gain and reaching full oral feeding time interval. *Iran J Nurs Midwifery Res.* 2016;21(2):202-206. doi:10.4103/1735-9066.178249.

32. Malhotra N, Vishwambaran L, Sundaram KR, Narayanan I. A controlled trial of alternative methods of oral feeding in neonates. *Early Hum Dev.* 1999;54(1):29-38. doi:10.1016/s0378-3782(98)00082-6.

33. Moreira CMD, Cavalcante-Silva R, Fujinaga CI, Marson F. Comparison of the finger-feeding versus cup feeding methods in the transition from gastric to oral feeding in preterm infants. *J Pediatr (Rio J).* 2017;93(6):585-591. doi:10.1016/j.jped.2016.12.008.

34. Israel-Ballard K, Coutsoudis A, Chantry CJ, et al. Bacterial safety of flash-heated and unheated expressed breastmilk during storage. *J Trop Pediatr.* 2006;52(6):399-405. doi:10.1093/tropej/fml043.

35. Israel-Ballard K, Chantry C, Dewey K, et al. Viral, nutritional, and bacterial safety of flash-heated and pretoria-pasteurized breast milk to prevent mother-to-child transmission of HIV in resource-poor countries: a pilot study. *J Acquir Immune Defic Syndr.* 2005;40(2):175-181. doi:10.1097/01.qai.0000178929.15904.95.

36. Murguia-Peniche T, Kirsten GF. Meeting the challenge of providing neonatal nutritional care to very or extremely low birth weight infants in low-resource settings. *World Rev Nutr Diet.* 2014;110:278-296. doi:10.1159/000358476.

37. Slutzah M, Codipilly CN, Potak D, Clark RM, Schanler RJ. Refrigerator storage of expressed human milk in the neonatal intensive care unit. *J Pediatr.* 2010;156(1):26-28. doi:10.1016/j.jpeds.2009.07.023.

38. Besser M, Jackson DJ, Besser MJ, Goosen L. How long does flash-heated breast milk remain safe for a baby to drink at room temperature? *J Trop Pediatr.* 2013;59(1):73-75. doi:10.1093/tropej/fms046.

39. Solanki K, Matnani M, Kale M, et al. Transcutaneous absorption of topically massaged oil in neonates. *Indian Pediatr.* 2005;42(10):998-1005.

40. Cleminson J, McGuire W. Topical emollient for preventing infection in preterm infants. *Cochrane Database Syst Rev.* 2021;5(5):CD001150. doi:10.1002/14651858.CD001150.pub4.

41. Soriano CR, Martinez FE, Jorge SM. Cutaneous application of vegetable oil as a coadjutant in the nutritional management of preterm infants. *J Pediatr Gastroenterol Nutr.* 2000;31(4):387-390. doi:10.1097/00005176-200010000-00011.

42. Imdad A, Rehman F, Davis E, et al. Effect of synthetic vitamin A and probiotics supplementation for prevention of morbidity and mortality during the neonatal period. A systematic review and meta-analysis of studies from low- and middle-income countries. *Nutrients.* 2020;12(3):791. doi:10.3390/nu12030791.

43. Panigrahi P, Parida S, Pradhan L, et al. Long-term colonization of a *Lactobacillus plantarum* synbiotic preparation in the neonatal gut. *J Pediatr Gastroenterol Nutr.* 2008;47(1):45–53. doi:10.1097/MPG.0b013e31815a5f2c.

Chapter 13

The Future of Neonatal Nutrition: Further Research and Investment, New Products

Josef Neu

Key Points

1. Many of today's nutritional guidelines for preterm infants are based on clinical judgment, an evidence base that relies on observational and randomized trials, and some basic scientific studies that aim to meet the needs of the mean of a population.

2. Technologies are being developed using artificial intelligence that will provide greater precision for meeting the more personalized needs of individuals.

Introduction

The paradigm of a healthy mother with good nutrition and her healthy term infant who breastfeeds for at least the first year after birth with minimal exposure to adverse environmental conditions is ideal. Mother's milk is personalized for her infant. Its composition undergoes dynamic fluxes over time and under various conditions, thus adjusting to the infant's needs. Unfortunately, this ideal is not met by a large portion of the world's population. Pregnant women and their fetuses are subject to their prepregnancy and intrapregnancy environments, which include nutrition, toxin exposure, genetic and epigenetic factors, and social influences. Many infants are born preterm and lack normal suck-swallow coordination and a fully developed intestine, negating the ability to directly feed from the breast. Various birth factors, as well as the mother's individual and social limitations, such as the need to work, influence ideal maternal–infant interactions, including breastfeeding; hence the ideal is not often achieved.

This chapter discusses how the challenges to meet this ideal are currently being addressed and the pathways for taking steps toward the ideal. A complete discussion of all these factors is beyond the scope of a single chapter; hence the chapter includes brief overviews on optimization of nutrition during pregnancy and lactation, nutrition for preterm infants, and enhancing the composition of commercial formulas toward that of breast milk.

Nutrition During Pregnancy and Lactation: Where Are We Now?

Nutrition plays a vital role during a woman's reproductive period and establishes the potential for health and risks for chronic diseases in their offspring throughout their lifetime.[1] Most women in the United States do not meet the recommendations for healthful nutrition and weight before and during pregnancy. Ways to overcome these problems have been addressed in a recent report[2] that provides background information on the physiologic rationale for dietary recommendations during pregnancy and lactation. Following is a summary of some of the major issues and recommendations in the report:

1. *It is critical that women's health status and nutrition is optimized not only during but also before pregnancy. This will contribute to optimal fetal growth, obstetrical outcomes, and long-term health in both mother and offspring.*
2. *Abnormal fetal growth patterns that include being small for gestational age (fetal growth restriction and macrosomia) are associated with maternal nutrition and increase the risk of later disease.*
3. *Diets that restrict any macronutrient should be avoided during pregnancy.*
4. *The optimal time to improve maternal body weight and nutrition-related lifestyle is well before conception occurs, but interventions may be more achievable during pregnancy.*
5. *Human milk consumption during infancy for term infants is associated with lower risks of chronic disease in later life. Many factors affect the composition of human milk including maternal adiposity and maternal diet. Exclusive breast feeding in women with gestational diabetes may mitigate the*

development of type 2 diabetes in the mother and childhood obesity in her offspring.
6. *All reproductive age women should have their balanced diet supplemented with optimal amounts of folic acid among other micronutrients at least 2 to 3 months before conception. This should be continued during pregnancy and at least the first 4-6 weeks after delivery.*

Strategies to address some of the major concerns related to nutrition in pregnancy and lactation were recommended in the same expert panel report.[2] These include:

- *Evidence-based educational approaches that focus on nutrition across academic clinical programs that emphasize multidisciplinary team approaches to management.*
- *Use of rapidly evolving technology to disseminate appropriate nutrition education that creates connections between scientists, policymakers, and the general population.*
- *Development of improved measures of maternal glucose concentration throughout pregnancy to establish glycemic patterns. Similarly, implementation of better methods to assess lipid availability and use by the fetus and, likewise, determine how to maintain maternal lipid concentrations in the "normal" range and at relatively constant concentrations with appropriate and successful maternal diets.*
- *Development of a better understanding of amino acid and protein needs of both fetus and mother during pregnancy.*
- *Development of methods to best feed the mother who is showing signs of fetal growth restriction or increased fetal fat mass.*

Precision Nutrition Prepregnancy and During Pregnancy and Lactation: The Future

Recognition of the issues and strategies cited in the expert panel report is of utmost importance. In addition to the strategies mentioned,[2] there are additional considerations related to rapidly developing technologies that provide opportunities for advancing care for mothers and their infants. With the increased recognition that one size does not fit all and the fact that individual factors may affect the overall nutritional status of the mother and infant, the concept of precision or personalized nutrition has become a topic that has received increasing attention. Fig. 13.1 shows some of the differences between current and future approaches.

Nutrient Intake Is Highly Individualized

Many of the current nutritional recommendations are based on population statistics and are focused on requirements that may be reasonable for a majority of the population. However, nutritional status is governed by numerous interacting genetic, physiologic, socioeconomic, cultural, and demographic factors. A problem with the one-size-fits-all approach relates to the fact that there is considerable variability as to how nutrients are absorbed

and metabolized.[3] Thus individuals often respond differently to the same nutritional intake. One study found that metabolic responses to food were highly individualized and that the gut microbiome was a key modulator of nutrient bioavailability. This influences postprandial responses and suggests a potentially informative strategy for developing personalized nutrition.[4] This study highlighted the importance of personalizing diet strategies to optimize nutrition. These strategies include the use of artificial intelligence and omics technologies that are rapidly changing the fields of medicine and nutrition.[5] There are several considerations related to precision nutrition that need to be considered. Of primary importance is that requirements for various nutrients may differ depending on phase of pregnancy.[6]

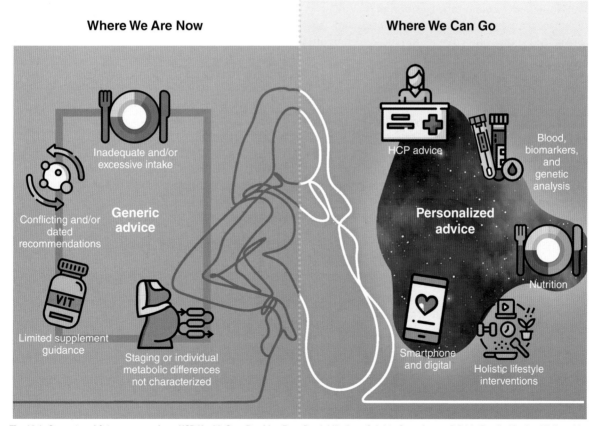

Fig. 13.1 Current and future approaches. *HCP*, Health Care Provider. From Derek Miketinas, Gabriele Gross, Lauren R Brink, Rosalind Davies, Nik Loveridge, Tonya M Bender, Hanqi Luo, Neil Fawkes, Neil. Optimizing Maternal Nutrition: The Importance of a Tailored Approach. Current Developments in Nutrition. Volume 6, Issue 9, September 2022

PRECONCEPTION

Maternal nutrition during the preconception period influences reproductive health and pregnancy outcomes.[6] Supplementation with folic acid for several months during the preconception period has been recommended.[7]

PREGNANCY

Women often do not prioritize future maternal health in advance of pregnancy. However, once pregnant, they are frequently more motivated to modify their diets. Thus pregnancy may act as a prompt to induce positive behavior change.[8] Due to the rate of fetal growth, published nutrient recommendations provide guidance regarding changes in protein and energy intakes during the different phases of pregnancy.[9]

LACTATION

Nutrient requirements during lactation depend on the ability to breastfeed, the stage of lactation, and the volume and composition of milk produced to support infant demand.[10]

It is generally accepted that demands for most nutrients and energy are higher than prepregnancy requirements. However, iron recommendations are lower during lactation because iron will not be lost due to amenorrhea during the first few months postpartum. Thus existing evidence supports the idea that precision approaches for maternal nutrition during the gestational period are important for both offspring and maternal health. Newer technologies such as multiomics and artificial intelligence are likely to play a role in refining our approaches in the future.[5]

Prematurity

Other chapters in this book discuss evidence-based practices currently used for nutrition of preterm infants. This chapter provides a brief discussion about personalized "precision" nutrition for preterm infants. Optimization of nutrition via a personalized approach for preterm infants constitutes a major challenge that not only provides the opportunity to enhance lifelong health for individuals but also has transgenerational consequences.[11,12]

It is critical to understand that preterm infants are not a homogeneous group. A preterm infant born at 23 weeks gestational age has nutritional requirements that differ markedly from one born at 32 weeks gestation. Factors that can alter a preterm infant's nutritional needs include prenatal nutrition, gestational age, severity of illness, cardiorespiratory status, mechanical ventilator support requirements, sepsis, thermoregulation, and use of catabolic drugs (most commonly corticosteroids).[13] Recent data suggest that sex plays a role in nutritional needs of preterm infants.[14] In attempts to meet these needs, there has been progress over the past few decades: specialized intravenous solutions, commercial formulas, milk fortifiers, addition of bioactive ingredients, and donor human milk (DHM) banks have been developed and refined. Population-based guidelines have been derived from these new developments and have been shown to meet the needs of some of these infants, but they marginalize others. Nutrition guidelines that take a one-size-fits-all approach will undernourish some infants, contributing to short-term adverse outcomes such as necrotizing enterocolitis (NEC), retinopathy of prematurity (ROP), bronchopulmonary dysplasia (BPD), late-onset sepsis (LOS), and growth failure. Overnutrition (imbalanced nutrition) for "catch-up growth" can lead to adverse lifelong and even transgenerational consequences, which include the metabolic syndrome.[15]

The monitoring of growth curves and serum markers such as albumin, blood urea nitrogen (BUN), and prealbumin is currently being used to respond to aberrant growth patterns, but too often this monitoring occurs after nutritional failure has begun, therefore providing little if any benefit for the prevention of adverse outcomes such as NEC, BPD, ROP, LOS, and/or growth failure. There is a need for objective evidence for individual risk of developing these outcomes before they start to occur.

The intestinal microbiome acts as an important intermediate in nutritional adequacy for the human host, such as in the biosynthesis of vitamins, short-chain fatty acids (SCFAs), and amino acids, as well as serving numerous protective roles for the host. When the composition and function of the microbiome becomes aberrant ("dysbiotic"), it can predispose the infant to several adverse outcomes such as BPD, NEC, ROP, LOS, and growth failure. Microbial interactions with the intestinal mucosal immune system, when unbalanced via dysbiosis, can induce systemic inflammatory responses exacerbating the potential to develop some of the adverse outcomes seen in preterm infants.[16-23] Evaluation of any single one of these omics (microbiome, metabolome, and inflammasome) will show pathophysiologic associations to disease. A multiomic evaluation approach holds the promise for higher-level predictive analytics, mechanistic information, the capability for biomarker discovery, and diagnostic application of these biomarkers for early personalized nutritional interventions. Recent studies support the value of longitudinal multiomic systems network analysis,[24-26] as well as the integration of these systems with machine learning.[27,28]

Enhancing the Composition of Commercial Formulas Fed to Preterm and Term Infants

Human milk contains bioactive substances and immune active factors that are important for infant health, growth, and development. Breastfeeding from the baby's own mother is the gold standard. The composition of mother's own milk changes dynamically under different environmental conditions and thus is thought to provide tailored nutrition for the infant.[29]

There is a high prevalence of infant formula feeding in the United States and many other countries. Manufacturers have begun to add to their formulas bioactive ingredients found in breast milk, including nucleotides, lactoferrin, and oligosaccharides, among many others.[30] Studies are needed to appropriately address the safety and efficacy of these substances when added to commercial formulas.[31] How to go about this in a safe and effective manner has been the topic of a recent workshop, the results of which have been published.[32]

Despite the addition of some of these substances to formulas, the resulting product is highly unlikely to provide the same activity and benefit as the infant's own mother's milk, which has a highly specialized matrix specifically formulated by natural selection over the past several thousand years. Furthermore, baby's own mother's milk is dynamic in its composition, including immunologic capability changes with differing environmental conditions, which will likely not be possible to duplicate.

Summary

Optimization of nutrition for mothers before and during pregnancy as well as during the lactation period is of utmost importance for the health of both mother and infant. For the infant, the benefits extend for a lifetime and likely even to future generations. Current evidence-based guidelines should continue to be used and refined. Newly emerging technologies will provide much greater precision that will offer guiding strategies for preemptive rather than reactionary nutritional strategies.

REFERENCES

1. Barker DJP. The developmental origins of adult disease. *J Am Coll Nutr.* 2004;23(suppl 6):588S-595S. doi:10.1080/07315724.2004.10719428.
2. Marshall NE, Abrams B, Barbour LA, et al. The importance of nutrition in pregnancy and lactation: lifelong consequences. *Am J Obstet Gynecol.* 2022;226(5):607-632. doi:10.1016/j.ajog.2021.12.035.
3. Rein MJ, Renouf M, Cruz-Hernandez C, Actis-Goretta L, Thakkar SK, da Silva Pinto M. Bioavailability of bioactive food compounds: a challenging journey to bioefficacy. *Br J Clin Pharmacol.* 2013;75(3):588-602. doi:10.1111/j.1365-2125.2012.04425.x.
4. Berry SE, Valdes AM, Drew DA, et al. Human postprandial responses to food and potential for precision nutrition. *Nat Med.* 2020;26(6):964-973. doi:10.1038/s41591-020-0934-0.
5. Berciano S, Figueiredo J, Brisbois TD, et al. Precision nutrition: maintaining scientific integrity while realizing market potential. *Front Nutr.* 2022;9:979665. doi:10.3389/fnut.2022.979665.
6. Savard C, Lemieux S, Weisnagel SJ, et al. Correction: Savard et al. Trimester-specific dietary intakes in a sample of French-Canadian pregnant women in comparison with national nutritional guidelines. Nutrients. 2018, 10, 768. *Nutrients.* 2019; 11(1):84. doi:10.3390/nu11010084.
7. Ami N, Bernstein M, Boucher F, Rieder M, Parker L. Folate and neural tube defects: the role of supplements and food fortification. *Paediatr Child Health.* 2016;21(3):145-154. doi:10.1093/pch/21.3.145.
8. Forbes LE, Graham JE, Berglund C, Bell RC. Dietary change during pregnancy and women's reasons for change. *Nutrients.* 2018;10(8):1032. doi:10.3390/nu10081032.
9. Marangoni F, Cetin I, Verduci E, et al. Maternal diet and nutrient requirements in pregnancy and breastfeeding. An Italian consensus document. *Nutrients.* 2016;8(10):629. doi:10.3390/nu8100629.
10. da Costa TH, Haisma H, Wells JC, Mander AP, Whitehead RG, Bluck LJ. How much human milk do infants consume? Data from 12 countries using a standardized stable isotope methodology. *J Nutr.* 2010;140(12):2227-2232. doi:10.3945/jn.110.123489.
11. Patel MS, Srinivasan M. Metabolic programming in the immediate postnatal life. *Ann Nutr Metab.* 2011;58 Suppl 2(suppl 2): 18-28. doi:10.1159/000328040.
12. Indrio F, Martini S, Francavilla R, et al. Epigenetic matters: the link between early nutrition, microbiome, and long-term

health development. *Front Pediatr.* 2017;5:178. doi:10.3389/fped.2017.00178.

13. Raiten DJ, Steiber AL, Hand RK. Executive summary: evaluation of the evidence to support practice guidelines for nutritional care of preterm infants—the Pre-B Project. *Am J Clin Nutr.* 2016;103(2):599S-605S. doi:10.3945/ajcn.115.124222.

14. Tottman AC, Bloomfield FH, Cormack BE, Harding JE, Taylor J, Alsweiler JM. Sex-specific relationships between early nutrition and neurodevelopment in preterm infants. *Pediatr Res.* 2020;87(5):872-878. doi:10.1038/s41390-019-0695-y.

15. Gounaris A, Sokou R, Panagiotounakou P, Grivea IN. It is time for a universal nutrition policy in very preterm neonates during the neonatal period? Comment on: "Applying methods for postnatal growth assessment in the clinical setting: evaluation in a longitudinal cohort of very preterm infants." Nutrients 2019, 11, 2772. *Nutrients.* 2020;12(4):980. doi:10.3390/nu12040980.

16. Underwood MA, Mukhopadhyay S, Lakshminrusimha S, Bevins CL. Neonatal intestinal dysbiosis. *J Perinatol.* 2020;40(11):1597-1608. doi:10.1038/s41372-020-00829-2.

17. Chen SM, Lin CP, Jan MS. Early gut microbiota changes in preterm infants with bronchopulmonary dysplasia: a pilot case-control study. *Am J Perinatol.* 2021;38(11):1142-1149. doi:10.1055/s-0040-1710554.

18. Li M, Liu S, Wang M, et al. Gut microbiota dysbiosis associated with bile acid metabolism in neonatal cholestasis disease. *Sci Rep.* 2020;10(1):7686. doi:10.1038/s41598-020-64728-4.

19. Gallacher D, Mitchell E, Alber D, et al. Dissimilarity of the gut-lung axis and dysbiosis of the lower airways in ventilated preterm infants. *Eur Respir J.* 2020;55(5):1901909. doi:10.1183/13993003.01909-2019.

20. Singer JR, Blosser EG, Zindl CL, et al. Preventing dysbiosis of the neonatal mouse intestinal microbiome protects against late-onset sepsis. *Nat Med.* 2019;25(11):1772-1782. doi:10.1038/s41591-019-0640-y.

21. Van Belkum M, Mendoza Alvarez L, Neu J. Preterm neonatal immunology at the intestinal interface. *Cell Mol Life Sci.* 2020;77(7):1209-1227. doi:10.1007/s00018-019-03316-w.

22. Skondra D, Rodriguez SH, Sharma A, Gilbert J, Andrews B, Claud EC. The early gut microbiome could protect against severe retinopathy of prematurity. *J AAPOS.* 2020;24(4):236-238. doi:10.1016/j.jaapos.2020.03.010.

23. Lu J, Claud EC. Connection between gut microbiome and brain development in preterm infants. *Dev Psychobio.* 2019;61(5):739-751. doi:10.1002/dev.21806.

24. van Bilsen JHM, Dulos R, van Stee MF, et al. Seeking windows of opportunity to shape lifelong immune health: a network-based strategy to predict and prioritize markers of early life immune modulation. *Front Immunol.* 2020;11:644. doi:10.3389/fimmu.2020.00644.

25. Dong Z, Wan D, Yang H, et al. Effects of iron deficiency on serum metabolome, hepatic histology, and function in neonatal piglets. *Animals (Basel).* 2020;10(8):1353. doi:10.3390/ani10081353.

26. Dougherty MW, Kudin O, Mühlbauer M, Neu J, Gharaibeh RZ, Jobin C. Gut microbiota maturation during early human life induces enterocyte proliferation via microbial metabolites. *BMC Microbiol.* 2020;20(1):205. doi:10.1186/s12866-020-01892-7.

27. Liebal UW, Phan ANT, Sudhakar M, Raman K, Blank LM. Machine learning applications for mass spectrometry-based metabolomics. *Metabolites.* 2020;10(6):243. doi:10.3390/metabo10060243.

28. Olin A, Henckel E, Chen Y, et al. Stereotypic immune system development in newborn children. *Cell.* 2018;174(5):1277-1292.e14. doi:10.1016/j.cell.2018.06.045.

29. Gridneva Z, George AD, Suwaydi MA, et al. Environmental determinants of human milk composition in relation to health outcomes. *Acta Paediatr.* 2022;111(6):1121-1126. doi:10.1111/apa.16263.

30. Salminen S, Stahl B, Vinderola G, Szajewska H. Infant formula supplemented with biotics: current knowledge and future perspectives. *Nutrients.* 2020;12(7):1952. doi:10.3390/nu12071952.

31. Indrio F, Marchese F, Beghetti I, Pettoello Mantovani M, Grillo A, Aceti A. Biotics in neonatal period: what's the evidence? *Minerva Pediatr (Torino).* 2022;74(6):672-681. doi:10.23736/s2724-5276.22.06968-3.

32. Callahan EA, Chatila T, Deckelbaum RJ, et al. Assessing the safety of bioactive ingredients in infant formula that affect the immune system: recommendations from an expert panel. *Am J Clin Nutr.* 2022;115(2):570-587. doi:10.1093/ajcn/nqab346.

Chapter 14

GI Surgical Conditions in the NICU

Emily Kristen Nes, Priyanka Verma Chugh and Tom Jaksic

Chapter Outline

Key Points

1. Long-term survival of children with intestinal failure has significantly improved with advances in management including the establishment of interdisciplinary intestinal rehabilitation centers.

2. A fundamental goal of intestinal failure management is weaning from parenteral nutrition (i.e., attaining enteral autonomy) while ensuring adequate growth and development.

3. There is a high mortality for spontaneous intestinal perforation (19%). Necrotizing enterocolitis requiring surgical intervention has a two-fold higher mortality (38%).

4. Hepatoprotective parenteral nutrition has been associated with decreased intestinal failure–associated liver disease and has improved survival; however, a majority of children with intestinal failure dependent on parenteral nutrition have persistent transaminitis.

5. For home parenteral nutrition patients, catheter-associated blood stream infections remain a major cause of morbidity and mortality. In addition to strict aseptic techniques and rigorous caregiver education, the institution of small molecule (e.g., ethanol) catheter locks appears to be of benefit.

6. Medical management of intestinal failure must address problems of oral aversion, gastroesophageal reflux disease, small bowel bacterial overgrowth, dysmotility, and mucosal inflammation.

7. The development of glucagon-like peptide 2 analogs, although costly, has shown promise in helping select patients achieve enteral autonomy.

8. Important aspects of the surgical management of short bowel syndrome are preserving intestinal bowel length and establishing intestinal continuity. In appropriate patients, autologous intestinal reconstruction can be considered.

9. The current overall patient survival of all types of intestine transplant is 60%. Over the past

decade, there has been a 64% reduction in pediatric intestine, intestine-liver, and multivisceral transplants. This probably reflects the improved outcomes of pediatric intestinal rehabilitation.

10. The advent of interdisciplinary pediatric intestinal failure centers has been associated with 5-year survivals of >90% for neonatal short bowel syndrome. Over three-quarters of these individuals will achieve enteral autonomy. A long lifespan is now expected; hence our focus must extend to optimizing neurodevelopmental outcomes and improving patient and family quality of life. Further, as this new cadre of complex pediatric patients enters adulthood, appropriate transitions of care become increasingly important. Currently, there are few adult analogs to pediatric intestinal failure centers.

Introduction

Short bowel syndrome (SBS) is a life-threatening condition that affects tens of thousands of children.[1] Historically, SBS or intestinal failure due to resection or bowel loss was a condition that was almost always fatal. However, over the past several decades survival has improved significantly.[1–5] The advent of parenteral nutrition (PN) in the 1960s reduced the number of deaths secondary to dehydration and malnutrition.[1,6] Although PN is lifesaving, duration of PN support has been shown to directly correlate with morbidity[7–9] and potentially life-threatening complications including intestinal failure–associated liver disease (IFALD), sepsis from central line–associated blood stream infection (CLABSI), and central venous thrombosis.[10–13] With decreased neonatal mortality in both term and preterm neonates, more children are at risk of certain diseases that predispose them to SBS and its associated complications.[14,15] The economic burden of this population is significant, with more than $500,000 in medical expenses in just their first year of life.[3,16] More recent advances in management including the establishment of interdisciplinary intestinal rehabilitation centers, improved hepatoprotective strategies, and CLABSI prevention protocols have resulted in long-term survival of >90%.[1,2,4,5,17,18] Interestingly, despite

these findings, a substantial proportion of providers still tend to recommend comfort care for neonates with significant bowel loss.[19] This is even more surprising as >75% of adolescents with neonatal onset SBS reach enteral autonomy (e.g., weaning fully from PN) with intestinal rehabilitation.[17]

Pediatric intestinal failure (PIF), a term that includes SBS, is a condition defined as a reduction in gut function that results in an inability to sustain growth, hydration, or electrolyte homeostasis.[1,2,20] SBS is the result of actual bowel loss or resection for acquired or congenital gastrointestinal diseases. Motility disorders (e.g., intestinal pseudo-obstruction) or mucosal defects (e.g., tufting enteropathy or microvillus inclusion disease) are causes of PIF that do not necessarily involve a diminution of bowel length.[1,20] A commonly used functional definition of PIF is PN dependence >90 days.[1,20–23] In 2021 the American Society for Parenteral and Enteral Nutrition (ASPEN) Pediatric Intestinal Failure Section suggested a consensus definition for PIF as dependence on PN for >60 days within a 74-consecutive day interval.[24] Percentage of predicted bowel length using established norms is available and is especially useful in patients who develop SBS after the neonatal period.[25] In animal models, the definition of SBS is usually a loss of 80% or greater of small bowel.[20,26] An alternative method to estimate the quantity of small intestine present is the plasma citrulline level. Citrulline is a free amino acid that is produced by the metabolism of glutamine and proline in the small intestinal mucosa and may be used as a biomarker that correlates with small bowel length and absorptive capacity.[20,27–30] Increased rates of CLABSI have also been associated with lower citrulline levels.[31]

To obtain current state-of-the-art outcomes, a detailed understanding of SBS, etiology, pathophysiology, and appropriate nutritional, medical, and surgical management strategies is essential.

Etiology

Common etiologies of pediatric SBS include necrotizing enterocolitis (NEC), intestinal atresias, gastroschisis, and malrotation with volvulus. Rarer causes of SBS include Hirschsprung disease extending into the small intestine, iatrogenic injuries (e.g., tumor resections), and trauma.[1,20]

NECROTIZING ENTEROCOLITIS

Epidemiology

NEC is a major cause of morbidity and mortality in neonates and the most common cause of PIF.[1,32,33] It is an umbrella diagnosis of similarly presenting, largely idiopathic disease processes that affect the neonatal intestine and hence specific subsets of NEC need to be considered separately. The classic form of NEC occurs in preterm neonates.

In a study with 71,808 very-low-birth-weight infants (≤1500 g), the incidence of NEC for neonates weighing between 501 g and 750 g was 12% with a decrease in incidence of 3% for each 250-g increase in weight.[34,35] Birth weight was the most significant predictor of mortality in this cohort.[34] A more recent study evaluating 473,895 very-low-birth-weight infants from 2006 to 2017 revealed a 4.1% and 5.1% decline in all-cause mortality of medical and surgical NEC, respectively.[32] Although this trend was encouraging, particularly in light of decreasing median birth weights for very-low-birth-weight neonates, the overall mortality for the last year of the investigation was still 16.8% for medical NEC and 31.6% for surgical NEC.[32] This same study also observed an overall reduction in NEC incidence, with medical NEC decreasing from 5.3% in 2006 to 3.0% in 2017 and surgical NEC decreasing from 3.4% in 2006 to 3.1% in 2017. The reason for this reduction in incidence and mortality may be secondary to use of human breast milk, careful feeding advancement, and antenatal corticosteroid use.[32,35–40] It is also important to note that although overall mortality has decreased, the mortality of very-low-birth-weight neonates with surgical NEC (receiving primary peritoneal drainage [PPD] or laparotomy) is still at least 30%.[41]

Term infants with NEC-like diseases have a considerably lower mortality.[35] In an analysis of 1629 such neonates, 45% of >2500-g birth weight neonates had a major congenital anomaly, most commonly gastrointestinal defects, followed by congenital heart defects and then chromosomal anomalies.[42]

Diagnosis

Bell's criteria have historically been used to define neonates with NEC, however these criteria are imprecise.[35] The Vermont Oxford Network (VON) has an alternative method for defining NEC. NEC diagnosis is determined at laparotomy, postmortem, or by specific clinical and radiologic criteria. NEC is clinically defined as the presence of one or more physical findings: bilious gastric aspirate or emesis, abdominal distension, or occult/gross fecal blood in the absence of an anal fissure and at least one diagnostic imaging finding: pneumatosis intestinalis, portal venous gas, or pneumoperitoneum.[32,35] The VON has historically differentiated NEC from spontaneous intestinal perforation (SIP) only if the neonate has had a laparotomy or at postmortem.

Pathophysiology

The pathophysiology of NEC is multifactorial. It is currently believed to be affected by two main factors: prematurity and microbial dysbiosis.[33,35,43] The intestinal epithelium provides a barrier against the external environment through epithelial cells and tight junctions.[44] Prematurity affects the tight junctions leading to increased permeability and bacterial translocation.[35] This causes a release of cytokines which in turn can cause microvascular constriction and intestinal ischemia.[35,43] The timing of NEC resembles that of retinopathy of prematurity and this similarity suggests that host maturity is a factor in the pathophysiology of NEC.[43] Microbial dysbiosis may also play a significant role in the pathogenesis of NEC.[33,35,43] The gut microbiome in premature infants has fewer bacterial species and microbial diversity with an increased proportion of pathogenic bacteria compared to full-term infants.[43] Many elements can alter the gut microbiome leading to microbial dysbiosis including antibiotics and the acid-base environment of the intestine.[37,43,45–47] Formulas can cause a higher intestinal pH compared to human milk and acidified formulas have been associated with a lower incidence of NEC.[35,43,45,46] It has also been described that the use of H2 blockers leads to increased *Proteobacteria* over *Firmicutes* and this may be important in the genesis of NEC.[33,43]

Clinical Presentation

The typical presentation of NEC is a preterm infant with feeding intolerance, abdominal distention, and bloody stools around 2 to 8 weeks after birth.[33,48] Abdominal radiographs are the standard imaging used to diagnose NEC. Pathognomonic signs include pneumatosis intestinalis and/or portal venous gas.[33] Abdominal ultrasound can also be used to evaluate peristalsis, intestinal wall thickness, presence of free fluid, decreased intestinal blood flow, and portal venous gas.[35,49] Laboratory tests may be of utility in supporting the diagnosis of NEC and assessing its progression. Common laboratory findings associated with NEC include thrombocytopenia, absolute neutrophil count (ANC) less than 1500 cell/μL, acidosis, and hyperglycemia.[35,50–52]

Management

Medical management of NEC includes broad-spectrum antibiotics, bowel rest and gastric decompression, initiation of PN, and supportive care.[35] Most neonates will recover with medical management alone, however 25% to 50% will require surgical intervention.[35,40] An absolute indication for surgical management of NEC is bowel perforation as indicated by free air. Clinical decompensation despite optimal medical management may also be an indication for surgery in an infant with NEC.

Operative approaches depend on the condition of the patient and clinician preference. A laparotomy with resection of necrotic bowel followed by proximal diversion is typical, but PPD is often utilized either as a stabilizing intervention or as attempted definitive management. In a recent multicenter randomized clinical trial of 310 premature infants with NEC or isolated intestinal perforation, there was no difference in death or neurodevelopmental impairment at 18 to 22 months corrected age between initial laparotomy versus PPD.[53] Primary anastomosis may also be done in stable patients with limited disease, while the clip and drop technique[54] may be used as a salvage operation in extensive NEC. For severe NEC, temporary silo closure of the abdomen to avoid the sequelae of abdominal compartment syndrome may be necessary. It is important to note that infants who survive after only receiving PPD likely have minimal NEC or SIP.[35] SIP differs from NEC in several ways. It usually presents as an isolated perforation without associated ischemia within 10 days of birth whereas NEC usually occurs between 2 and 8 weeks after birth.[48] In a study of 177,618 very-low-birth-weight infants from 2006 to 2010, infants with laparotomy-confirmed SIP had a mortality of 19% whereas laparotomy-confirmed NEC had a mortality twice that at 38%.[55]

INTESTINAL ATRESIA

Jejunoileal atresias may result in SBS with jejunal atresia being more common than ileal atresia.[56,57] The pathogenesis of jejunoileal atresia is thought to be a vascular accident *in utero* and associated anomalies are commonly not seen.[57,58]

Clinically, infants with jejunoileal atresia can have significant abdominal distention and multiple dilated loops of bowel on abdominal radiographs. A contrast enema may aid in diagnosing rare associated colonic atresias and more frequently reveal a microcolon consistent with a distal small bowel atresia. Isolated proximal atresias are not associated with a microcolon.[57]

There are four types of jejunoileal atresias. Type 1 has the intestinal wall in continuity, but there is a thin luminal blockage. Type 2 has a thin atretic cord connecting two ends of the intestine with no patent lumen. In Type 3, the bowel and mesenteric gap between the proximal and distal segments result in complete discontinuity. Type 3b is a variant in which the distal intestine has a spiral configuration around a single blood supply (retrograde flow through the ileocolic artery), called a *Christmas tree* (reflecting the garland on a Christmas tree) or *apple peal* deformity. Type 4 describes multiple atresia, sometimes referred to as a *string of sausages*. Type 3 and Type 4 atresias are most associated with SBS. Operative repair may be complicated by the size discrepancy between the dilated proximal segment and small, chronically obstructed distal segment. Tapering enteroplasty of the proximal segment is often needed and can help with dysmotility.[57]

GASTROSCHISIS

The incidence of gastroschisis in the United States has increased across all maternal age groups and is about 4.9 per 10,000 live births.[59] In a cohort of 4420 infants in the United States and Canada born between 2009 and 2014, survival to discharge home or alive in hospital at 1 year of age was 97.8%.[60] Gastroschisis is usually diagnosed on routine fetal ultrasound during the second trimester. Increased maternal serum alpha-fetoprotein (AFP) may also occur due to the passage of AFP from the fetus into the amniotic fluid and then in turn to the mother. Gastroschisis is usually right sided and has been attributed to disruption of the right terminal branch of the superior mesenteric artery (SMA) resulting in ischemia and necrosis causing a secondary abdominal wall defect. Another suggested explanation is a failure of the right umbilical vein to involute between 28 and 32 days gestation resulting in an abdominal wall defect secondary to vessel compromise and necrosis.[61] When an infant is born with gastroschisis, it is important to limit insensible fluid loss, prevent hypothermia, and protect the bowel from vascular compromise. Gastric decompression, fluid resuscitation, and broad-spectrum antibiotics are also commonly used in the management of gastroschisis.[61,62] There are several methods of achieving abdominal wall closure that depend upon defect size, associated anomalies, condition of the bowel and the patient, and ability to close the abdomen without impairing ventilation.[61,63,64] The abdominal wall can be primarily suture closed or placed in a silo for staged reduction and closure if primary closure cannot be safely performed. Silo reduction can be performed with use of a spring-loaded silo placed bedside in the NICU with serial reduction of the intraabdominal contents taking care not to cause bowel ischemia or impair ventilation.[62,63,65] Another method, the *sutureless closure*, uses the remnant umbilical cord to cover the abdominal wall defect followed by the application of an occlusive dressing.[63,66] Although overall survival for gastroschisis is excellent, nutritional morbidity is significant with the median time to achieving full enteral nutrition being 37 days.[60] In addition, 57% of infants are discharged at less than the 10th percentile weight for age.[60] Rare neonates, even with a full complement of small bowel, may need lifelong PN due to the inherent dysmotility that can accompany gastroschisis.

MALROTATION WITH MIDGUT VOLVULUS

Malrotation with midgut volvulus is a surgical emergency that if untreated results in extensive bowel loss. The estimated incidence of malrotation is 1 in 500 people based upon postmortem studies.[67] Malrotation is thought to be due to failure of normal intestinal rotation beginning at the fifth week of gestation. It involves a series of steps in which the bowel protrudes into the umbilical cord, undergoes a counterclockwise

turn around the SMA, and returns into the abdomen around the 12th week of gestation where fixation occurs. In malrotation, the right colon is abnormally positioned and may develop aberrant attachments to the right abdominal wall known as *Ladd's bands*. A narrowed mesenteric stalk creates a high propensity for volvulus.[68] The classic clinical presentation is that of an infant discharged home after birth who manifests bilious emesis. If suspected, an upper gastrointestinal series is the study of choice. If malrotation is present, the study shows incorrect positioning of the duodenal-jejunal junction, and volvulus is demonstrated as a complete obstruction of the duodenum or a "coiled spring" appearance of a partially obstructed twisted proximal small bowel. Significant bowel distension or indwelling tubes can distort the anatomy making definitive diagnosis of malrotation difficult. Computer tomography and ultrasound can also be used to diagnose malrotation by evaluating for inversion of the SMA and superior mesenteric vein (SMV). Duodenal dilation and "whirlpool sign" can also be seen in volvulus. However, a normal relationship between the SMA and SMV (with the SMV positioned to the right of the SMA) does not completely exclude malrotation and an upper gastrointestinal series may still need to be performed to confirm the diagnosis.[68] If malrotation is found immediate detorsion of the bowel is needed to avoid ischemia. This involves a counterclockwise untwisting of the midgut at the time of emergent laparotomy. Severe metabolic acidosis and hyperkalemia may be associated with detorsion. William Ladd first described his operation for malrotation in 1936 and it involves dividing Ladd's bands, widening the mesenteric base, and placing the cecum in the upper-left quadrant and the small bowel in the right abdomen. Commonly the appendix is removed as it is abnormally positioned and can cause difficulties with the timely diagnosis of appendicitis. Elective surgery for malrotation, to reduce the risk of volvulus via a Ladd operation, is now often performed laparoscopically.[69]

Short Bowel Syndrome Incidence

An estimation of the incidence of SBS is difficult due to variations in the definition of SBS, lack of complete follow-up, and challenges facing tertiary care centers in determining their study cohort due to complex referral patterns.[70] In a study of very-low-birth-weight preterm infants from 16 tertiary NICUs in the United States, the incidence of surgical SBS was 0.7% in 12,316 very-low-birth-weight infants and 1.1% in 5657 extremely low-birth-weight infants. In a study in Ontario Canada, the overall incidence of SBS was 24.5 per 100,000 live births. The incidence of SBS was higher for premature infants less than 37 weeks gestation compared to full-term infants: 353.7 per 100,000 versus 3.5 per 100,000 live births, respectively. Unfortunately, both studies are dated, and with the improved survival of premature infants the current incidence of SBS is likely higher.

Short Bowel Syndrome Clinical Presentation

Patients with SBS have as series of findings that tend to be stereotypic, including oral aversion, malabsorption of nutrients, cholelithiasis, strictures, reflux, vomiting, chronic diarrhea, IFALD, small bowel dysmotility, small bowel dilation, and bacterial overgrowth.[1]

Patients with severe SBS present have combinations of growth failure, dehydration, vomiting, and diarrhea. A central line for PN and gastrostomy tube (G-tube) or gastrojejunostomy tube (GJ-tube) for enteral supplementation and intestinal decompression are often necessary. Abdominal radiographs reveal small bowel dilation even without the presence of mechanical obstruction. This bowel dilation reflects the process of intestinal adaptation.[1,20] After significant bowel loss the remaining bowel undergoes structural and functional changes that increase absorptive capacity.[71] Histologically, there is an increase in villous height and crypt depth. Gross anatomic features include bowel dilation.[1] This dilation increases the absorptive capacity but can also lead to complications such as dysmotility and bacterial overgrowth.[20]

As a child grows, their intestines adapt and their caloric, protein, and fluid needs decrease on a per kilogram body weight basis. More than 75% of patients with SBS will eventually transition to full enteral nutrition.[20] This transition eliminates complications from PN and central venous access such as infection, sepsis, thrombosis, and IFALD, improving morbidity and mortality.[20]

Nutritional Management

A fundamental goal of intestinal rehabilitation is attaining enteral autonomy (independence from PN) while optimizing growth and development. Adequate nutritional support provides the appropriate quantities of fluids, protein, carbohydrates, lipids, electrolytes, vitamins, and trace minerals.[1,20] Evaluation of the child's weight, height or length, head circumference, and body mass index should be followed longitudinally compared with standardized growth charts. In cases where there may be changes in fluid status or organ mass, arm anthropometry may be needed to accurately assess body composition and lean body mass.[20]

ENTERAL NUTRITION

The timing and type of enteral nutrition has been shown to affect the rate of enteral autonomy. The provision of breast milk and amino acid (elemental) formula has been shown to promote more rapid enteral autonomy.[1,22] Breast milk contains long-chain fats, growth factors, amino acids, immunoglobulins, nucleotides, leukocytes, and other immune-protective factors that stimulate intestinal adaptation.[1,22,72] Several studies suggest breast milk is associated with a shorter duration of PN and decreased risk of IFALD in neonates with SBS.[3,22,73] If breast milk is unavailable, amino acid formulas are recommended over intact protein or protein hydrolysate formulas.[1] Since cell-mediated allergic enteritis is common in children with SBS, probably due to a compromised mucosal barrier, the amino acid formulas avoid peptide-mediated allergies.[20] In an animal model long-chain triglycerides have been associated with improved mucosal adaptation compared to medium-chain triglycerides.[22]

There are many benefits to enteral nutrition such as improved survival, enhanced adaptation, decreased complications, resolution of IFALD, and lower cost.[20,22,74] To prevent oral aversion, feeding by mouth is instituted as soon as it is feasible and safe. Placement of a gastrostomy tube allows for continuous or bolus supplemental enteral nutrition. Continuous feeds result in a lower volume of nutrients per unit time and may improve intestinal absorption and growth.[1,20] Feeding rate increases of 10 mL/kg/d are often used in neonates with SBS until a tolerance threshold is established. Our practice is if stool or stoma output is >2 mL/kg/d we hold enteral feeding advancement. The use of both loperamide and cholestyramine in selected neonates may reduce enteral losses. In cases of upper gastrointestinal dysmotility and vomiting, a gastrostomy tube may need to be converted to a gastrojejunostomy tube. The gastric portion of the feeding tube is placed to gravity for decompression and the jejunal portion is used for feeding. The disadvantage of gastrojejunostomy tubes is the need for replacement by radiology if dislodged and the concern for intussusception. In addition, potential absorptive surface area may be bypassed.[20] Erythromycin may improve gastric motility while cyproheptadine may increase gastric accommodation and appetite.[1,20]

Administration of prebiotics and probiotics is highly debated in PIF. Gastrointestinal colonization of probiotics (nonpathogenic anaerobic bacteria) has been described to prevent the attachment of pathogens, decreasing the likelihood of translocation and life-threatening infections.[75] Prebiotics (sugars that stimulate growth of probiotics) may also provide immunologic benefits.[76,77] There have, however, been reports of children with intestinal failure having catheter-associated bloodstream infections with both bacterial and yeast probiotics. The mechanism is unclear; however, there is concern for translocation or aerosolization of the organism and subsequent contamination of the line hub.[20] We have seen cases of lactobacillus sepsis in our SBS practice and do not use probiotics or prebiotics due to the risk of CLABSI.

PARENTERAL NUTRITION

If adequate growth cannot be achieved with enteral nutrition alone, PN should be initiated. Dr. Stanley Dudrick's seminal work showed that central intravenous nutrition or PN could be used to grow Beagle puppies into normal adult animals.[78] The first human use of central intravenous nutrition was in an infant with SBS secondary to intestinal atresia. PN is composed of amino acids, glucose, electrolytes, lipids, and trace minerals and vitamins.[20] A multidisciplinary team including pediatric surgeons, pediatric gastroenterologists, neonatologists, and specially trained dieticians, nurses, and advanced practice providers is needed for successful bowel rehabilitation.[1] Close

monitoring by such a team also facilitates the safe provision on PN at home if needed. Cycling allows for periodic time off PN infusion. The total amount of fluid and nutrients usually given over a 24-hour period is decreased or cycled over a shorter period. Care must be taken to monitor for episodes of hyperglycemia when starting PN and episodes of hypoglycemia when infusion is cycled. Cycling is not done if the serum glucose falls below 60 mg/dL after the halting of PN. Enteral nutrition during the time cycling off PN decreases the likelihood of hypoglycemia. In practice, cycling of infants weighing under 5 kg is not recommended due to the risk of hypoglycemia. Additionally, the presence of severe hepatic dysfunction may preclude cycling attempts even in larger neonates. This is thought to be secondary to impaired gluconeogenesis.

Complications of PN include CLABSIs, catheter breakage or thrombosis, metabolic bone disease, and IFALD.[1] The optimal treatment of IFALD is transitioning to full enteral nutrition, which on average is associated with a complete resolution of direct hyperbilirubinemia by 4 months in SBS neonates and eliminates the need for central venous access, the primary cause of sepsis in children with intestinal failure.[74] However, some children with intestinal failure are unable to transition to full enteral nutrition. In these cases, modification of lipid dose and consideration of lipid type can limit the extent of IFALD.[20,79] Conventional soy-based intravenous fats at >1 g/kg/d have been implicated in the development of IFALD.[1,20] This is thought to be due to excess phytosterols (e.g., stigmasterol), which are toxic to the liver.[80,81] Doses of lipid emulsion ≤1 g/kg/d have been shown to ameliorate IFALD. One prospective study using intravenous soybean lipid restriction to 1 g/kg/d in neonates with IFALD showed a decline in total bilirubin at a rate of 0.63 mg/dL/wk.[79,82] Essential fatty acid deficiency, however, may occur at these lower doses. Regular surveillance of complete fatty acid profiles is critical for children on restricted doses of lipids. Classic signs of essential fatty acid deficiency are a dry, scaly rash and elevated triene to tetraene ratios.[1,20] If lipid restriction is used, additional PN calories in the form of glucose are required to meet caloric requirements.[20]

A US Food and Drug Administration (FDA)–approved parental fish oil formulation at 1 g/kg/d demonstrated a reversal of hyperbilirubinemia in a majority of SBS patients after 5 months of therapy and was associated with a reduction in mortality.[83–85] Of note, parenteral fish oil contains insignificant amounts of phytosterols. This formula also has a low concentration of the essential fatty acids linoleic acid and alpha-linolenic acid; however, it does contain their downstream metabolites arachidonic acid and docosahexaenoic acid. In a study of 30 children with intestinal failure treated with parental fish oil as the only source of lipids for a median of 4.6 years, an elevated serum triene to tetraene ratio was not seen.[1,86]

Another commercially available lipid emulsion containing soybean oil (30%), medium-chain triglycerides (MCTs) (30%), olive oil (25%), and fish oil (15%) has recently been FDA approved for children. This combination lipid is usually administered at 2.0 to 3.0 g/kg/d. In a pilot multicenter blinded randomized controlled trial comparing this product with a soy-based lipid emulsion, infants who received the combination lipid product had significantly lower conjugated bilirubin than those who received a soy-based lipid emulsion.[80]

The impact of different lipid emulsions and lipid restriction on neurocognitive development, neuronal maturation, and cellular membrane composition and clinical outcomes in critically ill neonates is unknown and further long-term studies are needed.[1,3]

Our current practice in infants with SBS who are thought to require prolonged PN is to start the combination (soy, MCT, olive oil, fish oil) lipid emulsion at 2.0 to 3.0 g/kg/d. Biochemical markers are monitored and if the direct bilirubin is >2 mg/dL for 2 consecutive weeks in the absence of other causes (e.g., sepsis) we will strongly consider transitioning to a parenteral fish oil formula at 1 g/kg/d.

Hepatoprotective lipid strategies have been associated with decreased IFALD and improved survival. However, despite the use of hepatoprotective PN the large majority of SBS patients who are primarily dependent upon PN manifest persistent elevations in serum alanine aminotransferase (ALT) levels, which tend not to be seen in those successfully transitioned to full enteral nutrition.[87] Clinical vigilance and extended follow-up studies are necessary to determine the consequences of this latter finding. In our center, annual abdominal ultrasounds are performed on all SBS patients with a history of IFALD.

Transitioning from parenteral to enteral nutrition is started when a child is growing and tolerating enteral nutrition. The PN is weaned initially by decreasing the calories in the PN and then by skipping days of PN (while still meeting intravenous fluid requirements). An interdisciplinary team monitors the child's weight, height, and electrolytes closely to ensure adequate growth and hydration. Intravenous fluid boluses may be needed to maintain adequate fluid homeostasis. If growth remains adequate, more nonconsecutive days of PN are weaned until the patient is fully off intravenous nutrition.[20] Infants with intestinal failure have been able to achieve enteral autonomy even after many years on PN.[3] In a long-term retrospective study of 63 neonates with SBS, small intestinal length was found to be the primary predictor of weaning PN.[7] The median small intestinal length in patients with neonatal onset SBS fully weaned from PN (e.g., complete enteral autonomy) was 55 cm compared to 26 cm in those remaining on PN.[7] Other studies have shown that with intestinal rehabilitation, enteral autonomy can be achieved even in neonates with less than 20 cm of small bowel.[7,79,85,88] Interestingly neonates with NEC have an increased likelihood of weaning from PN when standardized for small bowel length.[89,90] This likely reflects the marked capacity of premature neonates to increase their small bowel length.

Greater proportions of remaining colon also favorably affect weaning from PN primarily due to improved fluid and electrolyte absorption.[1,79] The presence of an ileocecal valve has not been consistently associated with an improved capacity to attain enteral tolerance.[22] It is thought that the ileocecal valve is actually a marker for variable quantities of remaining terminal ileum. The more terminal ileum available the greater the propensity for maintaining its specialized absorptive roles (Fig. 14.1).[1]

Medical Management

ORAL AVERSION

Children with intestinal failure are at risk for oral aversion. This can be due to multiple interventions early in life such as endotracheal intubation or nasogastric tube feeding. There are often interruptions in oral feeding from multiple operations and nonnutritive

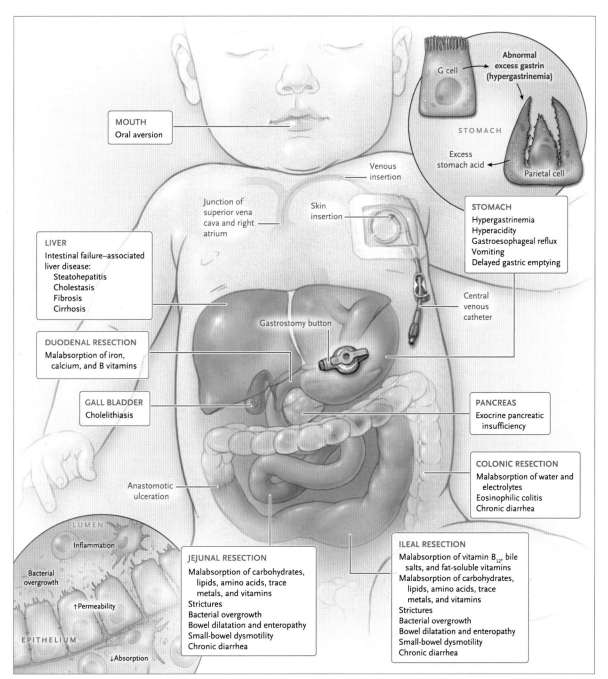

Fig. 14.1 Clinical manifestations of pediatric intestinal failure. There are numerous surgical, gastrointestinal, and nutritional manifestations of pediatric intestinal failure. Many children will have a central venous catheter for parental nutrition and a gastrostomy for enteral feeding access. Intestinal resection results in malabsorption and inflammatory complications that vary depending on the extent and location of the bowel resected. Dehydration, micronutrient and vitamin deficiencies, and electrolyte abnormalities are common.

sucking is inconsistently encouraged.[91,92] Many of these patients have associated motility disorders, reflux, vomiting, or loose stools that can be exacerbated by certain foods. This creates negative associations of oral intake with pain or discomfort.[91] The drive for hunger can also be diminished by the coexisting need for adequate nutrition supplementation using tube feeds or PN.[91,93] For those children who do have some oral feeding, it is often with elemental formulas, which alter their development of taste, and they may not engage with traditional table foods.[91]

Knowledge of this risk and early and consistent interventions with oral stimulation can decrease the likelihood of developing oral aversion. These patients should have evaluation with a feeding team including a speech-language therapist to ensure safety with oral intake and then rapid initiation of oral feeds. For those patients who do go on to develop oral aversion, investigating and improving upon modifiable etiologies of the food aversion, such as abdominal pain or vomiting, is essential. Once those have been addressed or ruled out, behavioral techniques such as exposing children to the sensation of a utensil at their lips and exploring various textures of foods should be utilized to overcome this aversion.[93,94]

GASTROESOPHAGEAL REFLUX AND HYPERGASTRINEMIA

In patients who have extensive small bowel resection, there can be a phenomenon of early postoperative hypergastrinemia. This may be due to loss of inhibitory molecules from the resected small bowel.[91,95] In patients with intestinal failure who do not have extensive bowel resection, there is still the risk of gastroesophageal reflux due to poor foregut motility.[96] These patients are managed with H2 blockers or proton pump inhibitors from an early age.[1,91] This is important not only to minimize risk of erosive esophagitis, but also to minimize downstream damage to remaining portions of the small bowel that might be impacted by the acidic contents.[96] While medications to control acid and reflux symptoms are important in these patients, they are not without risk as well. For example, long-term proton pump inhibitor use is associated with increased rates of gastrointestinal infection, small bowel bacterial overgrowth, metabolic bone disease, and renal toxicity.[97]

METABOLIC BONE DISEASE

Micronutrient malabsorption puts children with intestinal failure at risk of metabolic bone disease. In particular, vitamin D, calcium, and phosphorus deficiency can lead to decreased bone mineral density. Monitoring for low bone mineral density is important in this population during childhood, as this is a key time period for bone accrual. This can be done by using dual-energy X-ray absorptiometry (DEXA), which defines low bone mineral density as a z-score ≤ -2.0.[90] Osteopenia and osteoporosis are potential long-term complications if low bone mineral density is not addressed. Approximately 35% of pediatric patients with intestinal failure have low bone mineral density on DEXA and almost 30% have a history of fractures.[90] Yearly monitoring of bone mineral density with DEXA starting at age 5 is recommended.[98] This allows for early interventions to maximize bone mineral density.[99] The best treatment is weight-bearing exercise with normalization of calcium and 25-hydroxy vitamin D levels but there are challenges to adequately meeting patients' needs. Their enteral absorption can be decreased in SBS. Additionally, the parental provision of calcium in PN is limited by solubility constraints imposed by the simultaneous administration of calcium and phosphate.

CATHETER-ASSOCIATED COMPLICATIONS

Prolonged PN requires long-term indwelling central venous lines. A complication with a significant risk of morbidity and mortality is CLABSI. The rates of CLABSI in patients with intestinal failure have historically ranged from 2 to 7 infections per 1000 catheter days.[100,101] Prevention of CLABSI requires education of providers caring for the line and maintenance of strict aseptic technique.[1] This aseptic technique includes teaching caregivers hand hygiene, using chlorhexidine gluconate (CHG) skin preparation solutions and/or impregnated disks or dressings, and using clean tubing and caps on all supplies.[91,100,102] When compared to heparin locks, ethanol locks reduce the risk of CLABSI by 70%.[103] These techniques have decreased accepted CLABSI rates to 0.5 per 1000 catheter days, with improved outcomes from interdisciplinary intestinal failure programs.[104,105] Concern exists about the impact of ethanol on the integrity of central lines, so it is often used only with silicone lines and studies into the efficacy of 30% ethanol are ongoing.[102] Other solutions such as 4% tetrasodium ethylenediaminetetraacetic acid (EDTA) have been developed to add antibiofilm and antithrombotic properties to the antimicrobial properties of ethanol.[106] The risk of CLABSI is so significant in patients with intestinal failure that those with central lines who develop a fever of 38°C are evaluated for bacteremia and are treated empirically with antibiotics.[101,102]

The presence of long-term central lines also carries an increased potential for catheter-related thrombosis (CRT) in SBS patients. The presence of a line in and of itself creates endothelial damage and nonlaminar blood flow, while components of PN can be caustic. Further hypercoagulability from CLABSI or other thrombotic states can put these patients at even greater risk.[102,107] These thrombi usually occur at the tip of the line resulting in occlusion but may also progress to symptomatic deep vein thrombosis or pulmonary emboli.[102] The true incidence of CRT is not known due to variable screening practices but rates of CRT in patients with long-term indwelling central lines up to 50% have been reported.[102] Patients with intestinal failure and CRT are treated like all other patients with thrombosis with the use of anticoagulation. Currently, there are inadequate data regarding the appropriate use of prophylactic anticoagulation in SBS patients who require central lines. Repair, rather than automatic replacement of broken catheters, minimizes the number of line reinsertions and associated trauma to vessels.[102]

SMALL BOWEL BACTERIAL OVERGROWTH

Many patients with intestinal failure have altered anatomy and gut dysmotility that can result in reflux of colonic bacteria into the small bowel as well as small bowel dilation and stasis. This combination can result in overgrowth of bacteria within the small bowel, which can impair nutrient absorption. Patients with small bowel bacterial overgrowth (SBBO) present with bloating, nausea, vomiting, and poor tolerance of enteral intake. A common treatment strategy is to start cycled oral antibiotics in 7- to 10-day courses, once per month. Antibiotic choice varies and is empiric but at times may require trialing of different antibiotics in the setting of resistance. In cases of refractory to first-line antibiotic treatment, performing endoscopy with

duodenal aspirates to evaluate for predominant bacteria species can be useful to guide treatment.[1,108] Bacteria from aspirates that grow to $>10^5$ colony forming units (CFUs) are generally considered to be the species to target. The appropriate treatment of SBBO is critical, as it is associated with decreased symptoms and improved growth as evidenced by improved body mass index scores.[109]

INTESTINAL DYSMOTILITY

There are a wide spectrum of motility disorders in intestinal failure. In certain cases, such as in NEC, ischemic injury to enteric neurons or smooth muscle may have occurred, which can result in slow transit throughout the gastrointestinal tract. Gastroschisis is also known to be linked to underlying intestinal dysmotility. A subset of patients with gastroschisis, despite having theoretically adequate intestinal mass for absorption, have such significant dysmotility that they still require lifelong PN.[60] In other cases of intestinal failure, due to large segments of bowel resection, there can be rapid transit through the gastrointestinal tract. Once there has been confirmation that symptoms are not secondary to obstruction or stricture, medical treatment strategies can be employed. Prokinetic agents are used on a case-by-case basis and are balanced with the risk of side effects. Many of these agents are antibiotics such as erythromycin, which is a motilin receptor agonist, and may increase risk of antibiotic resistance. Erythromycin is of utility primarily in enhancing gastric motility; however, it is associated with tachyphylaxis. Cisapride, a prokinetic agent that works by enhancing acetylcholine release in the intestinal myenteric plexus, has had evidence of success in improving small bowel motility; however, patients require careful monitoring on this medication due to risk of prolonged QT interval, which can lead to torsades de pointes.[110] Cisapride can only be obtained on a compassionate use basis and is used extremely rarely because of its potentially fatal side effects.

In cases of rapid transit and high stool output, loperamide is a commonly used agent. Loperamide works on intestinal opioid receptors to slow intestinal transit, stool output, and water and electrolyte losses, with minimal systemic effects. In patients who do not have the ability to absorb bile acids, the presence of bile acids in the colon can lead to diarrhea. This type of diarrhea can be treated with cholestyramine, which sequesters the bile acids.[1,111] These medications have been used safely in neonates.

ANASTOMOTIC ULCERATION, INFLAMMATORY BOWEL DISEASE-LIKE SYNDROME

Ulceration at anastomosis sites is a known complication in intestinal failure. It happens more frequently in children and can be a major cause of morbidity and mortality with complications ranging in severity from iron deficiency anemia to massive bleeding, hypotension, and death. While the etiology of these ulcerations is not completely known, they are thought to arise from areas of poor bowel perfusion due to massive ischemia at time of initial bowel resection or secondary to bacterial overgrowth.[112] Anastomotic ulcers are usually considered when patients have an anemia that is refractory to iron supplementation. They are then generally diagnosed with upper endoscopy and colonoscopy. In older children with SBS and suspected gastrointestinal bleeding, capsule endoscopy may also be of utility to visualize areas of the intestine inaccessible to standard endoscopy; however, it has a risk of failing to pass, which may necessitate surgical intervention.[112–115]

In addition to isolated anastomotic ulcers, some children with intestinal failure go on to develop more extensive bowel inflammation and develop an inflammatory bowel disease (IBD)-like syndrome. The pathogenesis of this IBD-like syndrome is not yet well understood but may have to do with the altered gut microbiome seen in these patients, as demonstrated by an association with SBBO.[115,116]

The mainstays of treatment are enteral antibiotics for management of bacterial overgrowth and antiinflammatory medications such as mesalamine or budesonide.[112] If the ulcerations are associated with strictures or if there is significant bleeding resulting in hypotension, then endoscopic or surgical interventions may be necessary.[113] In severe cases of gastrointestinal bleeding, this may include laparotomy with on-table endoscopy to excise a bleeding lesion. Patients with an IBD-like syndrome might require even further antiinflammatory treatments such as biologics, and a specialist in IBD should be consulted for further management.[115]

GLUCAGON-LIKE PEPTIDE 2 ANALOGS

With the goal of enteral autonomy in mind, hormonal therapies have been studied to help improve adaptation of any remaining bowel. An example of such a medication that is commonly used is a glucagon-like peptide 2 (GLP-2) analog.[117] GLP-2 analogs work by binding to the GLP-2 receptor but with a longer half-life than endogenous GLP-2. This allows them to continue to stimulate the receptor, resulting in increasing villous height and crypt depth, promoting growth, and reducing apoptosis of enterocytes. These therapies also inhibit acid secretion, enhance motility and blood flow to the bowel, and overall improve absorption of nutrients and fluid.[118]

While long-acting GLP-2 analogs appear promising, there are important factors to consider when contemplating this therapy. They are only FDA approved for children over 1 year of age and are very costly. In pediatric studies with a primary outcome of a 20% reduction in parenteral fluid administration they were shown effective; however, only about 10% of patients achieved enteral autonomy after a 6-month treatment period.[117]

These medications are currently formulated as a once-daily subcutaneous injection. A longer-acting GLP-2 analog, administered once weekly, is currently being tested and may increase patient compliance.[119] All GLP-2 analogs can accelerate the growth of gastrointestinal malignancies and hence careful patient follow-up is mandatory.

Surgical Management

The most important aspects of the surgical management of SBS are the prevention and preservation of intestine (particularly small bowel). In certain cases, such as midgut volvulus, there is a potentially reversible process and care should be taken to diagnose and treat these conditions promptly.[91] If that is not feasible, it is essential to preserve as much bowel length as possible. This includes employing strategies such as temporary abdominal closures to obviate secondary abdominal compartment syndrome and second-look operations to reevaluate marginally viable bowel to salvage as much intestine as is feasible. Reestablishing bowel continuity as soon as is safely possible is associated with a more rapid progression to full enteral autonomy in neonates with SBS.[22] Distal enteral refeeding of mucous fistulas of NEC patients has been reported to improved outcomes.[120] In SBS neonates, other ancillary operations should also be considered and these are often done at the time of the reestablishment of bowel continuity. Placement of a gastrostomy tube allows for the provision of supplemental enteral nutrition and can also be used for gastric drainage as needed. In cases of poor gastric motility gastrostomy tubes can be converted to gastrojejunostomy tubes with the aid of interventional radiology to allow for both distal feeding and proximal drainage.[1] Baseline liver biopsies are also useful in older infants who require laparotomy.

SBS patients can evolve significant small bowel dilation, which may result in intestinal dysmotility, bacterial overgrowth, and reduced absorption.[1] Surgical procedures such as autologous intestinal reconstruction have been developed to ameliorate these issues. The longitudinal intestinal lengthening and tailoring (LILT) procedure is one such operation, and was described by Adrian Bianchi in 1980.[121] LILT is performed by splitting the small bowel longitudinally along the two leaves of its mesentery. Then the tubularized segments are reanastomosed end to end in an isoperistaltic manner. This is usually repeated multiple times. Another, more recently described and simpler procedure is the serial transverse enteroplasty (STEP) operation. In this procedure the bowel lumen is tapered and lengthened by a series of stapler applications placed perpendicular to the long axis of the bowel in an alternating manner. Both procedures lengthen and taper the bowel, demonstrate an improvement of enteral tolerance, and aid in weaning from PN.[122] A systematic review of the literature suggests that STEP has a lower mortality and decreased overall progression to transplantation compared to LILT.[123]

Over the past 30 years the surgical aspects of intestinal transplantation have been refined. The indications for pediatric intestine transplant are progressing severe liver disease, recurrent life-threatening central line infections, or impending loss of venous access.[124] The presence of cirrhosis, in and of itself, is not an indication for transplantation in pediatric SBS patients.[2] Children or adolescents with a very poor quality of life and little to no chance of attaining

enteral autonomy may also be considered. The 5-year transplant patient survival is approximately 60% with no differences in 5-year survival between isolated intestine and combined intestine-liver transplants.[125] There are significant risks associated with transplantation such as rejection, posttransplant lymphoproliferative disorder, and infection. Due to these issues, transplantation is considered more of a salvage option and rates of intestine transplant have been decreasing, likely due to the success of intestinal rehabilitation.[1,125,126]

Summary

Advances in management, especially the establishment of interdisciplinary intestinal rehabilitation centers, have significantly improved survival. Nutritional management focuses on hepatoprotective PN with the goal of enteral autonomy while ensuring adequate nutritional support and growth. Medical management focuses on management of symptoms such as reflux, SBBO, dysmotility, and inflammation. GLP-2 analogs, although costly, have shown promise in helping children with intestinal failure achieve enteral autonomy. Surgical management focuses on preserving bowel length, ensuring venous and enteral access, and establishing bowel continuity when clinically appropriate. Autologous intestinal reconstruction or transplantation is also an option in certain patients.

With the aging population of survivors with PIF, several challenges remain. Further evaluation of neurodevelopmental outcomes and quality of life is needed. In addition, as this population grows older, transition into adult care is imperative. With few adult interdisciplinary intestinal rehabilitation centers currently in place, establishment of adult centers is needed for this population to thrive.

REFERENCES

1. Duggan CP, Jaksic T. Pediatric intestinal failure. *N Engl J Med.* 2017;377(7):666-675. doi:10.1056/NEJMra1602650.
2. Fullerton BS, Sparks EA, Hall AM, Duggan C, Jaksic T, Modi BP. Enteral autonomy, cirrhosis, and long term transplant-free survival in pediatric intestinal failure patients. *J Pediatr Surg.* 2016;51(1):96-100. doi:10.1016/j.jpedsurg.2015.10.027.
3. Squires RHMD, Duggan C, Teitelbaum DH, et al. Natural history of pediatric intestinal failure: initial report from the Pediatric Intestinal Failure Consortium. *J Pediatr.* 2012;161(4):723-728. e2. doi:10.1016/j.jpeds.2012.03.062.

4. Modi BP, Langer M, Ching YA, et al. Improved survival in a multidisciplinary short bowel syndrome program. *J Pediatr Surg.* 2008;43(1):20-24. doi:10.1016/j.jpedsurg.2007.09.014.

5. Hess RA, Welch KB, Brown PI, Teitelbaum DH. Survival outcomes of pediatric intestinal failure patients: analysis of factors contributing to improved survival over the past two decades. sup.1. *J Surg Res.* 2011;170(1):27. doi:10.1016/j.jss.2011.03.037.

6. Wilmore DW. Factors correlating with a successful outcome following extensive intestinal resection in newborn infants. *J Pediatr.* 1972;80(1):88-95. doi:10.1016/S0022-3476(72)80459-1.

7. Fallon EM, Mitchell PD, Nehra D, et al. Neonates with short bowel syndrome an optimistic future for parenteral nutrition independence. *JAMA Surg.* 2014;149(7):663-670. doi:10.1001/jamasurg.2013.4332.

8. Christensen RD, Henry E, Wiedmeier SE, Burnett J, Lambert DK. Identifying patients, on the first day of life, at high-risk of developing parenteral nutrition-associated liver disease. *J Perinatol.* 2007;27(5):284-290. doi:10.1038/sj.jp.7211686.

9. Kubota A, Yonekura T, Hoki M, et al. Total parenteral nutrition–associated intrahepatic cholestasis in infants: 25 years' experience. *J Pediatr Surg.* 2000;35(7):1049-1051. doi:10.1053/jpsu.2000.7769.

10. Youssef NN, Mezoff AG, Carter BA, Cole CR. Medical update and pootential advances in the treatment of pediatric intestinal failure. *Curr Gastroenterol Rep.* 2012;14(3):243-252. doi:10.1007/s11894-012-0262-8.

11. Uko V, Radhakrishnan K, Alkhouri N. Short bowel syndrome in children: current and potential therapies. *Paediatr Drugs.* 2012;14(3):179-188. doi:10.2165/11594880-000000000-00000.

12. Mutanen A, Lohi J, Heikkilä P, Koivusalo A, Rintala RJ, Pakarinen MP. Persistent abnormal liver fibrosis after weaning off parenteral nutrition in pediatric intestinal failure. *Hepatology.* 2013;58(2):729-738. doi:10.1002/hep.26360.

13. Kocoshis SA, Merritt RJ, Hill S, et al. Safety and efficacy of teduglutide in pediatric patients with intestinal failure due to short bowel syndrome: a 24 week, Phase III study. *JPEN J Parenter Enteral Nutr.* 2020;44(4):621-631. doi:10.1002/jpen.1690.

14. Cole CR, Hansen NI, Higgins, RD, et al. Very low birth weight preterm infants with surgical short bowel syndrome: incidence, morbidity and mortality, and growth outcomes at 18 to 22 months. *Pediatrics.* 2008;122(3):E573-E582. doi:10.1542/peds.2007-3449.

15. Holman RC, Stoll BJ, Clarke MJ, Glass RI. The epidemiology of necrotizing enterocolitis infant mortality in the United States. *Am J Public Health.* 1997;87(12):2026-2031. doi:10.2105/AJPH.87.12.2026.

16. Spencer AU, Kovacevich D, McKinney-Barnett M, et al. Pediatric short-bowel syndrome: the cost of comprehensive care. *Am J Clin Nutr.* 2008;88(6):1552-1559. doi:10.3945/ajcn.2008.26007.

17. Han SM, Knell J, Henry O, et al. Long-term outcomes and disease burden of neonatal onset short bowel syndrome. *J Pediatr Surg.* 2020;55(1):164-168. doi:10.1016/j.jpedsurg.2019.09.071.

18. Oliveira CMDP, de Silva NT, Stanojevic S, et al. Change of outcomes in pediatric intestinal failure: use of time-series analysis to assess the evolution of an intestinal rehabilitation program. *J Am Coll Surg.* 2016;222(6):1180-1188.e3. doi:10.1016/j.jamcollsurg.2016.03.007.

19. Pet GC, McAdams RM, Melzer L, et al. Attitudes surrounding the management of neonates with severe necrotizing enterocolitis. *J Pediatr.* 2018;199:186-193.e3. doi:10.1016/j.jpeds.2018.03.074.

20. Jaksic T, Gutierrez IM, Kang KH. Short Bowel Syndrome. In: Coran AG, ed. *Pediatric Surgery.* 7th ed. Mosby; 2012:1135-1145.

21. Sondheimer JM, Cadnapaphornchai M, Sontag M, Zerbe GO. Predicting the duration of dependence on parenteral nutrition after neonatal intestinal resection. *J Pediatr.* 1998;132(1):80-84. doi:10.1016/S0022-3476(98)70489-5.

22. Andorsky DJ, Lund DP, Lillehei CW, et al. Nutritional and other postoperative management of neonates with short bowel syndrome correlates with clinical outcomes. *J Pediatr.* 2001;139(1):27-33. doi:10.1067/mpd.2001.114481.

23. Duro D, Kalish LA, Johnston P, et al. Risk factors for intestinal failure in infants with necrotizing enterocolitis: a Glaser Pediatric Research Network study. *J Pediatr.* 2010;157(2):203-208.e1. doi:10.1016/j.jpeds.2010.02.023.

24. Modi BP, Galloway DP, Gura K, et al. ASPEN definitions in pediatric intestinal failure. *JPEN J Parenter Enteral Nutr.* 2022;46(1):42-59. doi:10.1002/jpen.2232.

25. Struijs M.-C., Diamond IR, de Silva N, Wales PW. Establishing norms for intestinal length in children. *J Pediatr Surg.* 2009;44(5):933-938. doi:10.1016/j.jpedsurg.2009.01.031.

26. Chang RW, Javid PJ, Oh JT, et al. Serial transverse enteroplasty enhances intestinal function in a model of short bowel syndrome. *Ann Surg.* 2006;243(2):223-228. doi:10.1097/01.sla.0000197704.76166.07.

27. Fitzgibbons S, Ching YA, Valim C, et al. Relationship between serum citrulline levels and progression to parenteral nutrition independence in children with short bowel syndrome. *J Pediatr Surg.* 2009;44(5):928-932. doi:10.1016/j.jpedsurg.2009.01.034.

28. Rabier D, Kamoun P. Metabolism of citrulline in man. *Amino Acids.* 1995;9(4):299-316. doi:10.1007/BF00807268.

29. Crenn P, Coudray-Lucas C, Thuillier F, Cynober L, Messing B. Postabsorptive plasma citrulline concentration is a marker of absorptive enterocyte mass and intestinal failure in humans. *Gastroenterol.* 2000;119(6):1496-1505. doi:10.1053/gast.2000.20227.

30. Jianfeng G, Weiming Z, Ning L, et al. Serum citrulline is a simple quantitative marker for small intestinal enterocytes mass and absorption function in short bowel patients. *J Surg Res.* 2005;127(2):177-182. doi:10.1016/j.jss.2005.04.004.

31. Hull MA, Jones BA, Zurakowski D, et al. Low serum citrulline concentration correlates with catheter-related bloodstream infections in children with intestinal failure. *JPEN J Parenter Enteral Nutr.* 2011;35(2):181-187. doi:10.1177/0148607110381406.

32. Han SM, Hong CR, Knell J, et al. Trends in incidence and outcomes of necrotizing enterocolitis over the last 12 years: a multicenter cohort analysis. *J Pediatr Surg.* 2020;55(6):998-1001. doi:10.1016/j.jpedsurg.2020.02.046.

33. Neu J, Walker WA. Necrotizing enterocolitis. *N Engl J Med.* 2011;364(3):255-264. doi:10.1056/NEJMra1005408.

34. Fitzgibbons SC, Ching Y, Yu D, et al. Mortality of necrotizing enterocolitis expressed by birth weight categories. *J Pediatr Surg.* 2009;44(6):1072-1076. doi:10.1016/j.jpedsurg.2009.02.013.

35. Knell J, Han SM, Jaksic T, Modi BP. Current status of necrotizing enterocolitis. *Curr Probl Surg.* 2019;56(1):11-38. doi:10.1067/j.cpsurg.2018.11.005.

36. Quigley MA, Henderson G, Anthony MY, McGuire W. Formula milk versus donor breast milk for feeding preterm or low birth weight infants. *Cochrane Database Syst Rev.* 2007;(4):CD002971. doi:10.1002/14651858.CD002971.pub2.

37. Oddie SJ, Young L, McGuire W, McGuire W. Slow advancement of enteral feed volumes to prevent necrotising enterocolitis in very low birth weight infants. *Cochrane Database Syst Rev.* 2017; 8(8):CD001241. doi:10.1002/14651858.CD001241.pub7.

38. Grev J, Berg M, Soll R, Grev J. Maternal probiotic supplementation for prevention of morbidity and mortality in preterm infants. *Cochrane Database Syst Rev*. 2018;12(12):CD012519. doi:10.1002/14651858.CD012519.pub2.

39. Roberts D, Dalziel S. Antenatal corticosteroids for accelerating fetal lung maturation for women at risk of preterm birth. *Cochrane Database Syst Rev*. 2006;(3):CD004454. doi:10.1002/14651858.CD004454.pub2.

40. Berman L, Moss RL. Necrotizing enterocolitis: an update. *Semin Fetal Neonatal Med*. 2011;16(3):145-150. doi:10.1016/j.siny.2011.02.002.

41. Hull MA, Fisher JG, Gutierrez IM, et al. Mortality and management of surgical necrotizing enterocolitis in very low birth weight neonates: a prospective cohort study. *J Am Coll Surg*. 2014;218(6):1148-1155. doi:10.1016/j.jamcollsurg.2013.11.015.

42. Velazco CS, Fullerton BS, Hong CR, et al. Morbidity and mortality among "big" babies who develop necrotizing enterocolitis: a prospective multicenter cohort analysis. *J Pediatr Surg*. 2017;S0022-3468(17)30650-4. doi:10.1016/j.jpedsurg.2017.10.028.

43. Neu J, Pammi M. Pathogenesis of NEC: impact of an altered intestinal microbiome. *Semin Perinatol*. 2016;41(1):29-35. doi:10.1053/j.semperi.2016.09.015.

44. Shen L, Turner JR. Role of epithelial cells in initiation and propagation of intestinal inflammation. Eliminating the static: tight junction dynamics exposed. *Am J Physiol Gastrointest Liver Physiol*. 2006;290(4):577-582. doi:10.1152/ajpgi.00439.2005.

45. Bilali A, Galanis P, Bartsocas C, Sparos L, Velonakis E. H2-blocker therapy and incidence of necrotizing enterocolitis in preterm infants: a case-control study. *Pediatr Neonatol*. 2013;54(2):141-142. doi:10.1016/j.pedneo.2013.01.011.

46. Terrin G, Passariello A, De Curtis M, et al. Ranitidine is sssociated with infections, necrotizing enterocolitis, and fatal outcome in newborns. *Pediatrics*. 2012;129(1):E40-E45. doi:10.1542/peds.2011-0796.

47. Neu J. Necrotizing enterocolitis: the mystery goes on. *Neonatology*. 2014;106(4):289-295. doi:10.1159/000365130.

48. Clyman RI, Jin C, Hills NK. A role for neonatal bacteremia in deaths due to intestinal perforation: spontaneous intestinal perforation compared with perforated necrotizing enterocolitis. *J Perinatol*. 2020;40(11):1662-1670. doi:10.1038/s41372-020-0691-4.

49. Esposito F, Mamone R, Di Serafino M, et al. Diagnostic imaging features of necrotizing enterocolitis: a narrative review. *Quant Imaging Med Surg*. 2017;7(3):336-344. doi:10.21037/qims.2017.03.01.

50. Kenton AB, O'Donovan D, Cass DL, et al. Severe thrombocytopenia predicts outcome in neonates with necrotizing enterocolitis. *J Perinatol*. 2005;25(1):14-20. doi:10.1038/sj.jp.7211180.

51. Hällström M, Koivisto AM, Janas M, Tammela O. Laboratory parameters predictive of developing necrotizing enterocolitis in infants born before 33 weeks of gestation. *J Pediatr Surg*. 2006;41(1):792-798. doi:10.1016/j.jpedsurg.2005.12.034.

52. Christensen RD, Yoder BA, Baer VL, Snow GL, Butler A. Early-onset neutropenia in small-for-gestational-age infants. *Pediatrics*. 2015;136(5):E1259-E1267. doi:10.1542/peds.2015-1638.

53. Blakely ML, Tyson JE, Lally KP, et al. Initial laparotomy versus peritoneal drainage in extremely low birthweight infants with surgical necrotizing enterocolitis or isolated intestinal perforation: a multicenter randomized clinical trial. *Ann Surg*. 2021;274(4):e370-e380. doi:10.1097/SLA.0000000000005099.

54. Pang KKY, Chao NSY, Wong BY, Leung MWY, Liu KKW. The clip and drop back technique in the management of multifocal necrotizing enterocolitis: a single centre experience. *Eur J Pediatr Surg*. 2012;22(1):85-90. doi:10.1055/s-0031-1291287.

55. Fisher JG, Jones BA, Gutierrez IM, et al. Mortality associated with laparotomy-confirmed neonatal spontaneous intestinal perforation: a prospective 5-year multicenter analysis. *J Pediatr Surg*. 2014;49(8):1215-1219. doi:10.1016/j.jpedsurg.2013.11.051.

56. Virgone C, D'antonio F, Khalil A, Jonh R, Manzoli L, Giuliani S. Accuracy of prenatal ultrasound in detecting jejunal and ileal atresia: systematic review and meta analysis. *Ultrasound Obstet Gynecol*. 2015;45(5):523-529. doi:10.1002/uog.14651.

57. Rich BS, Bornstein A, Dolgin SE. Intestinal atresias. *Pediatr Rev*. 2022;43(5):266-274. doi:10.1542/pir.2021-005177.

58. Miscia ME, Lauriti G, Lelli Chiesa P, Zani A. Duodenal atresia and associated intestinal atresia: a cohort study and review of the literature. *Pediatr Surg Int*. 2019;35(1):151-157. doi:10.1007/s00383-018-4387-1.

59. Jones AM, Isenburg J, Salemi JL, et al. Increasing prevalence of gastroschisis—14 states, 1995–2012. *MMWR Morb Mortal Wkly Rep*. 2016;65(2):23-26. doi:10.15585/mmwr.mm6502a2.

60. Fullerton BS, Velazco CS, Sparks EA, et al. Contemporary outcomes of infants with gastroschisis in North America: a multicenter cohort rtudy. *J Pediatr*. 2017;188:192-197.e6. doi:10.1016/j.jpeds.2017.06.013.

61. Hunter A, Soothill P. Gastroschisis—an overview. *Prenat Diagn*. 2002;22(10):869-873. doi:10.1002/pd.414.

62. Nichol PF. Gastroschisis. *BMJ*. 2011;343:d7124. doi:10.1136/bmj.d7124.

63. Witt RG, Zobel M, Padilla B, Lee H, MacKenzie TC, Vu L. Evaluation of clinical outcomes of sutureless vs sutured closure techniques in gastroschisis repair. *JAMA Surg*. 2018;154(1):33-39. doi:10.1001/jamasurg.2018.3216.

64. Fraser JA, Deans KJ, Fallat ME, et al. Evaluating the risk of periumbilical hernia after sutured or sutureless gastroschisis closure. *J Pediatr Surg*. 2022;57(12):786-791. doi:10.1016/j.jpedsurg.2022.03.019.

65. Allin BSR, Opondo C, Kurinczuk JJ, et al. Management of gastroschisis: results from the NETS2G Study, a joint British, Irish, and Canadian prospective cohort study of 1268 infants. *Ann Surg*. 2020;273(6):1207-1214. doi:10.1097/SLA.0000000000004217.

66. Sandler A, Lawrence J, Meehan J, Phearman L, Soper R. A "plastic" sutureless abdominal wall closure in gastroschisis. *J Pediatr Surg*. 2004;39(5):738-741. doi:10.1016/j.jpedsurg.2004.01.040.

67. Green PA, Nicoara CD, Losty PD. Should all babies with oesophageal atresia have routine screening for midgut malrotation anomalies? A systematic review in search of evidence. *J Pediatr Surg*. 2022;57(4):655-660. doi:10.1016/j.jpedsurg.2021.06.005.

68. Lampl B, Levin TL, Berdon WE, Cowles RA. Malrotation and midgut volvulus: a historical review and current controversies in diagnosis and management. *Pediatr Radiol*. 2009;39(4):359-366. doi:10.1007/s00247-009-1168-y.

69. Ladd WE. Surgical diseases of the alimentary tract in infants. *N Engl J Med*. 1936;215:705-708. doi:10.1056/NEJM193610152151604.

70. Wales PW, Christison-Lagay ER. Short bowel syndrome: epidemiology and etiology. *Semin Pediatr Surg*. 2010;19(1):3-9. doi:10.1053/j.sempedsurg.2009.11.001.

71. Tappenden KA. Intestinal adaptation following resection. *JPEN J Parenter Enteral Nutr*. 2014;38(suppl 1):23S-31S. doi:10.1177/0148607114525210.

72. Pereira-Fantini PM, Thomas SL, Taylor RG, et al. Colostrum supplementation restores insulin-like growth factor -1 levels and alters muscle morphology following massive small bowel resection. *JPEN J Parenter Enteral Nutr*. 2008;32(3):266-275. doi:10.1177/0148607108316197.

73. Kulkarni S, Mercado V, Rios M, et al. Breast milk is better than formula milk in preventing parenteral nutrition–associated liver disease in infants receiving prolonged parenteral nutrition. *J Pediatr Gastroenterol Nutr.* 2013;57(3):383-388. doi:10.1097/MPG.0b013e31829b68f3.

74. Javid PJ, Collier S, Richardson D, et al. The role of enteral nutrition in the reversal of parenteral nutrition–associated liver dysfunction in infants. *J Pediatr Surg.* 2005;40(6):1015-1018. doi:10.1016/j.jpedsurg.2005.03.019.

75. Mack DR, Michail S, Wei S, McDougall L, Hollingsworth MA. Probiotics inhibit enteropathogenic *E coli* adherence in vitro by inducing intestinal mucin gene expression. *Am J Physiol.* 1999;276(4):G941-G950. doi:10.1152/ajpgi.1999.276.4.G941.

76. Schley PD, Field CJ. The immune-enhancing effects of dietary fibres and prebiotics. *Br J Nutr.* 2002;87(suppl 2):S221-S230. doi:10.1079/BJN/2002541.

77. Dilli D, Aydin B, Fettah ND, et al. The propre-save study: effects of probiotics and prebiotics alone or combined on necrotizing enterocolitis in very low birth weight infants. *J Pediatr.* 2015;166(3):545-551.e1. doi:10.1016/j.jpeds.2014.12.004.

78. Dudrick SJ. Early developments and clinical applications of total parenteral nutrition. *JPEN J Parenter Enteral Nutr.* 2003;27(4):291-299. doi:10.1177/0148607103027004291.

79. Fullerton BS, Hong CR, Jaksic T. Long-term outcomes of pediatric intestinal failure. *Semin Pediatr Surg.* 2017;26(5):328-335. doi:10.1053/j.sempedsurg.2017.09.006.

80. Diamond IR, Grant RC, Pencharz PB, et al. Preventing the progression of intestinal failure–associated liver disease in infants using a composite lipid emulsion: a pilot randomized controlled trial of SMOFlipid. *JPEN J Parenter Enteral Nutr.* 2017;41(5):866-877. doi:10.1177/0148607115626921.

81. El Kasmi KC, Anderson AL, Devereaux MW, et al. Phytosterols promote liver injury and Kupffer cell activation in parenteral nutrition-associated liver sisease. *Sci Transl Med.* 2013;5(206):206ra137. doi:10.1126/scitranslmed.3006898.

82. Cober M, Killu G, Brattain A, Welch KB, Kunisaki SM, Teitelbaum DH. Intravenous fat emulsions reduction for patients with parenteral nutrition–associated liver disease. *J Pediatr.* 2012;160(3):421-427. doi:10.1016/j.jpeds.2011.08.047.

83. Gura KM, Lee S, Valim C, et al. Safety and efficacy of a fish-oil-based fat emulsion in the treatment of parenteral nutrition-associated liver disease. *Pediatrics.* 2008;121(3):e678-e686. doi:10.1542/peds.2007-2248.

84. Puder M, Valim C, Meisel JA, et al. Parenteral fish oil improves outcomes in patients with parenteral nutrition-associated liver injury. *Ann Surg.* 2009;250(3):395-402. doi:10.1097/SLA.0b013e3181b36657.

85. Diamanti A, Conforti A, Panetta F, et al. Long-term outcome of home parenteral nutrition in patients with ultra-short bowel syndrome. *J Pediatr Gastroenterol Nutr.* 2014;58(4):438-442. doi:10.1097/MPG.0000000000000242.

86. Nandivada P, Fell GL, Gura KM, Puder M. Lipid emulsions in the treatment and prevention of parenteral nutrition-associated liver disease in infants and children. *Am J Clin Nutr.* 2016;103(2):629S-634S. doi:10.3945/ajcn.114.103986.

87. Keefe G, Culbreath K, Knell J, et al. Long-term assessment of bilirubin and transaminase trends in pediatric intestinal failure patients during the era of hepatoprotective parenteral nutrition. *J Pediatr Surg.* 2022;57(1):122-126. doi:10.1016/j.jpedsurg.2021.09.018.

88. Infantino B, Mercer DF, Hobson BD, et al. Successful rehabilitation in pediatric ultrashort small bowel syndrome. *J Pediatr.* 2013;163(5):1361-1366. doi:10.1016/j.jpeds.2013.05.062.

89. Sparks EA, Khan FA, Fisher JG, et al. Necrotizing enterocolitis is associated with earlier achievement of enteral autonomy in children with short bowel syndrome. *J Pediatr Surg.* 2016;51(1):92-95. doi:10.1016/j.jpedsurg.2015.10.023.

90. Khan FA, Fisher JG, Bairdain S, et al. Metabolic bone disease in pediatric intestinal failure patients: prevalence and risk factors. *J Pediatr Surg.* 2015;50(1):136-139. doi:10.1016/j.jpedsurg.2014.10.010.

91. Duggan CP, Gura KM, Jaksic T. *Clinical Management of Intestinal Failure.* United States: CRC Press; 2011.

92. Geertsma MA, Hyams JS, Pelletier JM, Reiter S. Feeding resistance after parenteral hyperalimentation. *Am J Dis Child.* 1985;139(3):255-256. doi:10.1001/archpedi.1985.02140050049020.

93. Byars KC, Burklow KA, Ferguson K, O'Flaherty T, Santoro K, Kaul A. A multicomponent behavioral program for oral aversion in children dependent on gastrostomy feedings. *J Pediatr Gastroenterol Nutr.* 2003;37(4):473-480. doi:10.1097/00005176-200310000-00014.

94. Nucci AM, Samela K, Bobo E, Wessel J, Section, ASPEN Pediatric Intestinal Failure Section. Complementary food introduction practices in infants with intestinal failure. *Nutr Clin Pract.* 2023;38(1):177-186. doi:10.1002/ncp.10883.

95. Cortot A, Fleming CR, Malagelada JR. Improved nutrient absorption after cimetidine in short-bowel syndrome with gastric hypersecretion. *N Engl J Med.* 1979;300(2):79-80. doi:10.1056/NEJM197901113000207.

96. Rybak A, Sethuraman A, Nikaki K, Koeglmeier J, Lindley K, Borrelli O. Gastroesophageal reflux disease and foregut dysmotility in children with intestinal failure. *Nutrients.* 2020;12(11):3536. doi:10.3390/nu12113536.

97. Dipasquale V, Cicala G, Spina E, Romano C. A narrative review on efficacy and safety of proton pump inhibitors in children. *Front Pharmacol.* 2022;13:839972. doi:10.3389/fphar.2022.839972.

98. Gatti S, Quattrini S, Palpacelli A, Catassi GN, Lionetti ME, Catassi C. Metabolic bone disease in children with intestinal failure and long-term parenteral nutrition: a systematic review. *Nutrients.* 2022;14(5):995. doi:10.3390/nu14050995.

99. Cuerda C, Pironi L, Arends J, et al. ESPEN practical guideline: clinical nutrition in chronic intestinal failure. *Clin Nutr.* 2021;40(9):5196-5220. doi:10.1016/j.clnu.2021.07.002.

100. Mohammed A, Grant FK, Zhao VM, Shane AL, Ziegler TR, Cole CR. Characterization of posthospital bloodstream infections in children requiring home parenteral nutrition. *J Parenter Enteral Nutr.* 2011;35(5):581-587. doi:10.1177/0148607111413597.

101. Eisenberg M, Monuteaux MC, Fell G, Goldberg V, Puder M, Hudgins J. Central line–associated bloodstream infection among children with intestinal failure presenting to the emergency department with fever. *J Pediatr.* 2018;196:237-243.e1. doi:10.1016/j.jpeds.2018.01.035.

102. Wendel D, Mezoff EA, Raghu VK, et al. Management of central venous access in children with intestinal failure: a position paper from the NASPGHAN intestinal rehabilitation special interest group. *J Pediatr Gastroenterol Nutr.* 2021;72(3):474. doi:10.1097/MPG.0000000000003036.

103. Jones BA, Hull MA, Richardson DS, et al. Efficacy of ethanol locks in reducing central venous catheter infections in pediatric patients with intestinal failure. *J Pediatr Surg.* 2010;45(6):1287-1293. doi:10.1016/j.jpedsurg.2010.02.099.

104. Nader EA, Lambe C, Talbotec C, et al. Outcome of home parenteral nutrition in 251 children over a 14-y period: report of a single center. *Am J Clin Nutr.* 2016;103(5):1327-1336. doi:10.3945/ajcn.115.121756.

105. Pironi L, Goulet O, Buchman A, et al. Outcome on home parenteral nutrition for benign intestinal failure: a review of the literature and benchmarking with the European prospective survey of ESPEN. *Clin Nutr.* 2012;31(6):831-845. doi:10.1016/j.clnu.2012.05.004.

106. Quirt J, Belza C, Pai N, et al. Reduction of central line–associated bloodstream infections and line occlusions in pediatric intestinal failure patients receiving long-term parenteral nutrition using an alternative locking solution, 4% tetrasodium ethylenediaminetetraacetic acid. *J Parenter Enteral Nutr.* 2021;45(6):1286-1292. doi:10.1002/jpen.1989.

107. Keefe G, Culbreath K, Staffa SJ, et al. High rate of venous thromboembolism in severe pediatric intestinal failure. *J Pediatr.* 2023;253:152-157. doi:10.1016/j.jpeds.2022.09.034.

108. Ching YA, Gura K, Modi B, Jaksic T. Pediatric intestinal failure: nutrition, pharmacologic, and surgical approaches. *Nutr Clin Pract.* 2007;22(6):653-663. doi:10.1177/0115426507022006653.

109. Culbreath K, Knell J, Keefe G, et al. Antibiotic therapy for culture-proven bacterial overgrowth in children with intestinal failure results in improved symptoms and growth. *J Pediatr Gastroenterol Nutr.* 2022;75(3):345-350. doi:10.1097/MPG.0000000000003501.

110. Raphael BP, Nurko S, Jiang H, et al. Cisapride improves enteral tolerance in pediatric short-bowel syndrome with dysmotility. *J Pediatr Gastroenterol Nutr.* 2011;52(5):590-594. doi:10.1097/MPG.0b013e3181fe2d7a.

111. Dicken BJ, Serg C, Rescorla FJ, Breckle, F, Sigalet D. Medical management of motility disorders in patients with intestinal failure: a focus on necrotizing enterocolitis, gastroschisis, and intestinal atresia. *J Pediatr Surg.* 2011;46(8):1618-1630. doi:10.1016/j.jpedsurg.2011.04.002.

112. Charbit-Henrion F, Chardot C, Ruemmele F, et al. Anastomotic ulcerations after intestinal resection in infancy. *J Pediatr Gastroenterol Nutr.* 2014;59(4):531-536. doi:10.1097/mpg.0000000000000472.

113. Fusaro F, Tambucci R, Romeo E, et al. Anastomotic ulcers in short bowel syndrome: new suggestions from a multidisciplinary approach. *J Pediatr Surg.* 2018;53(3):483-488. doi:10.1016/j.jpedsurg.2017.05.030.

114. Bass LM, Zimont J, Prozialeck J, Superina R, Cohran V. Intestinal anastomotic ulcers in children with short bowel syndrome and anemia detected by capsule endoscopy. *J Pediatr Gastroenterol Nutr.* 2015;61(2):215-219. doi:10.1097/mpg.0000000000000778.

115. Culbreath K, Keefe G, Nes E, et al. Factors associated with chronic intestinal inflammation resembling inflammatory bowel disease in pediatric intestinal failure: a matched case-control study. *J Pediatr Gastroenterol Nutr.* 2023;76(4):468-474. doi:10.1097/MPG.0000000000003718.

116. Wang F, Gerhardt BK, Iwansky SN, et al. Glucocorticoids improve enteral feeding tolerance in pediatric short bowel syndrome with chronic intestinal inflammation. *J Pediatr Gastroenterol Nutr.* 2021;73(1);17-22. doi:10.1097/MPG.0000000000003058.

117. Kocoshis SA, Merritt RJ, Hill S, et al. Safety and efficacy of teduglutide in pediatric patients with intestinal failure due to short bowel syndrome: a 24-week, phase III study. *J Parenter Enteral Nutr.* 2020;44(4):621-631. doi:10.1002/jpen.1690.

118. Jeppesen PB. Teduglutide, a novel glucagon-like peptide 2 analog, in the treatment of patients with short bowel syndrome. *Therap Adv Gastroenterol.* 2012;5(3):159-171. doi:10.1177/1756283x11436318.

119. Eliasson J, Hvistendahl MK, Freund N, Bolognani F, Meyer C, Jeppesen PB. Apraglutide, a novel glucagon-like peptide-2 analog, improves fluid absorption in patients with short bowel syndrome intestinal failure: findings from a placebo-controlled, randomized phase 2 trial. *JPEN J Parenter Enteral Nutr.* 2022;46(4):896-904. doi:10.1002/jpen.2223.

120. Lau EC, Fung AC, Wong KK, Tam PK. Beneficial effects of mucous fistula refeeding in necrotizing enterocolitis neonates with enterostomies. *J Pediatr Surg.* 2016;51(12):1914-1916. doi:10.1016/j.jpedsurg.2016.09.010.

121. Bianchi A. Intestinal loop lengthening—a technique for increasing small intestinal length. *J Pediatr Surg.* 1980;15(2):145-151. doi:10.1016/S0022-3468(80)80005-4.

122. Iyer KR. Surgical management of short bowel syndrome. *J Parenter Enteral Nutr.* 2014;38(1):53S-59S. doi:10.1177/0148607114529446.

123. Frongia G, Kessler K, Weih S, Nickkholgh A, Mehrabi A, Holland-Cunz S. Comparison of LILT and STEP procedures in children with short bowel syndrome—a systematic review of the literature. *J Pediatr Surg.* 2013;48(8):1794-1805. doi:10.1016/j.jpedsurg.2013.05.018.

124. Kaufman SS, Atkinson JB, Bianchi A, et al. Indications for pediatric intestinal transplantation: a position paper of the American Society of Transplantation. *Pediatr Transplant.* 2001;5(2):80-87.doi:10.1034/j.1399-3046.2001.005002080.x.

125. Horslen SP, Smith JM, Weaver T, Cafarella M, Foutz J. OPTN/SRTR 2020 Annual Data Report: Intestine. *Am J Transplant.* 2022;22 Suppl 2:310-349. doi: 10.1111/ajt.16992.

126. Lee EJ, Smith JM, Mazariegos GV, Bond GJ. Pediatric intestinal transplantation. In: *Seminars in Pediatric Surgery.* 2022:151181. doi:10.1016/j.sempedsurg.2022.151181.

Chapter 15

Multiomic-Based Therapeutics: The Future

Josef Neu

Chapter Outline

Key Points

1. Integration of different "omics" such as microbiome, metabolome, and proteome provides opportunities to more closely evaluate mechanisms of action leading to disease processes as well as provide biomarkers for future diagnostics and therapeutics.
2. Technologies are being developed using artificial intelligence that will provide greater precision for meeting the more personalized needs of individuals.

Introduction

The past three decades have witnessed a revolution in the medical sciences. Contributing to this are advances in *omics*, a rapidly evolving, multidisciplinary and emerging field that encompasses the central dogma of biology, which describes the process of gene transcription and translation that produces proteins acting as biological catalysts and key gatekeepers of metabolic pathways (Fig. 15.1).

Each omic layer individually may provide important information about associations between omic and phenotypic variants. For example, one can associate a high relative abundance of the phylum *Proteobacteria* in the intestine with the development of bowel necrosis in preterm neonates.[1] However, associations alone may not provide strong enough causal or mechanistic evidence for development of predictive or diagnostic biomarkers, strategies for prevention, or therapeutic measures. Another well-known problem is that a genomic variant may be detected in several individuals but only a small number of individuals with that variant express the phenotype. Full or dampened expression may require environmental exposures, the results of which may be detectable by downstream omic evaluation, which may include

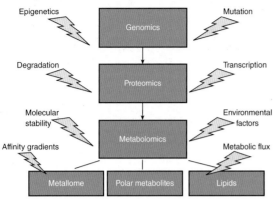

Fig. 15.1 Omic flow via the central dogma.

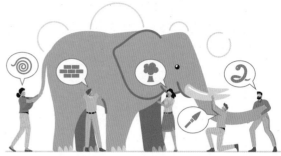

Fig. 15.2 "Six Blind Men from Indostan." From blind men of indostan and multiomics - Bing images. https://www.bing.com/images/search?view=detailV2&ccid=WUCIN2Cd&id=4C0EC886251C261B72F51BDC65F4074DF0979141&thid=OIP.WUCIN2Cdh7IJ_A1JBvzqdwHaEP&mediaurl=https%3a%2f%2fth.bing.com%2fth%2fid%2fR.5940a537609d87b209fc0d4906fcea77%3frik%3dQZGX8EOH9GXcGw%26riu%3dhttp%253a%252f%252f4.bp.blogspot.com%252f-b0B83VjlfWo%252fUUOIPBCiRbI%252fAAAAAAAAB9g%252fecRXjNcSX3o%252fs1600%252fblind_men_and_the_elephant.jpg%26ehk%3d9AqAUJMnrt5TA5mv0zkR0N2h91QidS0koHltnRysCm8%253d%26risl%3d%26pid%3dImgRaw%26r%3d0&exph=516&expw=900&q=6+blind+men+and+the+elephant+indostan&simid=608026924222123021&FORM=IRPRST&ck=4854BAEAE5002CFEE8A4FB16849E35F5&selectedIndex=13&qpvt=6+blind+men+and+the+elephant+indostan&ajaxhist=0&ajaxserp=0

transcriptomics (gene expression), *proteomics* (gene translation), *epigenomics* (gene amplification or silencing), and *metabolomics* (small molecules that often act as effectors of various metabolic processes). It is to be noted that such analyses require powerful computational methods. These artificial intelligence methods are evolving alongside the rapid development of multiomics.[2–6]

This chapter provides a brief review of the current understanding of this rapidly emerging area with the caveat that it is a new field with many examples of successful applications and therapeutics still under intense investigation. This is a field that likely will change our current paradigms of medical practice into an approach that is more individualized, precise, not based on population statistics, and proactive rather than reactive.

Individual Omics

Expression of genetic information is highly variable and depends on environmental exposures. Stress, antibiotic use, nutrition, and other modifiable factors play important roles and the effects of these cannot be evaluated by simply interpreting the sequence of the original DNA template. The Hindi parable of "The Six Blind Men from Indostan" (Fig. 15.2) provides an apt caveat to our current evaluation of single omics rather than their integration. Each of the blind men was asked to feel a portion of a structure they did not know was an elephant. One felt the side and was convinced this was a wall. Another felt the tusk and was convinced this was a spear. Another felt the tail and stated this was a rope, and so on. They dogmatically

argued what they felt and their conclusions but were not able to identify the elephant for lack of integration and agreement.

Similarly, in our scientific endeavors we have problems with each individual omic stratum and are beginning to recognize that focus on one represents simple associations rather than a holistic scheme. Integration of these using bioinformatic techniques can yield systems biology networks that provide mechanistic patterns that can be used to relate these different layers to causality and mechanisms. A summary of the individual omic layers (aka individual blind men) is provided in Table 15.1.

An in-depth discussion of all these technologies is beyond the scope of this chapter. Instead, three will be emphasized in more detail: genomics, proteomics, and metabolomics.

Genomics

The technologies associated with genomics and the description of the Human Genome Project have resulted in DNA amplification and sequencing that is being applied to the various taxa of life, including microbes. Not only have these technologies emerged

TABLE 15.1	**Some Major Omics Technologies**
Technology	**Description**
Genome	The basic template of DNA. Technologies can identify genetic (DNA) variants associated with diseases.
Microbiome	Allows for accurate quantitative determination of microbial taxa, their abundance, and their diversity that can be associated with healthy and diseased states.
Transcriptome	Examines RNA levels transcribed from DNA templates. A small amount of RNA is transcribed for protein synthesis; a much larger amount is encoded for other purposes, which may be implicated in disease.
Proteome	Quantifies peptides that may be used as disease biomarkers.
Metabolome	Detects and quantifies small molecules that include carbohydrates, amino and fatty acids, and other products of cellular metabolism. Abnormally high or low levels may predict disease.
Epigenome	Characterizes modifications of DNA or DNA-associated proteins.

From Pammi M, Aghaeepour N, Neu J. Multiomics, artificial intelligence, and precision medicine in perinatology. *Pediatric Res*. 2023;93(2):308-315. doi:10.1038/s41390-022-02181-x.

rapidly, but their associated costs have decreased dramatically. Despite the excitement generated by genomics, there are limitations. The presence of a gene does not necessarily indicate its influence on the phenotype. Transcription of RNA can be modified by epigenetic factors, degradation, splicing and silencing, protein synthesis and degradation, protein folding, and environmental influences that control enzymatic production of small molecules (metabolites).

Proteomics

Proteomics is the large-scale study of proteins—vital parts of living organisms with many functions, such as the formation of structural fibers of muscle tissue, enzymatic digestion of food, and synthesis and replication of DNA. Instrumental technologies upon which proteomics are based include chromatography coupled to mass spectrometry and nuclear magnetic resonance spectroscopy. These technologies aid in determining not only protein amino acid sequence (translational product) but also posttranslational modifications such as acetylation, which may markedly alter the protein's function.

Metabolomics

Metabolomics is the large-scale study of small molecules, commonly known as *metabolites*, within cells, biofluids, tissues, and organisms. These are largely evaluated by mass spectroscopy or nuclear magnetic resonance techniques. Collectively, these small molecules and their interactions within a biological system are known as the *metabolome*. They may be substrates or products of the reactions modified by the proteome via various environmental conditions. Metabolites are considered one of the most sensitive of the omic markers that relate to the phenotype. The presence or absence of certain metabolites may be indicative of genetic diseases, infections, metabolic illnesses such as diabetes, organ dysfunctions, and cancers. The myriad of metabolites, however, makes analysis challenging. This also underlines the importance of refining technologies that clarify the information contained in this highly important downstream omic layer.

Examples of Multiomics

A major goal of biomedical research in the newly emerging area of precision medicine is to identify accurate, early indicators of disease. Ascertaining this goal holds promise for the detection of early stages of disease development and the prevention or slowing of disease progression. This could be accomplished through lifestyle interventions and more effective and preventive pharmacologic or nutritional treatments. Following are some general examples in medicine, as well as more specific examples that relate directly to neonatology.

PHARMACOGENOMICS

Gene variations play an important role in determining a person's response to medication. This can markedly affect the safety and effectiveness of a particular medication. Currently, most medications are developed in a one-size-fits-all manner. This can lead to potentially unsafe use of a drug or poor efficacy for some individuals.

Pharmacogenomics can proactively distinguish drug responders from nonresponders, which can assist in selecting the most ideal therapy for a patient. For example, genome interrogation techniques have identified biomarkers for several cardiovascular drugs to prevent stent thrombosis in patients who require stent placement after an acute coronary syndrome.

Warfarin is an anticoagulation agent used to treat and prevent venous thromboembolism as well as to prevent stroke in patients with atrial fibrillation. Warfarin is metabolized by the hepatic enzyme protein CYP2C9. Variations in CYP2C9 play a role in variations in warfarin responses and are genetic determinants of dosing. Evaluation of this variant prior to administering warfarin may protect against detrimental side effects or provide important information related to dosing.

While still in its infancy, pharmacogenomics has been useful in precision medicine and individualizing patient care. Further advancements including development of big data and artificial intelligence technologies may become increasingly accessible in the coming years.

CANCER DIAGNOSIS AND MULTIOMIC APPROACHES

Despite numerous success stories, exclusive characterization of the genome of an individual is often not sufficiently predictive of their risk of developing cancer, nor of their likelihood to respond to treatment or their cancer recurrence risk. Different omics methodologies assess different parts of the complex pathophysiology of disease development and progression, and the analysis of just one omic subset provides a skewed, biased, and incomplete picture of the underlying biology. However, given the wide range of data that can be generated from tissue samples to characterize differences between normal and diseased cells and tissues, how does one select the most meaningful omic data types to generate (limited primarily by cost and tissue availability), and more importantly, how does one integrate the resulting multiple omic datasets to obtain a comprehensive picture of the underlying biological processes? These processes are developing rapidly. Following is a brief discussion of two approaches that have been used.

The first approach looks at the various analytes (transcripts, proteins, metabolites, epigenetic factors) in the context of known (reported) pathways and mechanisms. For this, prior knowledge of molecular pathways for a certain disease is needed.

The second approach is initially agnostic of existing knowledge of pathways and network interactions in cells and tissues. It looks for correlations across multiple datasets to identify molecules/analytes that are changing in a correlated manner. This approach is unbiased but can discover novel molecules and pathways essential for the disease process. Computational techniques for these complex integrated analyses are needed in interpretation of obtained co-expression networks or clusters of multiomics analytes.

Multiomics in the Intestine

The complexity of the microbial environment of the intestinal tract is discussed in detail in Chapter 3. It is becoming clear that simply providing the relative abundance, diversity, and genetic potential of microbes in this ecosystem is of interest but may not provide enough information for understanding the overall environment and functional interactions of the intestinal tract under various circumstances, such as term versus preterm infants, those delivered via C-section versus vaginal delivery, and those being fed mother's milk, donor milk, or commercial formula.

Thus newer approaches are being utilized and further developed. These employ metaomics approaches, including 16S rRNA gene sequencing, metagenomics, metatranscriptomics, metaproteomics, and metabolomics, which directly examine the phylogenetic markers, genes, transcripts, proteins, or metabolites from the samples. Each one of these by itself can be informative, revealing significant associations between the gut microbiome and human diseases, including obesity, diabetes, inflammatory bowel disease (IBD), cardiovascular disease, and various cancers.

When evaluating the composition of the microbiome, for example, it has become clear that it differs among individuals and is affected by various factors such as diet, lifestyle, and host genetics. Thus each patient's microbiome will respond differently to therapeutic treatments, and we currently cannot accurately predict these responses in advance.

However, these shortcomings can at least be partially alleviated by using metaomics approaches such as metatranscriptomics and metaproteomics and by integrating the data obtained from each omics layer (Fig. 15.3).[2] Metagenomic sequencing of

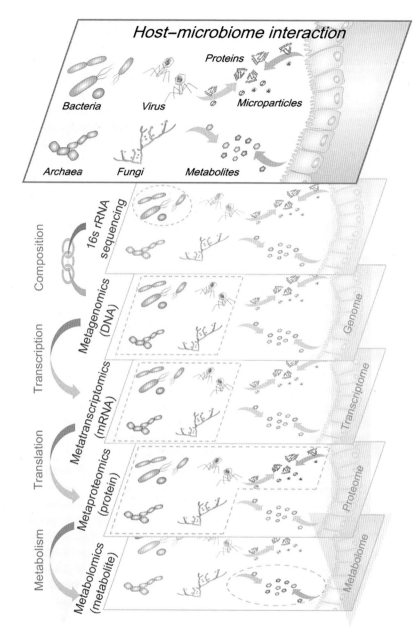

Fig. 15.3 Integration of multiomic information. From Zhang X, Li L, Butcher J, Stintzi A, Figeys D. Advancing functional and translational microbiome research using meta-omics approaches. *Microbiome.* 2019;7(1):154. doi:10.1186/s40168-019-0767-6.

hundreds to tens of thousands of samples was recently carried out in large-scale projects studying the role of the microbiome in human disease. Included among these are studies on early-onset type 1 diabetes, IBD, prediabetes, and colorectal cancer.

These studies employed longitudinal and/or multiomic experimental designs, which enabled better characterization of the dynamic changes and functional activities of the microbiome during disease progression.

Data processing tools are increasingly being developed for all these multiomic layers. Detailed discussion of these tools is beyond the scope of this chapter but can be found in various reviews.

The fecal metabolome is an important endpoint readout of biological processes originating from the gut microbiome. Identified metabolites in fecal metabolomics can include those derived from the microbiota (e.g., lipopolysaccharide and butyrate) or the host (e.g., antimicrobial peptides). Co-metabolism of the host and microbiome may also produce various metabolites. Imbalance of metabolites has been associated with disease.

Integration strategies transform each omic dataset independently into a simpler, less dimensional and less noisy representation, and decreases heterogeneity between omic datasets. The transformed and combined representation can then be analyzed using classic machine learning models. Fig. 15.4 aptly demonstrates differences between single omic associations with phenotype (IBD) versus an omic integration approach.[7,8]

The top of Fig. 15.4 shows single omic integrations leading to secondary mechanisms and random therapies, which is suboptimal. The bottom shows omic integration with resulting information that includes primary mechanisms, detection of specific biomarkers, and individualized personalized therapies.

APPLICATION TO NEONATOLOGY

Several serious outcomes in preterm neonates are amenable to multiomic and artificial intelligence analyses. Recognition, prevention, and treatment of necrotizing enterocolitis (NEC) is a major problem because of lack of definition. What is called "NEC" is not a discrete disease but rather a diagnosis that pertains to several different, more discrete entities. Multiomic approaches are being proposed along with the use of artificial intelligence to differentiate the different forms of intestinal injury being termed "NEC."[9] Once these have been differentiated into more discrete clusters of intestinal injury and dysfunction, each cluster can be

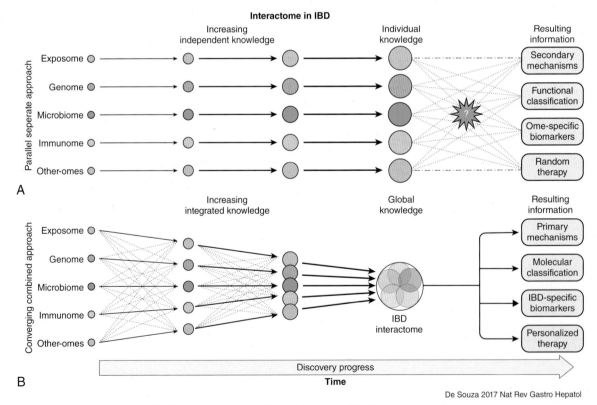

De Souza 2017 Nat Rev Gastro Hepatol

Fig. 15.4 Single omics versus multiomic integrations. *IBD,* Inflammatory bowel disease.

more intensively interrogated for predictive biomarkers, which can in turn be utilized for early detection, leading to personalized nutritional and pharmacologic preventive strategies.

PRECISION NUTRITION

One of the greatest challenges in neonatology is how to optimize the timing and composition of nutrition in preterm infants. Guideline-based approaches have been developed that may be adequate for many of these infants, but a significant percentage require a more personalized (precision) approach. The one-size-fits-all approach is not appropriate for all these infants. The infant's sex, *in utero* growth restriction, previous exposure to medications, and maternal stressors may all be important factors that necessitate personalization.

In the past, the physician's intuition and best opinion available guided therapeutics. Currently, more evidence-based approaches are being used that rely largely on population-based data, which do not optimize nutrition for all infants. Fig. 15.5 shows three different infants, all with markedly different phenotypes, who are likely to have major differences in their multiomic profiles. Current nutritional assessment relies considerably on growth curves, but for these three infants, more than growth is obviously required for preemptive nutritional strategies. Thus precision-based nutritional strategies that leverage newly developed integration of multiomics, systems biology, and artificial intelligence as applied to each of these infants in a precision-based approach should significantly improve their short-term and lifelong health outcomes

Summary and the Future

Integration of metatranscriptomics, metaproteomics, and metabolomics with metagenomics holds the promise of enhancing our understanding of disease pathogenesis as well as providing predictive biomarkers and preventive interventions.

There are tremendous opportunities for enhancing patient outcomes that technological advances integrating multiomics and clinical datasets with modern computing platforms have brought forth. The advances and capabilities have the potential to bring about paradigm shifts in how we practice in the fields of perinatal and neonatal medicine.[2–6]

Is there a role for precision nutrition in neonatology? How do we best nourish these infants?

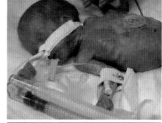

25-week AGA

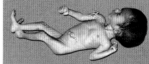

38-week IUGR

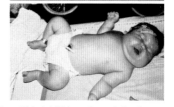

38-week LGA

Past	Present	Future
Intuition medicine	Evidence-based medicine	Precision medicine
Signs and symptoms	Clinical trials	Algorithms

Fig. 15.5 The need for precision nutrition. *AGA*, Appropriate for gestational age; *IUGR*, intrauterine growth restricted; *LGA*, large for gestational age.

SELECTED REFERENCES

1. Pammi M, Cope J, Tarr PI, et al. Intestinal dysbiosis in preterm infants preceding necrotizing enterocolitis: a systematic review and meta-analysis. *Microbiome*. 2017;5(1):31.
2. Zhang X, Li L, Butcher J, Stintzi A, Figeys D. Advancing functional and translational microbiome research using meta-omics approaches. *Microbiome*. 2019;7(1):154.
3. Neu J. Multiomics-based strategies for taming intestinal inflammation in the neonate. *Curr Opin Clin Nutr Metab Care*. 2019;22(3):217-222.
4. Pammi M, Aghaeepour N, Neu J. Multiomics, artificial intelligence, and precision medicine in perinatology. *Pediatr Res*. 2023;93(2):308-315.
5. Taddei CR, Neu J. Editorial: Microbiome in the first 1000 days: multi-omic interactions, physiological effects, and clinical implications. *Front Cell Infect Microbiol*. 2023;13:1242626.
6. Stelzer IA, Ghaemi MS, Han X, et al. Integrated trajectories of the maternal metabolome, proteome, and immunome predict labor onset. *Sci Transl Med*. 2021;13(592):eabd9898.
7. Borren NZ, Ananthakrishnan AN. Precision medicine: how multiomics will shape the future of inflammatory bowel disease? *Curr Opin Gastroenterol*. 2022;38(4):382-387.
8. de Souza HSP, Fiocchi C, Iliopoulos D. The IBD interactome: an integrated view of aetiology, pathogenesis and therapy. *Nat Rev Gastroenterol Hepatol*. 2017;14(12):739-749.
9. Neu J. Necrotizing enterocolitis: the future. *Neonatology*. 2020;117(2):240-244.

Index

Note: Page numbers followed by "f" refer to illustrations; page numbers followed by "t" refer to tables; page numbers followed by "b" refer to boxes.